# The secret battle

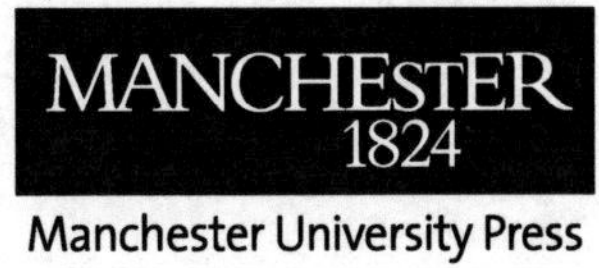


Manchester University Press

**Cultural History of Modern War**
*Series editors*

Peter Gatrell, Max Jones, Penny Summerfield and Bertrand Taithe

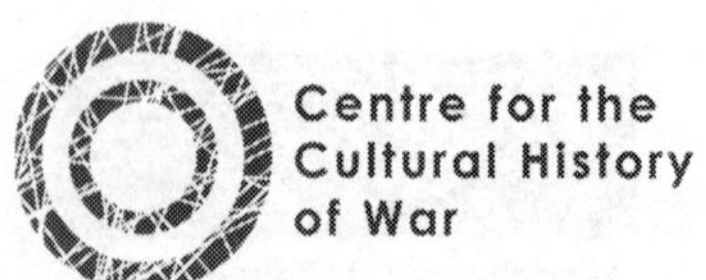

# The secret battle

## Emotional survival in the Great War

~

MICHAEL ROPER

Manchester University Press
Manchester and New York
distributed in the United States exclusively by Palgrave Macmillan

Published by Manchester University Press
Oxford Road, Manchester M13 9NR, UK
and Room 400, 175 Fifth Avenue, New York, NY 10010, USA
www.manchesteruniversitypress.co.uk

Distributed in the United States exclusively by
Palgrave Macmillan, 175 Fifth Avenue,
New York, NY 10010, USA

Distributed in Canada exclusively by
UBC Press, University of British Columbia, 2029 West Mall,
Vancouver, BC, Canada V6T 1Z2

British Library Cataloguing-in-Publication Data is available

Library of Congress Cataloging-in-Publication Data is available

ISBN 978 0 7190 8386 0 paperback

First published by Manchester University Press in hardback 2009

This paperback edition first published 2010

Printed by Lightning Source

In memory of my grandparents, Robert Henry Roper (1896–1980) and Alice Victoria Roper (1897–1987)

# Contents

# List of figures

# Preface

This book is about the battle for emotional survival of young British civilian soldiers on the Western Front in the First World War, and the part played by their families in that battle. The relationships with loved ones at home, it contends, were a source of practical survival skills and support, and played a crucial role in sustaining the morale of this largely young, amateur army. These relationships were conducted during the war through letters, parcels and other long-distance means, but drew their strength from a much longer history, whose legacy could be seen not only in the soldier's domestic skills and memories of home, but in his deepest states of mind. It is these deep ties whose character and manifestations this book explores – especially those between mothers and sons – for trench warfare not only turned these young soldiers into men, it also made them anxious and homesick. Many yearned for their mothers.

In researching and writing about these men and their families I have inevitably drawn on my own experiences of family life. I started research on the book in 2000, the year that my daughter Alice was born. Becoming a parent has shown me the emotional importance of food, clothing, warmth and rest, things that we sometimes take for granted, as some Edwardian mothers and sons, although less insulated from the necessities of survival than we are today, also did before the war. When I took Alice to visit her relatives in Australia at the age of two and a half, breezily confident of my ability to manage on my own with her, I soon discovered the depth of the maternal tie. Separated from her mother, Alice's sleeping bag became her 'baggy', to be carried everywhere and at all times, as it sometimes still is five years later when she is tired or feeling uncertain of herself. Bringing up children has shown me too how the most primitive parts of our personalities co-exist with more mature ones; so that my son Thomas, now five, moves in a matter of seconds between the baby enjoying the reverie of his mother in early morning cuddles in bed, and the street-wise boy who on a freezing Autumn morning insists that he will only wear his football strip. There was of course little 'pre-teen' culture among the Edwardian soldiers who are the subjects of this book, but in the stresses of war they experienced particularly violent psychic movements between the child and the adult. The character Paul Bäumer in Eric Maria Remarque's classic First World War novel *All Quiet on the Western Front* sums up their split position: 'We are like children who have been abandoned and we are as experienced as old men.'[1]

If this study is influenced by my becoming a parent, it is also informed by being a son in a family which has been divided for the past quarter-century and more between Britain and Australia. Having arrived in Britain in my mid-twenties on a Commonwealth Scholarship, convinced that my stay would be temporary, I know something of what it feels like to be separated from parents and siblings, and the equally intense pleasures and disappointments of keeping in touch. My sister Cath and niece Ally, my father Stan Roper, step-mother Robyn Roper and mother Ailsa Roper have kept up steadfast connections during our long separation; not so much via letters nowadays, but through phone calls, emails and photos by attachment, and in birthday presents for cousins and grand-children that almost always arrive on time. What has been gained today in synchrony and the vividness of image or sound is lost in touch and permanence, the letter (as my own archives and those of many an Edwardian mother attest), being a uniquely tangible sign of the loved one.

There is a direct connection to the First World War in my family, which the Epilogue explains. This, as much as any strictly historical concern, has inspired my concern to investigate the emotional experience and impact of the war. My grand-father served in Gallipoli and Palestine, and I well recall him in his middle seventies, writing his memoirs at the roll-top desk in the lean-to behind the kitchen. We heard a lot about his war, and even amid the quiet and leafy suburbs of Melbourne, something of its turmoil was communicated to us. So if this book is concerned to rescue the 'war generation' from sometimes unthinking assertions of victim-hood, and to show the emotional survival of men like my grand-father for the victory it was, it is at the same time equally concerned with the costs, and with the shadow which the First World War has cast over families like mine for nearly a century.

During my research for the book I have gained from the insights of innumerable people. Audiences at Cambridge, the Institute of Historical Studies, and at the Universities of Kent, Monash, Newcastle and Oxford have helped refine the ideas. I am unusually lucky in being based at the University of Essex, which retains relatively strong inter-disciplinary links, and I have gained especially through conversations with my colleagues in the History Department, Sociology Department and the Centre for Psychoanalytic Studies. Peter Evans, the late Ian Craib and Bob Hinshelwood all inspired me to think more deeply about psychoanalysis. I owe many intellectual debts to the PhD and MA students I have taught at Essex, among them Chris Corr, Penny Da Costa, Rachel Duffett, Wendy Gagen, Ana Ljubinkovic (who also did some valuable research for me on patterns of family correspondence at the Imperial War Museum) and Helen Peters. Their enthusiasms and insights have helped shape the project.

Staff at the Imperial War Musuem have proven unfailingly helpful, being a model of how an archive should function, and under the domed roof of the old Bethlem asylum they have provided me with among the most moving experiences in my research career, handling the fragile pages of letters home, written in now faint, supposedly indelible, pencil. Thanks go also to the librarians at the Liddle Collection at the University of Leeds, John Rylands Library at the University of Manchester, and Churchill Archives at Cambridge.

I would like to thank the Arts and Humanities Research Council for funding this project with matching leave during 2004–5, the Research and Enterprise Office at Essex for financial support from its Research Promotion Fund and the Department of Sociology for funding travel, conference and other research expenses. It would not have been possible to finish the book without the generous study leave provided by the University of Essex.

Colleagues and friends have proven a constant source of insight. Andrew Briggs, himself a child psychotherapist, has given me the benefit of a clinician's insight, something which is sometimes missing from historical discussions of psychoanalysis, which can suffer from being theoretically over-rarefied. Peter Barham, Beatrice Clarke, Mark Connelly, Santanu Das, Jeremy Krikler, Anne McElroy, Ailsa, Cath and Stan Roper read and commented upon parts of the manuscript. Anthony Fletcher has been a great help throughout, not least by giving me access to the letters of his grand-father Reggie Trench, but also through sharing his own research and insights with me. So too has Delle Fletcher, Reggie's daughter, who wrote to me on more than one occasion to fill in some family history of the father she barely knew. Francesca Bion was kind enough to show me the original draft of Wilfred Bion's 1919 war memoirs, a text which has inspired many of the ideas in this book. My colleagues at Essex, among them Rowena Macaulay and Sue Aylott, gave me access to private family collections, and I enjoyed the companionship of Sean Nixon during a visit to the battlefield sites and war cemeteries around Ypres in November 2006, where he took many excellent photographs.

An early draft of the book was read by Leonore Davidoff, Sean Nixon, Lyndal Roper, Nick Stargardt and John Tosh, and I owe them all a debt that extends well beyond their fertile commentaries in the margins. I hope that they will feel this book is strengthened by my engagement with their thoughts. I'm especially grateful to Nick Stargardt and Lyndal Roper, who volunteered for a second round of reading and editing, and who have made it possible for me to complete the project amid other unduly pressing demands. Along with my nephew Sam, Lyndal and Nick constitute my extended family on this side of the world, and their company is treasured.

I am deeply grateful for the generosity of families in giving me permission to reproduce extracts from papers at the Imperial War Museum to which they hold the copyright. In many cases my request for permission resulted in conversations and letters that told me a great deal more about the person concerned than I had gleaned from the papers alone. I would like to thank Donald Anderton for the papers of E. H. Anderton; Harriet Chipperfield for the papers of A. J. Arnold; Rosemary Chorley for the papers of A. G. Baker; Peter Arnold for the papers of O. H. Best; Mike Bickersteth for the papers of the Bickersteth family; the Trustees of the Imperial War Museum for the papers of A. P. Burke; Mrs D. M. Brady for the memoir of J. Brady; Michael Brown for the papers of S. E. Brown; Harry Carter, for the papers of H. Carter; Gill Hinson for the papers of W. C. Christopher; the Trustees of the Imperial War Museum for the papers of J. A. C. Clarke; Sheila Roome for the papers of T. Corless; David Brown for the memoirs of F. J. Cornes; Sue Aylott for the papers of S. J. Dawson; Audrey Fenton for the papers of D. H. Fenton; Andy Fortune for the memoirs of G. Fortune; Jocelyn Hemming for the papers of R. K. Foulkes; Jennifer Keeling for the papers of A. Gibbs; Helena Hague for the papers of H. W. Hague; Susan de Courcy Rolls for the memoirs of E. J. Harrison; Leeds University Library for the papers of A. Hooper, K. Hooper and L. Hooper; Joyce Hoyle for the papers of W. Hoyle; Dick Hubbard for the papers of A. H. Hubbard; Tom Leland for the papers of H. J. C. Leland; Leeds University Library for the papers of I. McLeod; Annie Page and Mrs M. Solon for the papers of E. C. Mercer; Roger Middlebrook for the papers of J. B. Middlebrook; Rose Hunt for the papers of C. Miller; Susan Martin for the papers of R. D. Mountfort; Lesley Bratton for the papers of H. A. Munro; E. Coleman for the papers of G. W. Nightingale; Edward Nugee for the papers of G. T. Nugee; Trevor Campbell Smith for the papers of H. S. Payne; Kathleen Margaret Clarke for the papers of E. J. Poole; Charles Adrian Ramsdale for the papers of C. Ramsdale; Peter Robinson for the papers of M. Robinson; Patricia Clarke for the papers of R. D. Russell; Sally Woodrow for the papers of H. J. Savours; Phil Morgan for the papers of P. Smith; Nicola Kent for the papers of W. B. P. Spencer; Mrs S. Marriott for the papers of A. H. Swettenham; C. F. J. Thompson for the papers of A. Thompson; Audrey Timpson for the papers of L. Timpson; the University Librarian and Director, John Rylands Library, The University of Manchester for the papers of K. Tynan; A. Urwick for the papers of L. Urwick; Phil Gunyon for the papers of P. E. William; the University Librarian and Director, John Rylands Library, The University of Manchester for the papers W. M. Wills; and J. Giappone for the papers of S. Wootton.

Every effort has been made to trace copyright holders and the author and the Imperial War Museum would be grateful for any information which might help to trace those whose identities or addresses are not currently known. It has not proven possible to trace the copyright holder for the papers of H. F. Bowser; R. W. Brierley; S. E. Brown; G. Carpenter; B. F. J. Chapman; E. F. Chapman; J. M. Connor; W. A. Goodwin; R. Gwinnell; L. Hall; C. D. Hanman; W. T. Hate; A. Higginson; M. Holroyd; E. R. Hutt; A. Knight; E. Marchant; J. H. Merivale;

N. R. Russell; J. H. Standrick; D. Starrett; A. G. Steavenson; N. A. Taylor; T. Thorpe; J. D. Tomlinson; M. Webb; F. Wollocombe and N. Woodroffe.

My final thanks go to Anne McElroy, my partner, for helping keep a space in our busy lives for the book to grow, but who never allowed me to become entirely lost to it either; and who in that way has greatly enriched the emotional connections it seeks to make with families in wartime.

## Note

1 E. M. Remarque, *All Quiet on the Western Front* (London: Vintage, 1996), p. 88.

# List of abbreviations

Imperial War Museum (IWM)
Liddle Collection, 1914–18, Leeds University Library (LC)

# Introduction

On 7 August 1918, the eve of the Battle of Amiens, Captain Wilfred Bion was ordered to manoeuvre his Company's tanks into position. Their route lay across the river Luce, over a bridge whose repair Bion had just supervised, a difficult task as the bridge was shelled every evening by the Germans. As Bion walked ahead of his tanks, guiding them towards the river, their engines in low gear so as to conceal the noise of their preparations, he experienced a powerful sensation. Listening intently for the bombardment that must surely be unleashed once the Germans discovered their movements, he was momentarily overcome:

> The strain had a very curious effect; I felt that all anxiety had become too much; I felt just like a small child that has had a tearful day and wants to be put to bed by its mother; I felt curiously eased by lying down on the bank by the side of the road, just as if I was lying peacefully in someone's arms.

This description comes from a memoir which Bion wrote in 1919 and dedicated to his mother and father 'In place of letters I should have written!'[1] After the Second World War he would become a leading psychoanalyst in Britain, whose writings focused on the infant's most primitive fears and the mother's capacity to respond to them, a capacity for which he coined the term 'containing'. The description that Bion gave his parents, therefore, anticipated his later psychoanalytic concerns by some forty years. It related a moment of intense fear, in which he was thrown back to a child-like state, and longed for the comfort of a mother. Bion, in August 1918, had found a substitute by nestling against the roadside bank, reviving the feeling of being held in another's arms. Other men would seek solace in dug-outs and funk holes, or by pressing their bodies to the ground. 'My one desire was to hug closely to mother earth', wrote Private Norman Gladden, recalling the experience of going over the top at Ypres in 1917.[2]

In 2003, Harry Patch was interviewed for a BBC programme, 'The Last Tommy'. Then aged 105 and among the last handful of British survivors of the war, he told of the mortally wounded man he came across after going over the top at Pilckem Ridge in 1917. The man was from another company in his Battalion, the 7th Duke of Cornwall's Light Infantry:

> I was with him in the last seconds of his life. Then he went from this life, to whatever is beyond . . .
>
> . . . And when that fellah died, he just said one word: 'Mother.' It wasn't a cry of despair. It was a cry or [*sic*] surprise and joy. I think – although I wasn't allowed to see her – I am sure his mother was in the next world to welcome him. And he knew it. I was just allowed to see that much and no more. And from that day until today – and now I'm nearly 106 years old – I shall always remember that cry and I shall always remember that death is not the end.

For almost ninety years this vision of the dying man calling out to his mother remained with Harry Patch. He had not talked about it earlier in his life, but he would 'always remember' the man's injuries, his chest and stomach torn 'all to pieces' by shrapnel.[3]

Even national enmities grew less important when a man was this close to death. Henry Williamson recalls a German boy, crushed by a tank, moaning '"Mutter, Mutter, Mutter", out of ghastly grey lips.' A British soldier, hit in the leg and sitting nearby, took the man's hand and told him 'All right, son, it's all right. Mother's here with you'.[4] The Dutch war cartoonist Louis Raemaekers, renowned for his ultra-patriotic and anti-German depictions, broke with convention in his sketch of a dying English soldier being comforted by a German soldier. A man in a Pickelhaube kneels beside a child-like figure, looking into the startled clear eyes. One hand nestles against the youth's head and his soft locks of hair, the other takes his hand. The caption reads 'Is it you, Mother?'[5] A French soldier (*poilu*) writing in a trench newspaper recalled the mutilated arms of the wounded, stretched upward and searching for someone to hold them:

> And there, right by my side, a monotone,
> A childish cry that groans, intoning,
> 'It hurts! Maman . . . Maman . . . Oh God I'm going to die!'[6]

Soldiers *in extremis* harked back to the earliest relationships of their lives, even when they were contemplating a death which would bring shame on their families. At 7.45 p.m. on 4 January 1917, whilst playing cards with some fellow officers, the twenty-one-year-old Sub Lieutenant Edwin Dyett was told that he would be executed the following morning for desertion. He was joined by a Padre and with hours to go he wrote a final letter to 'Dearest Mother Mine.' He apologised for the mistakes, but without the comfort of the Padre, 'I should not be able to write myself.' He hoped that his mother would keep up correspondence with 'my friend' the Padre, who had given him such 'kind support'. Dyett left all his personal effects to his mother, but wanted her to pass on half the sum to the 'poor girl' who had been his sweetheart. 'Give dear Dad my love and wish him luck', he wrote. 'I feel for you so much and I am sorry for bringing dishonour upon you all.' He closed his letter asking God to 'protect you all now and for evermore. Amen.'[7]

This book is about the relationships between British men on the Western Front and their families, particularly their mothers. It seeks to account for the scenes described above; to ask *why* it was that, in General Seeley's words 'when men die of dangerous wounds, in almost every case "mother" is the last word that crosses their lips'.[8] What do such scenes reveal about the emotional experience of the war and the role of loved ones in sustaining men psychologically? The book's title, *The Secret Battle*, is taken from a remarkable novel written in 1917 by the future Liberal parliamentarian, A. P. Herbert, while he was convalescing from a shrapnel wound.[9] Herbert's novel describes the struggle of a conscientious young officer, Harry Penrose, serving first at Gallipoli and then on the Western Front, to keep going in the face of fear which becomes more and more debilitating. Penrose is accused of running back up the line during battle, Court Martialled, and eventually shot for cowardice although, as the final words in the novel proclaim, 'he was one of the bravest men I ever knew'.[10] Herbert based his novel partly on personal experience, but also on the plight of Edwin Dyett, who had been a fellow officer in the Royal Naval Division and whose treatment at the hands of the military authorities had angered Herbert. Dyett was one of just three officers on whom the death sentence was passed, among a total of around 350 British and Commonwealth soldiers executed during the war.[11] Their fates were exceptional, but the 'secret battle' for emotional survival was not, being fought by every young man who saw active service on the Western Front. Most, unlike Dyett, found ways to get through it, and so this book asks: in a war that was unprecedented in the scale of its violence, on what familial and emotional resources did these young men draw?

The Great War was a uniquely deadly conflict in British military history. It brought about a 'new kind of armed confrontation', with large civilian armies opposing each other locked into trenches, using increasingly mechanised and deadly weapons.[12] It was violent even by comparison with the Second World War. An average of 457 British men were lost each day in the First World War, compared with 147 in the Second World War.[13] Around one in eight British soldiers was killed and one in four was wounded.[14] Because most casualties were due to snipers and long-range armaments, the infantry soldier in trenches was more often the victim than the perpetrator of violence.[15]

The immersion in violence was intense and prolonged. The British soldier square-bashing at the dreaded 'Bullring' Base Camp in Étaples had an early intimation of mass death, for in one corner of this camp was a cemetery with some 12,000 dead.[16] In a 'noisy' sector of the Western Front it would not be long before a man got a close-up view of a corpse. On his first tour of the trenches, Roland Leighton followed the splashes of blood on the duck-boards left by a man from his own regiment, killed when he put his head above the parapet. Leighton blamed the victims of snipers for not keeping their heads down, but ironically, it was probably a sniper's bullet that later killed him.[17] After Jim Tomlinson's company arrived in the firing line at Hill 60 following the British attack of mid-April 1915, he tried to shift a sandbag that was 'always being tripped over when we . . . went by. When I had lifted it up I found a shoulder + top half of an arm under neath [*sic*]. I soon reported the sandbag + ran to the Sergeant for some chloride of Lime. All along were pieces of body.'[18] Just as disturbing as the dead were the victims of artillery fire who – like Harry Patch's comrade – suffered severe wounds but did not die immediately. Those who looked on would never forget such scenes.

Violence was all around them, but it was random and unpredictable. Tomlinson wrote to his mother of one such death after their spell in the gruesome trenches at Hill 60 when his company went into reserve trenches. The fighting died down and as they waited to move back up towards the firing line, Tomlinson commented to his friend Vic how quiet it was. Vic replied:

> 'its better to be quiet whilst we are moving up'. The last word just left his lips when a stray bullet hit him in the left lung. He clutched at his chest, reeled and fell back. I knelt down beside him, his nose and mouth was bleeding furiously.[19]

At no moment – even the most apparently quiet – was safety guaranteed. 'Unknown fortune', as one put it, kept them alive.[20] The man who appeared most at risk could escape scot-free whilst his better-protected comrade did not. Percy Smith survived a heavy bombardment with his 'head & shoulders above the parrapit [*sic*]' throughout, whilst the Sergeant who had 'been beside me . . . cursing & swearing only a few moments before, had his arse blown off.' Smith was at a loss to know how to explain his survival to his parents; he kept 'expecting Fritz to spot me but I did not get a scratch which was a miracle.'[21] As George Mosse puts it, the 'encounter with mass organized death' was the defining feature of the war.[22] Its emotional impact, and the long-term scars of it in memories, dreams and behaviour, would spread well beyond the veteran to affect his parents and siblings, his children and even his grand-children.

The effects of violence were all the greater because these were young men. Much has been made of the 'boy soldiers' who enlisted under-age, but in fact this was a fighting force composed largely of the young: 70 per cent of those who served in the war were under thirty, while around 40 per cent were under twenty-four.[23] Anyone over twenty- three, remarked Donald Hankey, was 'an "old man"'.[24] The men who commanded British soldiers in the field – particularly the volunteer officers – were also young.[25] Wilfred Bion was barely in his majority when he lay down on the bank at Amiens, temporarily overwhelmed by his responsibilities. Ernest Smith's friend Ford was considered too old at thirty to become a subaltern, the age limit among the Artists' Rifles in early 1915 being twenty-seven.[26] When a forty-year-old schoolmaster was posted to Captain Greenwell's Company as a Second Lieutenant, Greenwell – who was himself only twenty-two – wondered what on earth to do with the man. 'I can't put him with a boy half his age', he explained to his mother, 'though I am myself young enough to be his son.'[27] Recruitment was targeted at unmarried men. When the so-called Derby Scheme of voluntary registration was introduced in 1915, married men were promised that they would not be called up until all eligible bachelors had entered the services, and indeed the first Conscription Bill of January 1916 excluded them.[28] Although married men were conscripted on the same basis as single men after April 1916, bachelors predominated.[29] They bore the brunt of the casualties: it is estimated that around two-thirds of the men killed in the war were single.[30]

Faced with unpredictable and horrific violence, these young civilian soldiers depended on two kinds of relationship. One tie was to their families and particularly their mothers. For the 'war generation' born in the 1890s and in their late teens or early twenties when they joined up, mothers were the key link to life beyond the war. Among the Imperial War Museum's collections of sons' correspondence from the Western Front there are almost six times as many letters to mothers as to fathers. Second Lieutenant Arnold Hooper summed up the importance of mothers: 'I said when I saw my mail the other day to a chap standing near. In the long run who is it that writes every mail and who always writes a good letter? Why one's Mother. One's first friend.'[31]

The other source of support was their fellow soldiers. 'The daily comradeship of my pals, whether in or out of the line, gave me strength' wrote the machine gunner George Coppard.[32] Family ties are sometimes seen as the antithesis of comradeship in histories of the war; and indeed, it would be hard to imagine an environment more alien from the homes many of these men had left than the Western Front. Stuart Cloete's view is widely quoted:

> Impossible to believe. That other life, so near in time and distance, was something led by different men. Two lives that bore no relation to each other. That was what they felt, the bloody lot of them.[33]

These men may have *felt* that their mental worlds were split between the civilian and the soldier, but home and the trenches were structurally connected and inter-dependent. Each revolved around basic bodily needs such as food and water, shelter, warmth and rest. Many of the skills needed to survive on the Western Front were domestic. Families and comrades, moreover, depended on each other in all sorts of ways, from the parcels that would be shared out among friends, to the home visits paid by men to their friends' parents on leave. The home and battle fronts were linked through families, and it was mothers who often managed the networks between them, effectively underwriting the war effort. The 'maternal' and the 'military' were allied, the habits of home helping soldiers to adapt to Army life.

At the same time, however, although family ties often remained strong, war also put them under immense stress. Veterans sometimes enacted on their loved ones and carers the violence to which they had been subjected. Just weeks after her husband returned home from a war hospital, Beatrice Munson petitioned for him to be re-admitted. He had 'repeatedly been making wild threats to thrash her, to murder the doctor at the war hospital and to drown himself.'[34] Soon after being sent back to England suffering from shell-shock, Herbert Asquith smashed a vase in a house where he and his wife Cynthia were guests. Feeling in pieces himself, he could not bear to be in 'a house with its roof on'. Cynthia feared that Herbert might not stop at smashing the bric-a-brac, but would vent his fury on their host's face and she might even have feared for her own safety.[35] Social order in post-war Britain, Susan Kent has argued, would depend on the strengthening of marriage and the drawing of women into caring relationships as a means of 'making peace'. It fell upon mothers, sisters and wives to minimise 'the provocations of men to anger'.[36] Soldiering might have domesticated men, but equally, the emotional damage wrought by the war showed itself in their home lives.

By studying the course of family relationships through the war and into peacetime, this book shows how these twin stories, of the love and support given to young men on the Western Front, and the anger, bitterness and disappointment when they returned, were connected. My thinking has been influenced by two distinct, although related, approaches to the emotional history of the war. On the one hand there are those who argue that the encounter with violence undid the civilising process. Bernd Weisbrod, in his essay on the German author and trench-soldier Ernst Jünger, describes a 'weakening capacity for empathy.'[37] George Mosse argues that pre-war mores became irrelevant when killing was on a mechanised scale. The war gave free rein to 'primitive, instinctual, and violent' impulses that had hitherto been restrained; the soldier ended up 'holding life cheap'. He returned from the war full of hatred and 'numb . . . in the face of human cruelty and the loss of life'.[38] Kent reaches a similar conclusion, arguing that many people in Britain felt that the war had exposed 'aggression, destructiveness, and violence' as 'inherent characteristics of masculinity'.[39]

For Paul Fussell and Eric Leed, the effect of the war was less one of brutalisation than of alienation. They describe how the frontline soldier became 'estranged' from home.[40] During the war families could have little real knowledge of the hardships men faced, a fact reflected in their frequently inappropriate and ineffectual efforts at support. One of the reasons why so many men broke down afterwards, claims Leed, is that during the war they had often idealised home as a point of continuity amidst the disruption they encountered on the battlefields. The reality of return, however, released 'funds of repressed anger and bitterness'.[41] This viewpoint, which emphasises the emotional separation between soldiers and civilians, has obtained the status of historical fact in some quarters. One study, for example, states baldly that 'one of the most devastating consequences of fighting the war was combatants' discovery that the concept of "home" no longer existed'.[42]

On the other hand, partly in response to the view that there existed an 'emotional chasm' between the home and battle fronts, German, French, British and Australian historians have become interested in what actually happened to family relationships during the war. What kind of contact, they ask, did men keep with their loved ones, and did the moral compass of home retain any meaning?[43] Working on personal correspondence from Austria and Germany, Christa Hämmerle has demonstrated its importance for loved ones separated by the war, and has shown too that officials recognised the role played by the Army postal service in sustaining morale on the war and home fronts. The Austria-Hungarian Army postal service carried in the order of 9.9 million items of post each day, and postage was free for all letters to and from the front. [44] A study of wartime letters, Hämmerle concludes, reveals not a chasm but the 'mutual dependence and the interconnectedness of differing modes of perception and experience.'[45] In a study of French correspondence, Martha Hanna finds that, rather than growing more distant, family bonds became stronger as people concentrated their attention on the closest members of the family.[46] Audoin-Rouzeau, in his study of French trench newspapers, found that wives and families were the second most common topic of discussion, and that the importance of home 'grew ever greater as time passed.'[47] '[C]lose bonds with the home front' co-existed with the 'anomie of the battlefields', Audoin-Rouzeau and Becker conclude, in *1914–1918. Understanding the Great War.*[48] Joanna Bourke has shown how much British soldiers valued the ties with home, and her conclusion that the 'gulf between civilians and servicemen was not as wide as historians have sometimes portrayed it', is shared by Ilana Bet-El in her study of conscripts.[49] Stressing the continuing links with home and their importance for the soldier's morale, these historians implicitly argue against his brutalisation.

This study, focusing as it does on the relationships between mothers and sons, also demonstrates the emotional significance of home for the trench soldier. It was not just dying, but any number of terrifying experiences, that might cause a man to cry out for his mother. Terror threw men back to the memory of those who had cared for them from the earliest moments: it made them regress. The men in this study were, after all, barely adults, whose closest emotional ties remained in many cases with their mothers. Yet it was not just in these extreme moments that men relied on their mothers. Their spirits were buoyed, even when they were safe behind the lines, by the letters and parcels that came from home and particularly from their mothers. Mothers played an important part in the practical tasks of day-to-day survival. A study of mothers and sons, therefore, is revealing not only about the secret battle to hold together that went on inside men's heads, but about another, less dramatic and sometimes unnoticed secret battle: the one fought by families as they tried to make their sons more comfortable and help them cope with the traumas of trench warfare. This battle would not end with the war, but would continue afterwards as sons became husbands and fathers, and were cared for by wives as well as mothers.

Part I of the book, 'Mothers and sons', investigates the hidden history of what mothers did to support their sons during the war. They sent letters and parcels by the thousand. A building covering five acres, said to have been the largest wooden building in the world, was constructed in Regent's Park in 1915 to handle parcels to the front, and eventually even it was found inadequate to deal with the volume of traffic.[50] The Home Depot, which sorted mail to every unit, had a staff of 2,500 by the end of the war, most of them women.[51] Much of the traffic handled by the Home Depot originated from families. Mothers cooked their sons' favourite foods. They supplied socks and underwear. They sent blankets, helmets, scarves, jerkins, overcoats and mittens when the weather turned cold. They sent remedies for the ubiquitous louse, for boils, blisters and sores, diarrhoea and constipation. They kept sons supplied with soap, toothpaste and toothbrushes. The rank-and-file soldier and his officer alike relied on home and mothers for support. 'You honestly have no idea what letters are out here', wrote Second Lieutenant Ralph Bickersteth to his mother, 'They are <u>the</u> link to home life and England. When the mail arrives the rush to the mail bag is just like a rugger scrum – the Colonel leading!'[52] Eric Marchant wrote of how 'We all look forward each day to the postbag, as the great event of the day.'[53] After spending four days in heavy snow in trenches near St Quintin, Second Lieutenant Wilfred Owen snuggled up in bed to open his parcel from home. He inspected each item in turn before falling asleep. 'It was like a look in at Home to burrow into that lovely big box and examine all the loving presents.'[54] Matt Webb's appetite for his mother's cakes could not be sated after living on bread and jam for four days: 'anything sent from you through kindness of heart I am sure I shall never be tired of.'[55] The most intimate signs of home could appear in the mail. Second Lieutenant Edward Chapman returned the quarter-pound kitchen weight that arrived with his parcel, it having fallen in by accident, perhaps as his home-baked cakes were packed or as his family weighed the parcel to calculate the postage.[56] Having sent her son Richard a pudding, Mrs Foulkes asked him to return the basin. He replied that he would do his best, though it was difficult to send parcels back home.[57] When re-decorating the family home, Charles Ramsdale's mother sent him swatches of their new kitchen wallpaper.[58] Some might interpret these offerings as signs of civilian incomprehension of life in the trenches, but this was the stuff of home itself, and it offered the most direct contact short of going on leave. Historians, transfixed as they are by the written word and the drama of the trenches, have sometimes overlooked the significance of these ordinary domestic objects – now vanished – in conveying maternal love. Niall Ferguson's list of seven 'carrots' that kept men going in the war includes food, warm clothing, leave and leisure, all of which depended on the support of families. The traffic in mail which made this support possible and which sustained the links with home, rather than being seen as crucial to survival, goes under the category of leisure.[59] Keith Grieves is surely right to assert that an efficient Army postal service is the key to understanding 'the resilience of the British soldier on the Western Front after 1916.'[60]

Part II of the book, 'Mothering men', is about comradeship and the relations between maternal care and military survival. The rank-and-file soldier existed in a domestic world. He was responsible for keeping his kit in order. He would sew on buttons and patch uniforms using a needle and thread from his 'housewife'. If he wanted warm food or a hot drink in the line, he heated it up on a brazier or tommy cooker. He was responsible for his own iron rations, which could be eaten only on the officer's say-so, and he tried to keep aside a bit of extra food for lean times. He carried and kept clean his own eating and drinking utensils. The experience of looking after themselves on the Western Front heightened these men's awareness of domestic matters, putting them all, in a sense, in mother's shoes.

Officers also had responsibilities that, although going under military labels such as 'maintenance of morale', were essentially domestic. They had to make sure that the men were kept warm, dry, clean and well-fed. Housed more comfortably and safely in the line than the men in dug-outs and billets, military efficiency nevertheless demanded that they were attuned to the men's living situation. Cold could kill a man, as Wilfred Owen discovered in his first experience of trench warfare, lying in snow on the exposed Redan ridge in the teeth of a blizzard.[61]

Civilian soldiers did not possess the deep knowledge of Army routines on which the Regular soldier could fall back, but they did have experience of their own families and households, and mothers liked to give advice. Sam Dawson, an Army cook, used his mother's recipes, and prepared his men's food with the wooden spoon she had sent him. '[S]hould like to see you making your tarts', she wrote.[62] The upbringing of the 'war generation' provided their resources for survival in the war. Comradeship did not supplant home ties. These men's identities, as Bourke argues, 'remained lodged within their civilian environment'.[63]

At the same time, the approach taken by Bourke and others, which rightly demonstrates the inter-connections between the fronts, can tend to down play the mis-understandings, tensions and sometimes the outright hostility which could flare up between soldiers and their loved ones. Soldiers only had to sew on their own buttons because their womenfolk were not there to do it for them; and writing home did not actually get them out of the trenches. The traffic in letters and parcels, the movement of women towards the front line to work as VADs and nurses, or the backward movement of soldiers to Blighty on leave or as casualties, did not create a united wartime community. Try as they might to imagine themselves in the other's position, Susan Grayzel surely goes too far when she asserts that letters and home leave enabled people 'to transcend the gender-bound categories – to bridge the gap between divided fronts – in which they had been placed.'[64] To conclude this is to set too much store by the rhetoric of keeping in touch, and not enough by the emotional experience of separation, which was felt equally by the soldier and his loved ones.

A further problem with approaches that stress the ties between loved ones, and downplay the extent to which the war brutalised men, is that they tend to restrict themselves to the war experience, when families were separated and men were prone to homesick longings. They rarely investigate in detail the family situations that these men left, or the ones they returned to after they were demobilised. They can assume an unproblematic return to the bosom of the family. But was it the case that men 'breathed more freely once they returned home'?[65] In a recent and accomplished study of the Pals' battalions in Liverpool, Helen McCartney argues that the ties with home were so strong that, on their return, men were simply able to pick up the threads of their lives where they had left off. They 'successfully merged back into civilian life, their pre-war ambitions and interests substantially intact.'[66] The men who filled the ranks of the Liverpool Territorial battalions in McCartney's study were older than most and many had established careers and families of their own before joining up. Even among these mature adults the idea that violence could be forgotten seems improbable, but for the subjects of this study, who were unmarried and mere youths when they signed up, it is untenable. Such studies have little to say about the state these men were in at the war's end. They can assume that there was an 'unexpectedly smooth transition from war to peace', and that 'no cultural or psychological rupture had taken place.'[67] What it felt like to have seen a man 'ripped from his shoulder to his waist', as Harry Patch did, or to have the brains of a best mate splattered over one's tunic, trousers, and breakfast, as happened to George Coppard, is little considered. [68]

The middle-class recruit who had entered the Army straight from school, or the ranker who had been serving an apprenticeship or in a clerical post before joining up, grew to manhood during the war. He had seen and endured things on the Western Front that his sisters and brothers, mother and father could only imagine. When Greenwell published his wartime letters to his mother, he prefaced his volume with the remark that it traced his 'development from the immature subaltern to the veteran of the later years.'[69] Coppard, demobbed from the war just after his twenty-first birthday, described how the 'youth had become a man but with only the capabilities of a youth to meet adult realities in civvy street.' Now an adult, the only civilian identity he knew was that of a child.[70]

The studies produced in the 1970s by Paul Fussell and Eric Leed were attuned to precisely these kinds of questions about what it felt like for young veterans to return as civilians to a society of which they had no adult experience, and with the effects of violence still raw. For Leed, the return not only meant the 'collapse of the idealized home' but in many cases the 'counter-idealisation' of comradeship, a kind of nostalgia for the military life.[71] Fussell traced the development of a binary mentality of 'us' and 'them', through which the veteran's perception of the post-war political and personal world was framed. For Mosse, the psychological effects of unassimilated violence were played out in a post-war politics of bitterness and hatred. Weisbrod, in a similar spirit, shows how wartime violence provided the basis for Ernst Junger's post-war vision of a virile warrior race.[72] All these historians concur in seeing the veteran's anger as a powerful force. The issues they raise about the emotional damage of war are addressed in Part III, 'Falling apart'. This investigates what it meant psychically to be subjected to the sustained violence of the Western Front, and asks how this violence revealed itself once the men were actually back, and 'home' was no longer an abstract ideal but a day-to-day reality. It shows how women were drawn into managing the veteran's depression and mood swings, and explores the limits – psychological and practical – of support.

Despite the assertions in Fussell, Leed, Mosse and others about the negative effects of the war on domestic relationships, in fact families remain in the shadows even in these studies. When these historians mention 'home', what they generally mean is the nation-state or civil society, not the family. The targets of veteran anger, says Leed, were 'those in authority', the profiteer, the puffy generals and the politicians who continued the war.[73] 'Home' for these historians is primarily a *political* entity and not, as most veterans probably imagined it, a shorthand for loved ones, bricks and mortar, a garden or a neighbourhood, perhaps a local landscape.

Even Susan Kent, who in *Making Peace* focuses explicitly on gender, never pauses to ask what actually went on in households around Britain at the end of the war after soldiers were demobilised. Her analysis stays at the level of public discourse, and her conclusion that women were made to bear the strain of the war, re-civilising the veteran, is therefore little more than conjecture. 'Sexual antagonism' there may have been in post-war writings, but what was happening was that the violence that had been put into the soldier during the war, in the form of shells and bullets, was being projected into those around him afterwards; and these were people whom he loved and upon whom he depended. Kent's analysis sees only the conflict and not the intimacy of domestic relationships. The hatred that veterans vented on officials in the demobilisation riots of the first half of 1919 and in the Peace Day ceremonies was less ambivalent than on the domestic scene, where veterans also wanted to be cared for. It was in lived relationships within the home, as much as in public rhetoric or political action, that the war's deepest emotional effects were played out.

The anger felt by so many veterans, far from being a rejection of their loved ones, was a way of trying to get through to them. Poems such as Wilfred Owen's 'S.I.W.' and Siegfried Sassoon's 'Glory of Women' and 'Their Frailty' are often cited as examples of misogyny, but the label gives no hint of the close affection these men had for their own mothers.[74] Owen's 'S.I.W.' explores the convention that mothers would be shielded from the full horror of trench warfare. The poem ends with the lines 'With him they buried the muzzle his teeth had kissed,/And truthfully wrote the Mother, "Tim died smiling."'[75] 'SIW' comments on the mother's supposed ignorance about life in the line: only a soldier, it suggests, would understand that a rictus was often to be found on a man who had shot himself through the head. Women's naivety is also the theme of Sassoon's *Glory of Women* which ends with a vision of a German mother 'dreaming by the fire', knitting socks for her son while 'His face is trodden deeper in the mud'.[76] The title of *Their Frailty* applies to those women whose interest in the war extends no further than the fate of their own loved one, and whose support for the war had allowed it to continue. The poem ends 'Mothers and wives and sweet-hearts, – they don't care/So long as He's all right.'[77]

But these war poems did not just blame and disparage mothers. They also appealed to them for help. Attacking women's romantic ideas about war, and confronting them with horror, was as much a means of arousing sympathy as of expressing disillusionment. The war poetry echoed the tone of many letters home from the front, which acknowledged the convention that mothers must be protected, but which were written nonetheless to get under their skin. Shortly after he returned to the front in late September 1918, one of Wilfred Owen's men was shot through the head and bled to death on Owen's shoulder. Owen said he would refrain from worrying his mother, but his brief description of the death pulled her inescapably onto the scene: 'Of whose blood lies yet crimson on my shoulder where his head was – and where so lately yours was – I must not now write.'[78] In declaring their refusal to write about it, sons drew their mothers' attention to horror, and made them anxious.

* * *

In part, historians have found it difficult to write the emotional history of the war because it gave rise to contradictory emotional states: aggression as well as tenderness, cruelty and care, fascination and fear. As Frederic Manning remarked in *Her Privates We*, 'The extremities of pain and pleasure had met and coincided too.'[79] Historians of the war, however, have lacked concepts that can accommodate the contrary character of emotions. Hence there remains something of a gap between those who demonstrate the humanity of the trench soldier in the face of mechanised destruction, but largely overlook his aggression, and those who extrapolate his anger and disenchantment from the intimate settings – the letter, and home itself – in which they were often expressed.

Trying to comprehend Manning's extremities in relation to one another goes some way towards reconstructing the emotional experience of the war. It allows us to see feelings that had often been split off from one another as part of the same psychic reality.

This book arises from around a decade and a half of reading in psychoanalysis. Although for the most part it avoids explicit theoretical discussion, psychoanalytic ideas inform the whole account. Psychoanalysis, through its concern with the unconscious effects of extreme emotional experience, has helped me to understand the impact of trench warfare on the mind. It has also helped me with the methodological problem of how to discern states of mind from the often oblique clues given in letters, diaries and memoirs. Psychoanalysis highlights the emotional and symbolic importance of maternal support during the war, of food as a source of psychic as well as physical nourishment; and of the stomach as a site of pollution, pain and protest as well as pleasure. It sensitises us to the ways in which physical ailments, and the trench soldier's reports about them, could express his spirits. Its focus on early experiences allows us to view the behaviour of these young soldiers, separated from home, through the prism of their individual upbringings and the wider emotional dynamics of Edwardian families. It gives us insights into how the war became lodged in memory afterwards, and how its effects were enacted on loved ones.

Psychoanalysis has, lastly, proven indispensable to me because the emotion that dominated people more than any other during the war was anxiety; and psychoanalysis is itself, particularly in its Kleinian variety, centrally concerned with anxiety. Anxiety for Klein is related to the very earliest experiences of the infant, when it does not have a sense of the boundaries of its body, and is subjected to a myriad of sensations, from within and without, that it cannot comprehend and cannot control. What extreme anxiety did to these young men was to throw them back to the position of the small child, who needs its mother to assuage its terror. The cry for his mother of the French *poilu* as he lay dying; or Bion's attempt to comfort himself in the roadside at Amiens, suggest how anxiety could reduce them to infancy. Indeed, Bion's very description of waiting for battle to commence at Amiens enacts a regression, from the young officer, through the exhausted child, to the tiny babe in arms. He begins by referring to a desire to 'be put to bed by . . . mother'; and ends with the feeling of 'lying peacefully in someone's arms'.[80]

Military historians have recently been questioning the emphasis on horror in accounts of the First World War. They have argued that the story of trenches mired in horror is a myth, and that it became installed only in the middle of the twentieth century. It was a *post*-war phenomenon more than a contemporary experience. Moments of anxiety, they suggest, were relatively few and far between. For the most part, soldiers spent their time in the back areas, doing 'bull', parading, or on the march. These historians argue that we need to consider other emotions in the life of the soldier apart from anxiety, such as boredom, the pleasure of comradeship and the thrill of combat.[81] It is true that most infantry soldiers were only in front-line trenches for relatively short periods of time, typically four days, although in battle the proportion was likely to increase.[82] They normally moved in a cycle between the firing line, the support line some 70–100 yards back with its deep dug-outs and Company Headquarters, and the reserve lines.[83] Looking back over his diary for 1916, Carrington concluded that he had participated in twelve 'tours' of the trenches. He had spent 101 days 'under fire', sixty-five of which were in front-line trenches. The infantry soldier was often on the move: Carrington estimated that he packed up his goods around eighty times during 1916, usually prior to a route march.[84] He might be 'at rest' behind the lines in billets. When 'at rest', the Army kept men busy parading, cleaning uniforms and kit and transporting supplies to the front lines. Far from being terrified, they were often bored and resentful. The normal experience of the trenches was not of fighting, but of simply holding the line. Most British soldiers probably only participated in two or at most three attacks during their military service. Carrington had twelve tours in the trenches during 1916, four of which involved him in action, while on a fifth occasion he took part in a failed trench-raid.[85] Some men never went 'over the top' during the whole of their military service. Wilfred Owen's introduction to the trenches, being bombarded for four days whilst stuck in a half-flooded dug-out ahead of the British front line, was exceptional.[86] More usually, the trench soldier spent his time peering out into No Man's Land for signs of German movements, fetching and carrying supplies, or shovelling muddy soil into sandbags.

Despite being more often out of the line than in, and more often holding the line than attacking, time in the trenches wore men down. F. E. Noakes reckoned that, though going over the top was more dangerous, it 'was probably less of a strain on the nerves, because less protracted, than life in the trenches.' Far from familiarity 'deadening my sense of peril', his fear increased with every trip back up the line. He felt '"windy" during most of the time I spent in the line.'[87] Fear nagged at them and sometimes broke to the surface. Sentries, exhausted from standing on the fire step and peering hour after hour into the gloom, sometimes opened fire on comrades returning from patrols or raiding parties.

Shelling frayed the nerves. During a barrage one man was heard calling for his mother in a 'thin, boyish voice', his cries giving way to screams as the thunderous explosions continued around him.[88] Roland Mountfort, on one of his first sentry duties, got down from the firing step and crouched in the bottom of the trench when shells began falling thick around them. He was 'in a terrible funk, + judging from the faces I noticed, was not unique in that.' The 'row shakes you to pieces', he added.[89] Shelling was felt with an intensity that made it more like a physical blow than a sound. It became, as Santanu Das puts it, 'something tangible'. Robert Graves tried to describe it in an interview for *The Listener* in 1971, but 'You couldn't; you can't communicate noise.'[90] Many men found that the longer they were at the front the more edgy they became when under shell-fire. They would say they had 'wind-up', a phrase that appeared as quickly in the war as it became out-dated afterwards. The officer Graham Greenwell, who had been five months in trenches, explained the feeling to his mother, suggesting as he did so, the derivation of the word: 'The row these things make is incredible and I can hear nothing but the low whistle of heavy shells; every puff of the wind startles me and I feel as nervous as a cat. It is the sitting still throughout a solid day listening the whole time to shells and wondering if the next one will be on the dug-out or not which is so unnerving.'[91] The sudden resumption of shelling might send a man into a spin. One of Geoffrey Thurlow's fellow officers, on being awoken by a 'crump' ('crump' was another term coined during the war and described the explosion of a heavy shell) scrambled into the pouring rain in bare feet. The scattered furniture in his dug-out revealed his frantic attempts to get out.[92]

Terror might be momentary, but it could make the heart race even in quiet moments behind the lines. It could come out of the blue.[93] A single, stray shell hit a man who was walking in woods near Poperinghe, taking his head off. Having survived the frontline during Hooge in 1915, he died behind the lines.[94] The father of the historian of trench warfare, Denis Winter, 'saw a man shot in the stomach miles from the front when a bullet ignited in the heat of a brazier.'[95]

The war broke into veterans' sleep decades afterwards. Private Hyder had a recurrent nightmare, based on his actual experience, when he shot dead a badly wounded German whom he heard dragging himself along the passage to his pillbox: 'still at night comes a sweat that wakes me by its deadly chill to hear again that creeping, creeping.'[96] The structure of Manning's autobiographical novel *Her Privates We* shows how battle, and the aftermath of it, would come to dominate their feelings. Most of the action in the novel takes place behind the lines, marching, parading and searching for food and warmth. But it opens with the disturbing visions of Private Bourne as he lies awake in his tent after battle, thinking of 'one man shot cleanly in his tracks and left face downwards, dead, . . . another torn into bloody tatters.' Bourne tries to put these scenes from his mind, but they are destined to reappear in his sleep.[97]

Horror and dread were certainly not the only emotions that soldiers experienced, but at the same time, war's pleasures were rarely unalloyed. Comradeship, for example, gained some of its intensity from anxiety. It was *because* conditions in the trenches were so primitive, and because men had looked onto horrible scenes together, that they needed each others' help and comfort, and felt separated from civilians. Comedy could itself be a product of terror: when a dud shell landed amidst Edwin Vaughan's party, he and his runner burst into hysterical laughter. The runner had 'tears rolling down his face' at the sight of one of the officers, 'upside down, bent almost double with his head pressed into the earth, his great bespectacled face white with fear and streaked with mud.'[98] Even the lust for killing cannot be separated from anxiety. Men might feel a 'subtle thrill' when opening fire on some Germans, or a sense of 'exaltation' or 'elation' at surviving battle unharmed, but these emotions drew their strength from fear.[99] A man who seemed positively intoxicated by slaughter, such as Ernst Jünger (who describes the anticipation of killing in *The Storm of Steel* as 'one of the very few moments that I can call truly happy') was reacting to terror. Jünger himself thought so, regarding the 'voluptuousness of blood' felt by the trench soldier as a defence, a 'release from a heavy and unbearable pressure' of fighting for one's life.[100]

Both fear and fascination impelled the soldier, newly arrived in the trenches, to take a close look at a corpse, which was for many, their first face-to-face encounter with the dead.[101] They wanted to know what it meant to kill, and what it meant to be killed. The military psychiatrist W. H. R. Rivers noted the compulsion, and thought it was a way of inuring themselves to the 'utmost rigours and horrors of warfare' which were to come.[102] Harry Penrose in *The Secret Battle* shows 'undisguised interest' when discovering his first Turkish corpse on arriving in trenches at Gallipoli.[103] The pocket diary of Gunner William Hate shows the heady mixture of feelings he experienced after going up the line at Neuve Chapelle. He was keen to see the damage his bombardment had inflicted: 'go to the support trenches + take photos see many gruesome sights go back loaded with officers souvenirs.'[104] Charles Carrington had to wait six months in France before viewing his first German corpses, though he had often seen men hit. He was 'fascinated' by their 'horrid plumpness', the skin on the faces stretched tight over cheeks and brows, the bodies 'bursting out of their clothes'. His Sergeant boasted of having 'pulled the teeth out of one of them and made a necklace of them.'[105]

Gape as they might at the grotesque forms of the dead, the excitement and intensity of war at the same time exhausted and disturbed them. Carrington scorned the 'self-pitying school' of memoir writers, wanted people to know that his generation had gone to war with their eyes open, and insisted that he, 'like so many young men', had 'enjoyed being a soldier on the whole'.[106] Yet he too, by his own description, was 'nervously exhausted' after Passchendale.[107] Guy Nightingale wrote extraordinarily graphic accounts to his mother and sister from Gallipoli, relishing the violence. He commented witheringly on the new officers too soft to take it, but perhaps ultimately nor could Nightingale, for he took his own life in the 1930s.[108] The myth of horror did not arise through the cultural manipulation of unusually 'sensitive and imaginative' literary men, but arose from the actual situation of the infantry soldier.[109]

The concept of 'emotional experience' is one that will recur throughout this book when describing the reactions of soldiers and their families. Like some other concepts to which I refer in the forthcoming chapters, it has been used by both veterans and psychoanalysts. The war, observed Guy Chapman in the 1966 preface to his wonderful memoir *A Passionate Prodigality* (first published in 1933), was 'a long emotional experience with extreme heights and depths.' Chapman's memory was not just of the loss of 800 men and thirty-two officers –casualties which amounted to the entire strength of the Battalion by the end of the war – but of comradeship too. In terms that resonate with those of the neo-Kleinian D. W. Winnicott, Chapman explained that in the book he was 'preoccupied with an attachment, the sentiment of belonging to a living entity, and of course, its death.'[110] His memoir was a way of exploring the deep identification he had felt with his Battalion, a bond that was not weakened but conditioned and intensified by loss.

The term 'emotional experience' would also be used by Wilfred Bion in his psychoanalytic writings from the late 1950s, but whereas Chapman used his memoir to bring to the surface, and mentally work through, the emotional heights and depths of the war, Bion was more concerned with times when the mind was overwhelmed and thinking became impossible. 'Emotional experience' was for Bion a matter of 'sense impressions' – such as touch, smell, sight and so on – and how they were handled within the mind. Not all emotional experiences, especially those of acute anxiety, could be processed, and were consequently not 'available for conscious . . . thought'.[111] These undigested sensations were experienced as concrete matter, as 'things in themselves'. Unprocessed, they continued to work away within the unconscious, revealing themselves in psychic disturbances, such as 'acting out', or in psychosomatic illnesses. In psychotic states, Bion argued, the very awareness of the difference between an emotional experience in the external world, and the internal apprehension of it, was itself obliterated.[112]

For the young men of the war generation, schooled as many were in the Edwardian idea of the 'stiff upper lip', the gap between emotional experience and what was actually conscious to them, let alone what they felt they *ought* to communicate in letters home, was large. Fear made them want to run from battle, but cowardice was shameful. They wanted their mothers but they were soldiers and men, and mothers needed to be kept in good cheer. In any case, maybe it was better to keep a lid on things. Letters home frequently hint at mental struggles such as these. Although it is true that many said more about their situation than is sometimes assumed given military censorship, it is equally true that many of their deepest emotions were not self-evident to them then or to us now as historians. Emotions were just as often unconsciously *enacted* in letters, as deliberated upon.

An eminent historian of the First World War has recommended that scholars should be cautious of retrospective accounts by veterans because many are tainted by memory and the myth of horror. He summarises the typical contents of interviews: 'Up to my neck in muck and bullets; rats as big as footballs; the sergeant major was a right bastard; all my mates were killed.'[113] He directs us instead to contemporary sources, the rich collections of diaries and letters in archives such as the Imperial War Museum and Liddle Collection, because 'the closer we get to events the better our chance of finding out how people really felt.'[114] But proximity to events does not mean the sentiments expressed in letters or diaries were transparent. What these men experienced was sometimes too disturbing to take in; the very ability to think was under attack. Bringing events to mind and writing about them threatened to repeat them: the capacity to symbolise, to translate emotional experience from raw impulses into words, and thus to contain and mediate it, was damaged. In Captain Herbert Leland's account, written as the shells fell about him (a more contemporaneous account would be hard to imagine), the jokey tone scarcely conceals his terror of being rent apart, which was less evoked than *performed* in the very writing: 'Oh – Damn these shells. I am quite unable to write coherently. One has just dropped, and lifted me off my biscuit box!!!' 'Oh! Such a crump has just fallen. Mud, dust, splinters of wood all over me, but I am hanging on to this piece of paper.'[115] Only a scrap of paper, his one connection to home, kept Leland sane amidst the shellfire, and if he lost his grip on it, he might not hold together.

Retrospective accounts are generally more reflective about the emotional experience of war than the letter or diary. It was not just that writers were liberated from the constraints of military censorship, but that, at the time of experience, language had tended to function as a primitive vehicle for ejecting raw and intolerable sense impressions. Experiences such as Leland's, scrawled on paper, were not wholly constituted in language. Time was needed before a coherent narrative could be constructed.[116] For veterans like Guy Chapman or A. P. Herbert, writing about the war was thus often a form of auto-therapy, an attempt to try and process the tumultuous sensations that had violently forced themselves into them. Other veterans would never be capable of this level of mental functioning.

The sensations conveyed in letters, by comparison with memoirs, were relatively undigested and are often now opaque to us, forcing us to read between the lines. What Freud calls 'parapraxes' – slips of the pen, grammatical errors, contradictions, repetitions and so on – give the merest glimpse of emotional states. In some cases, it is the very protestation of good spirits that suggests all was not well. In others, reports of rashes and boils, eczema, or tummy problems expressed their distress. Ailments could be discussed in letters home, when poor spirits might not. Food was a common topic of conversation; their appetites seemed insatiable.[117] Some reported dreams, but did not pause over their meanings. If letters, being close to the moment of experience, conveyed something of 'how people really felt', it was often more than the writers themselves intended, and sometimes in spite of their efforts at concealment. The real value of letters as psychological sources becomes fully evident once we accept that emotional states are not wholly conscious, and take into account what is hinted at, unspoken, or unspeakable. Without an appreciation of the unconscious impact of the war, it is difficult to fathom how the seeming war-monger Nightingale could end up committing suicide; why the battle-hardened professional soldier Leland was admitted to the Special Hospital for Officers in Palace Green in late 1917; how the young tank-commander Bion became a psychoanalyst who devoted his professional career to regression and psychotic states; why men always felt hungry and why they complained about Army food; or why the mud, rats and slaughter of the Western Front loomed larger than life in their memories in old age.

* * *

Men of the war generation venerated their mothers with a frankness and intensity that now, in a post-Freudian age, can make us squirm. Wilfred Owen signed off his first letter home after joining his platoon in France in verse:

> The favourite song of the men is
> 'The Roses round the door
> Makes me love Mother more'
> They sing this everlastingly.
> I don't disagree. Your very own W.E.O. x[118]

Owen presented this as an observation on his men's sentiments, but of course in putting their verse at the end of his letter, he sang his own mother's praises. From her home in Twickenham, Alice Swettenham sent her son Alf a postcard depicting a vase of flowers, beside which was printed in verse, a 'greeting from Home/to my Son, who's so dear'. On the back is a message whose brevity makes the written hand all the more powerful: 'With much love from Mother.'[119] In Spring 1915, as he prepared for a second stint on the Western Front, Stephen Brown sent his mother a postcard from Sheerness. It depicts a soldier, quill pen poised in hand, lost in thought, and the caption reads: 'I am thinking of you.' Brown's own feelings at this point were rather less composed than the image suggested, however, as the message scrawled on the back reveals: 'Just a few lines to let you know that I am quite well I am for the front on Teusday [sic] But if you write to the Commanding [officer] and say I am only seventeen it will stop me from going get it here before Teusday for I cannot get a pass to come and see you don't forget from Stephen'.[120] Many of the images and expressions used by rank-and-file soldiers in their letters are formulaic, even commercial. In reacting against the sentimentality, however, we fail to take seriously the motives that animated

Edwardian people in sending and keeping them. Families resorted to stereotypes as a means of conveying deep and authentic feelings, feelings that conjoined an abstract idea of motherhood to actual mothers.[121] Swettenham hung on to the postcard from his mother: it was among the few personal effects that were returned to his family. Brown's postcard pleading for his mother to keep him away from the fighting must have haunted her, for he was killed on 10 May 1915 just weeks after he reached France, but she kept it and perhaps for all its note of desperation, she valued it as a sign of the depth of his attachment to her. Correspondents drew on the public conventions of emotional expression but made them their own, and got their message across. The ranker Bert Chapman, an apprentice printer from London conscripted into the army, experimented with verse:

> You say Flo misses me.
> Gee: so do I miss you all.
> Very much so at times.
> Well I suppose 'it' will soon be over,
> At least lets [*sic*] hope so.
> I haven't any news Mother Dear, bar that I am alright. So I must pack.[122]

The sentiments that Chapman expressed, missing everyone at home, wishing for the war to end, and reassuring his mother, are repeated in many letters home. They are generic, but no less profound and intensely felt for that, and they meant so much more to the writer and recipient than the assemblage of stock phrases itself appears to suggest. To use such letters as historical sources, we need to analyse their cultural codes so as to bring out the powerful emotions that are often implicitly expressed, or that lie within what appears to be mere cliché.

A distinctive feature of psychoanalysis is that it understands the emotional experience of adults in terms of relationships within early life. Because of this psycho-historians are often criticised for being reductive. In the popular jibe, mothers are always to blame. There are obvious problems with an approach which seems to presume that emotional survival during the war owed something to the adequacy of mothering. For one thing, the assertion that a man's capacity to endure the Western Front was influenced by the quality of his early relationships is difficult to assess since we rarely have direct evidence of his childhood. This book, in contrast, argues that the violence to which men were exposed in the First World War was itself deeply traumatising. In so doing, it goes against those military historians who argue (in an analysis unwittingly influenced by a popular version of Freudianism) that the mental turmoil of Robert Graves, Richard Aldington, Siegfried Sassoon and others was due less to the horror of the war itself than to 'sexual problems deriving from their education and repressive home environment.'[123]

How then might we draw on the insights of psychoanalysis without being reductive in this way? Freud's work – especially as it developed through and after the war – has been a fertile source of insight in studies of the First World War. In his pessimistic essay, 'Thoughts For the Times on War and Death', written early in 1915, Freud asks how it was that mass destruction could be instigated by societies that had hitherto been considered among the most advanced in human civilisation. The civilised European had been living 'psychologically speaking, beyond his means' in believing that he had tamed evil.[124] The lesson for Freud was that the instincts of life and death, love and aggression, bore an intimate relation to one another, a point which is telling for this study, concerned as it is with the co-existence of violence and love. Freud's work on mourning has also been taken up in studies of how the war was commemorated. Jay Winter, for example, in his work on war memorials, looks at the role played by traditional symbols and collective rituals in mediating loss, and hence in helping the wartime bereaved separate from the dead.[125] Freud's work on trauma has also been important, especially his essay 'Beyond the Pleasure Principle', which, perhaps partly in response to the plight of shell-shocked soldiers, asked why it was that the victims of traumatic neurosis felt compelled to re-visit and repeat, in their dreams and talk, the source of their disturbance.[126]

Freud's insights on love and hate, loss and trauma, also inform this account, but it makes use of Kleinian theories as well. This is partly due to its subject matter: it is concerned with mothers and sons, and Kleinian theory focuses on the source of psychic life in the relationship with the mother. As a result, emotions for the Kleinian are not perceived as self-contained and individual, but as generated in human conduct and thus as always relational. Emotional states are incited by and fostered through communication – conscious and unconscious – with others. For Guy Chapman, it was the close attachments among the men in his Battalion, and their eventual fates, which made him want to write about the war. Chapman's memoir exemplifies Bion's theoretical formulation: '[a]n emotional experience cannot be conceived of in isolation from a relationship.'[127] Bion's ideas about how anxiety was experienced within individuals came from thinking about the mother and baby, and the communication between them. Anxiety was not a sensation felt by the baby autonomously, but passed back and forth, and either tolerated and made recognisable by the mother, or resisted and thrown back, and so made unintelligible. The baby's emotions were not distinct from the mother's way of handling them, that is, her capacity to receive and to take in its psychic states, or what Bion called the capability of 'reverie'.[128]

The relational character of emotions means that *who* a son was writing his letter to had a direct bearing on the kinds of experiences he related. What he felt in writing home to his mother was not necessarily what he felt when writing to a sister or sweetheart, and different again from his state of mind when writing to a father or fellow soldier. The person being imagined and addressed brought some states to mind, suppressed others and left yet others unthought. This book has little to say about gambling, drunkenness or visiting prostitutes, though these experiences were common enough on the Western Front. It has more to say about trench foot than about venereal disease, and less about killing than the fear of dying. Its themes and omissions reflect the kinds of emotional states that were brought into play in correspondence with mothers. The neglected topics were not merely a matter of conscious censorship, but reflected the longer histories of subjectivity – of confession, silence and conflict – between mothers and sons. It was often with their mothers that they had shared their most vulnerable feelings as children, or at least had expected to, and this expectation would re-surface during the war. As a result, men sometimes found that their spirits grew poorer when writing to a mother. 'I think I ought to close now as the more I write the worse I feel so au Revoir mother dear', wrote Second Lieutenant Harold Hague after a splash of liquid mustard gas had led to 'exema [*sic*] breaking out on my face.'[129] Frank Wollocombe apologised because 'my letters have been a bit melancholy lately, but I haven't felt so in the least since I have been out. I like it much better than the awful old training days in England'.[130] What the psychoanalyst Paula Heimann states as a guide for the clinician, might hold true for the historian reading a young soldier's letter home: '*who is speaking, to whom, about what, and why now?*'[131]

It is a common criticism of the use of psychoanalysis in history that we cannot put the dead 'on the couch'. We do not possess the analyst's intimate knowledge of the client, gathered from sessions over weeks, even years. We do not have direct evidence of childhood and we cannot test our interpretations on our subjects as a psychoanalyst would. This study is not a psycho-history, however. In contrast to a psycho-history, it focuses on the psychological states that the war itself gave rise to, rather than seeing these states primarily as reproductions of an original childhood drama. Nor does it view the battle-stressed soldier or the grieving mother as exemplifying a particular psychological process or pathology. I am more concerned here to place the emotional experience of the war within a cultural context – one which, for example, put great store by mothers as emotional and moral beings, and prized dutifulness in sons – and to track the longer emotional impact of the war into peacetime and civilian life. To put it another way, this account treats the war itself as the primary psychic drama, and is just as concerned with consequences as with origins.

Psychoanalysis helps reveal the connections between emotions that were exalted by the Edwardians and which they wrote constantly about, and others that they found deeply uncomfortable and did not easily express. It points us towards the relations *between* love and hate; generosity and envy; courage and cowardice; grief and triumphalism; selflessness and aggression. In a society where mother-love was so greatly prized, it is important to bring these other emotions out from the shadows. For, as Priscilla Roth suggests, 'our capacity to experience the precious ones (pity, grief, love and so on) is intimately, causally related to the ways we have of coping with the others. That is, our capacity to experience love is related to the ways we have of dealing with our hatred.'[132] Historians of the war have been rightly concerned to sympathise with the battle-stressed soldier or the grief of the bereaved mother, but sympathy can easily lead us to ignore the underbelly of these states, with the result that we end up conspiring in the idealisations of our subjects. Psychoanalysis, with its attention to the unconscious, allows us to identify with the human situations of Edwardian mothers and sons, but without lapsing into lurid repetitions of horror or unreflective sympathy, both of which actually numb us to pain.

Lastly, psychoanalysis helps push beyond some rather rigid frameworks that have emerged within some recent cultural histories of the First World War, which have been characterised by a concern with the social conventions surrounding emotions such as loss, fear and aggression. This work has shown how emotions are situated within the wider culture, and has rightly highlighted the opacity of personal sources. It has demonstrated how in wartime, the most private and intimate feelings, such as bereavement, are harnessed and managed by the state in ways that make it possible, even in the face of mass deaths, to keep fighting.[133] At the same time, such work can result in rather a flat conception of subjectivity, as if emotion consisted of little more than linguistic codes. Emotional states are always, of course, mediated through the culture. It is true, as Carol Acton points out in her study of grief in modern warfare, that the bereaved mother was a 'discourse user', but in focusing on the operation of narratives such as honour and pride on the 'grieving subject', the pain of loss threatens to be rationalised away.[134] Paradoxically, despite the professed intention to explore the relations *between* public discourse and private feeling, the emphasis in such texts on the power of language to shape emotion means that the two can become conflated. Psychoanalysis, which focuses on the states of mind that emerge within human relationships, provides a less linguistically driven way of thinking about emotions and about how they are expressed. It helps sustain an important analytical distinction between emotional experience and its representation, while at the same time guarding against the abstraction of emotion into semantics.

* * *

The sources used in this study include around eighty collections of wartime correspondence between unmarried men and their families, and forty published and unpublished memoirs of the war. In each collection I have examined the totality of family correspondence, so that, for example, letters to mothers can be compared with those to brothers, sisters, fathers and other relatives. Most of the letters are housed at the Imperial War Museum (hereafter, IWM). Rich though these collections are, the vast majority consist of letters from sons to their mothers. Examples of mothers' letters are hard to come by. Sometimes all we have is a last letter, returned with the son's personal effects after his death. Reciprocal correspondence is even rarer, constituting only around twenty of the collections which I targeted. Hence reconstructing the mother's situation has been difficult. I have sometimes relied on the son's own queries and replies, and sometimes on notes scrawled by mothers on their sons' letters. I have had to cast the net wide to include the diaries and letters of mothers, daughters, aunts and even grand-parents; memorial books; oral history interviews with daughters and sons of the war generation; and inscriptions on gravestones.

The collections of letters used in the study are from both rank-and-file soldiers and their officers, but hardly in proportion to the ratio of 50–60:1 that was typical in the infantry. In addition to the cases of reciprocal correspondence, around forty of the collections are from rank-and-file soldiers; and twenty-four from junior officers including Second Lieutenants, Lieutenants and Captains, most of whom were volunteers, Territorials or conscripts. The officers' letters are usually longer and often more numerous than the rankers'. The fifty-six letters that Ernest Smith wrote to his mother between December 1914 and his death in December 1915 inevitably reveal more of his war experience than the four letters and seven postcards that Stephen Brown sent his mother between September 1914 and April 1915. With some exceptions, we know less about the rank-and-file soldier's family and daily routines than we do about his officer's, although the brevity of the ranker's letter can make its emotional power all the greater. Memoirs can be a useful corrective to the elite bias in letters, and the IWM contains many examples from rank-and-file veterans, often written in the 1960s and early 1970s once they had retired, and public interest in the ordinary soldier's experience of the war was increasing. These have been drawn on in conjunction with the oral history project, 'Family Life and Work Experience Before 1918', which contains information about family life before and after the war from across the class spectrum of British society.[135] Interviews and memoirs constitute an important source for Chapter 4, 'Learning to care', which is about family backgrounds, and Chapter 7 on 'The return of the soldier'; after which of course men were usually at home and no longer needed to keep in touch through letters.

It is difficult to avoid an element of bias towards the better-off. Even the rankers whose letters figure in this study were probably better educated, and more literate, than most, their dutifulness in writing home, or later composition of a memoir, being itself a sign of respectability. To take one example, the diary of Alfred Hale, though it gives fascinating insights into the life of a soldier-servant, is hardly the product of a typical batman. Hale was a gentleman, a bachelor with independent means and a woman who kept house for him while he, in effect, kept house for his officers.[136] In the case of rankers' families the difficulties of access are particularly great. Although the study contains examples of middle-class mothers' reactions to having sons away at the front, the evidence for poorer families is fleeting and often refracted through the accounts of their children.

* * *

If in part this book, based largely as it is on writing, draws disproportionately on accounts from the better-off, at the same time it sets out not only to investigate the social backgrounds of the well-off, but of the clerk, the industrial worker, the agricultural labourer and the casually employed poor. In answering the question: How did men survive emotionally?, it looks as much to social as to psychological resources: the physical environment of the home; roles and responsibilities within the household; income; family size; and the links between families, neighbourhoods and other social networks. In so doing, it pursues lines of inquiry familiar to some gender and military historians. John Bourne and Ilana Bet-El, for example, have asked about the features of working-class culture that helped the rank-and-file soldier cope with the hardships of life in the trenches.[137] This study takes their analysis a step further, by looking at the economic and social dynamics of working- and middle-class households in relation to their *emotional* dynamics.

Differences in social background matter, for as Jay Winter has observed of British soldiers in the First World War, 'Their "England" was envisioned as a very local and particular place, bounded in many cases by the streets they knew, and the daily lives they led.'[138] Unconscious conflicts and defences were not the only things that conditioned a man's capacity to hold together under the pressure of trench warfare. Where a man had lived and what his living conditions were like before the war; what kind of work he had done, if any; how much income he had been bringing home; how used he was to living independently and to 'roughing it'; all these things help explain how – and to what extent – he became habituated to Army life. Most soldiers missed their homes, but what 'home' was, how it sustained his spirits and what kind of support it could provide, was not universal. The urban ranker's relatively fluid household, with its traditions of mutual help, provided a different kind of model for survival in the trenches than the service relationships typical in large middle-class homes.

Ideas of socialisation or of 'place', however, do not capture fully the emotional quality of the ties to families and how these were transplanted to the trenches. When a man imagined the local landscape or his family's house, the scene was usually peopled by his loved ones. The sense of place made human attachments feel the more vivid. When Sarah Jane Dawson passed recipes on to her son, she was not just helping him to add some variety to the diets of the men in his platoon, but to recreate the taste of home. Often the family resources that men drew on were not deliberately copied, as Mrs Dawson's recipes were, but unconscious, and resorted to automatically. Bion writes of nestling in the ground 'as if' he was in lying in a mother's arms, but in more extreme circumstances the difference between original relationships and wartime facsimiles became blurred. The mortally wounded man was not aware of acting 'as if' towards a mother, but felt as if he were actually back in her arms. Emotional reactions drawn from family relationships were reproduced. Comradeship might not just approximate, but itself be based on domestic intimacies. This is suggested by S. Rogerson, whose war years had been happy ones; 'the clue', he thought, was that 'we were all comrades . . . we saw love passing the love for women of one pal for his half section.'[139]

Whilst on the one hand the survival skills of wartime depended on particular family and class cultures, on the other, many of the emotional experiences of soldiers and their families were more commonplace than is sometimes assumed. Within both social and military histories of the Great War, the thrust in recent years has been contrary to this. The emphasis has been on disaggregating groups and investigating in fine detail the effects of social class, regional background, gender, type of military service, rank and type of military unit. Diversity is the order of the day. The British people, Janet Watson tells us were 'fighting different wars.'[140] Keith Grieves, in his study of Sussex in the war, has asserted that attention to the local throws into question 'undifferentiated monolithic descriptions of the impact of war.'[141] Differences there undoubtedly were, yet it is also surprising how far, when looking at the soldier's reactions to the post, his avid reading of the local papers, or the support given to him by local comfort funds and families, the local chimes in with the larger picture. For the Sussex soldier, so close to the Western Front that his family could hear the big guns if the wind was in the right direction, the propinquity of home to the war was particularly 'ridiculous'; but the Welsh miner missed home none the less for being further removed.[142]

In the military literature, the stereotype of the Tommy is equally in question. John Horne has stressed 'the relativity of combat experience'.[143] Conscripts, Bet-El reminds us, remained deeply immersed in the civilian lives they had been required to leave, while McCartney sees rankers of the Liverpool Territorials, who questioned Army procedures and cast a critical eye on their officers, as keeping up the habits of the pre-war clerk and manager.[144] Of all the variables in military experience, rank is seen as the fundamental point of division among British regimental soldiers. Whether the literature deals with the daily routines of trench life, popular culture and leisure, or shell-shock, the assumption is that the ranker and the officer, having been socialised in different environments, had different subjectivities.

This stress on different subjectivities can be traced right back to the war. In his essay 'War-Neurosis and Military Training', W. H. R. Rivers noted the different dispositions of officers and men in their reactions to danger, and hence the different kinds of neuroses they suffered. The ranker was less able to control his survival instinct when in danger, and hence he had 'fewer scruples about giving expression to his fears'. He was more likely to exhibit primitive survival mechanisms such as freezing, mutism, or other hysterical symptoms.[145] He was closer to the child in terms of his psychological development. As Rivers put it, the 'characteristic of the uneducated person is that the mental outlook of the adult life does not differ appreciably from that of childhood'.[146] By comparison the mental life of the officer was 'more complex and varied'.[147] His public school had given him a more complete education in repression than the ranker, and he was liable to go on in the face of fear until physically and mentally exhausted. His symptoms – tremors, nightmares, sweats, fatigue and lack of concentration – were signs of the mental effort to repress traumatic memories. Thus for Rivers there existed two 'entirely different mechanisms' of war neurosis, regression accompanied by hysterical symptoms on the one hand; and repression accompanied by neurasthenia on the other.[148] These stemmed from the different socialisation of officers and men – particularly education – but were also a product of more deep-rooted emotional dispositions and mental capacities.

When officers and men commented on each other's characters and habits, it was often to note their differences. J. G. Fuller quotes the ranker Burrage on his officers: 'they were only with us, not of us, and they cannot get inside our skins.'[149] Guy Chapman felt equally alien from his men, though conscientious in the care of them:

> Did any of us know you? Ever pierce your disguise of goose-turd green, penetrate your young skin and look through you to learn the secret which is the essential spirit, the talisman against the worst that fate can offer? No. That was yours. As you would have said: 'Gawd knows; but 'E won't split on a pal.' So you still remain a line of bowed heads, of humped shoulders, sitting wearily in the rain by a roadside, waiting, hoping, waiting – but unknown.[150]

Crushed together in trenches, the geographical segregation that had insulated social classes from each other in civilian life was vastly reduced. Officers and men were brought face-to-face with the things that made them different. Rankers looked on enviously at the officers' hampers from Harrods and their duty-free whisky, and officers wondered at how the men, suffering the cold and wet on a diet of bully beef and hard biscuits, managed to stay cheerful.[151]

It is undeniably the case that rankers and officers were typically brought up within different familial cultures. Even within the middle classes there were large variations, from the small, tight-knit families and emotionally intense relationships characteristic of the lower middle class, to the large households and emotional distance between parents and children often found in the wealthier sections of the upper middle class.[152] There was not a single family structure and, in addition to class, relationships between sons, their parents and siblings varied according to family size and place in birth order, region and religion. Much depended too on individual personalities. Moreover, the different military responsibilities of officers and rankers meant that they needed to draw on different capacities from their home lives. Officers owed a duty of care to their men and many felt the stress of being responsible for others' lives, while rankers had to put up with being given orders that were frequently pointless and harsh, and which exposed them to deadly risk, by men who they sometimes thought – with good reason – wet behind the ears. Yet, despite the differences within and between classes in the way that children were raised, and consequently in the way that these young civilian soldiers reacted to army life, there were also some important similarities. When the country rector's son Edward Chapman joined the 20th Royal Fusiliers as a Second Lieutenant in August 1916, he found that some of the men in his charge were older, and from more prosperous backgrounds, than he. Half the men in his platoon had private incomes and had joined up early in the war, the 20th having been one of the Public School Battalions, and the other half were young, 'average Tommies, mostly Cockneys', who had been drafted in since the Somme began. The men in Chapman's platoon might have varied in age, wealth and military experience but, having travelled with them from the Base Camp to the front line, Chapman felt that after all 'there is perhaps not such a very great difference between them.'[153]

What Chapman had come to feel through being with this body of men was the common humanity of the 'gentleman ranker' and the poor urban recruit. His observation should make historians cautious, for in emphasising only difference, we risk de-humanising those who left less elaborate psychological records. We may end up reproducing Rivers' idea that the ranker had a 'simpler mental training' which led him to cope with trench warfare using more psychologically 'crude solutions' than his officer.[154] It would be all too easy to conclude from the discursive style of many officers' letters that they had indeed a richer, more developed emotional life than the ranker. But as Julie-Marie Strange has commented of grief in nineteenth-century working-class culture, 'verbal eloquence is only one of many representations of feeling', while less voluble reactions, such as resignation, can be 'mistaken for indifference or a lack of humanity'.[155] Rather than assume constitutional differences in the capacity for feeling, this study demonstrates the greater opportunities of the middle-class family for its expression, being better educated, more used to keeping in touch via letters, and with drawing room desks or dug-out benches, leisure and a measure of solitude to facilitate their writing. In the process of deconstructing supposedly monolithic interpretations of the war, as historians of the war are being counselled to do, another form of essentialism, based on the class scripts of Edwardian Britain, is rehabilitated.

This book seeks to establish the commonality of emotions like fear, anger, love, and loss in war, whilst at the same time showing how they took shape according to particular class and family cultures and idioms of expression. Looked at from the point of view of emotional survival, the similarities are as striking as the differences. The terror of trench warfare was experienced by both rankers and officers, and indeed was felt to have constituted a powerful bond between them. Both yearned for their families, and depended on them for comfort and support. In the face of danger they reacted with the same psychic mechanisms: both the officer Bion and the dying French *poilus* were regressed. The same can be said for mothers. Many felt the enervating effects of worry about loved ones at the front, though they did not all possess the same ability, or the desire, to express it in writing. The contents of their parcels provide eloquent markers of wealth and social status, but the impulse to want to protect and give succour transcended class boundaries. Each felt equally deep pain at the loss of a son.

Psychoanalysis is used in this study, not to delineate absolute differences in subjectivity, but to identify common features in the emotional reactions of soldiers and their loved ones to the war. In the pursuit of these reactions, I have drawn upon published fictional accounts of the war in addition to memoirs. Historians usually treat the two genres separately, the one having to pass muster in terms of being faithful to actual events, the other allowing the author to move beyond what he witnessed personally. It is striking how many veterans opted for fiction: Siegfried Sassoon (who, significantly, makes George Sherston an orphan in his trilogy); the Australian veteran Frederic Manning who lost his commission in the Royal Irish Regiment due to his drinking; Richard Aldington, for whom fiction permitted a savage satire of the Edwardian bourgeoisie; the subaltern R. H. Mottram who gained in fiction the freedom to write about the war not just from the soldier's perspective but from that of the woman behind the lines; and the ex-doctor Warwick Deeping who had an immensely successful career after the war as a middlebrow novelist. A. P. Herbert took just weeks to complete *The Secret Battle*, upset by the treatment of Edwin Dyett, and suffering from the 'most horrible and extraordinary nightmares'.[156] He had taken part in the same attack at Beaucourt in November 1916 in which Dyett was accused of desertion, when 415 rank-and-file soldiers went into battle and only twenty answered roll-call after dark. Herbert was one of only two officers in his Battalion to survive.[157] These war novels have more than the ring of personal experience about them, which suggests that fiction was being used not so much to create a work of fiction about the war from the outside, as to explore events and emotional states that *had* been their own, but which still felt difficult to acknowledge. The secrets of the war – the dread and helplessness that contradicted the Edwardian ideal of the soldier, and the fury which traduced domestic ideals – could emerge in fiction in a way that limited personal exposure or the imputation of failure.[158] Fiction could permit a certain freedom to reflect upon and digest emotional experiences that, in a more obviously personal account such as a letter, written soon after the event, were more likely to have been communicated unconsciously. The following chapters convey this psychological journey as it was undertaken by the war generation, from the mental assault of trench warfare, sometimes barely capable of expression in letters home, to the memoir or autobiographical novel, often composed in a domestic setting, yet nonetheless still caught up in the violence of war.

## Notes

1 W. R. Bion, *War Memoirs 1917–19* (London: H. Karnac, 1997), p. 3, p. 122.
2 N. Gladden, *Ypres 1917* (London: William Kimber, 1967), p. 131.
3 Interview with Harry Patch, 'World War One, The Last Tommy Gallery', http://www.bbc.co.uk/history/worldwars/wwone/last_tommy_gallery_03.shtml. Accessed 13 June 2007. The programme was shown in November 2005 to mark Remembrance Day.
4 Quoted in G. Robb, *British Culture and the First World War* (Basingstoke: Palgrave, 2002), p. 155.

5 L. Raemaekers, *The Great War. A Neutral's Indictment: one hundred cartoons* (London: Fine Art Society, 1916), plate 75.
6 S. Audoin-Rouzeau, *Men at War 1914–1918. National Sentiment and Trench Journalism in France during the First World War* (Oxford: Berg, 1995), p. 80.
7 Shot at Dawn Website, 'Shot Unjustly, Unlawfully', http://www.shotatdawn.org.uk/page15.html. Accessed 5 May 2007.
8 Quoted in D. Winter, *Death's Men. Soldiers of the Great War* (London: Penguin, 1979), p. 200.
9 R. Pound, *A. P. Herbert. A Biography* (London: Michael Joseph, 1976), p. 53.
10 A. P. Herbert, *The Secret Battle* (Thirsk: House of Stratus, 2001), p. 141.
11 http://www.shotatdawn.org.uk/page15.html. Accessed 5 May 2007.
12 S. Audoin-Rouzeau and A. Becker, *1914–1918. Understanding the Great War* (London: Profile Books, 2002), p. 20.
13 Audoin-Rouzeau and Becker, *1914–1918*, pp. 22–3.
14 J. M. Winter, *The Great War and the British People* (Basingstoke: Macmillan, 1985), p. 72.
15 Audoin-Rouzeau and Becker, *1914-1918*, p. 25, p. 39.
16 Winter, *Death's Men*, p. 73; R. Aldington, *Death of a Hero* (London: Consul, 1965), p. 138.
17 A. Bishop and M. Bostridge, (eds.), *Letters From a Lost Generation. First World War Letters of Vera Brittain and Four Friends* (London: Abacus, 1999), p. 226.
18 J. D. Tomlinson to brother Ted, 17 April 1915, IWM 87/51/1.
19 J. D. Tomlinson to mother, 26 April 1915.
20 W. B. P. Spencer to mother, 3 January 1915, IWM 87/56/1.
21 P. Smith to mother and dad, 18 September 1917, IWM 01/21/1.
22 G. Mosse, *Fallen Soldiers. Reshaping the Memory of the World Wars* (Oxford: Oxford University Press, 1990), p. 3.
23 Winter, *The Great War and the British People*, p. 83.
24 D. Hankey, *A Student in Arms* (London: Andrew Melrose, 1917), p. 106.
25 The Territorial soldier Private Ellison described the Kitchener's Army battalions as full of 'inexperienced youths with commissions.' Quoted in H. McCartney, *Citizen Soldiers. The Liverpool Territorials in the First World War* (Cambridge: Cambridge University Press, 2005), p. 50.
26 E. K. Smith to mother, 16 February 1915, *Letters Sent From France. Service with the Artists' Rifles and the Buffs, December 1914–December 1915* (London: J. Cobb, 1994), p. 23.
27 G. Greenwell, *An Infant in Arms. War letters of a Company Commander 1914–1918* (London: Allen Lane, The Penguin Press, 1972), p. 143. Roland Leighton thought subalterns over thirty were 'too old'. A. Bishop, with T. Smart (eds.), *Vera Brittain. War Diary 1913–1917, Chronicle of Youth* (London: Victor Gollancz, 1981), p. 204.

28 N. Gullace, *The Blood of Our Sons. Men, Women and the Renegotiation of British Citizenship in the Great War* (Basingstoke: Palgrave, 2002), p. 111; T. Wilson, *The Myriad Faces of War. Britain and the Great War, 1914–1918* (Cambridge: Polity, 1986), pp. 168–9.
29 See Wilson, *The Myriad Faces*, pp. 396–401.
30 J. M. Winter, 'Forms of Kinship and Remembrance in the Aftermath of the Great War', in J. M. Winter and E. Sivan, *War and Remembrance in the Twentieth Century* (Cambridge: Cambridge University Press, 1999), p. 42.
31 A. Hooper to L. Hooper, quoted in L. Hooper to K. Hooper, 30 September 1915, LC, DF066.
32 G. Coppard, *With A Machine Gun to Cambrai. A Story of the First World War* (London: Cassell, 1980), p. 109.
33 E. Leed, *No Man's Land. Combat and Identity in World War I* (Cambridge: Cambridge University Press, 1979), p. 2. Leed takes the quotation from Fussell.
34 P. Barham, *Forgotten Lunatics of the Great War* (New Haven: Yale University Press, 2004), p. 171.
35 C. Asquith, *Diaries 1915–18* (London: Hutchinson, 1968), p. 78.
36 S. Kent, *Making Peace. The Reconstruction of Gender in Interwar Britain* (Princeton, NJ: Princeton University Press, 1993), p. 99.
37 B. Weisbrod, 'Military Violence and Male Fundamentalism: Ernst Jünger's Contribution to the Conservative Revolution', *History Workshop Journal*, Vol. 49, (Spring 2000), p. 77.
38 Mosse, *Fallen Soldiers*, p. 163, p. 159.
39 Kent, *Making Peace*, p. 99.
40 P. Fussell, *The Great War and Modern Memory* (Oxford: Oxford University Press, 1975), pp. 86–7.
41 Leed, *No Man's Land*, pp. 188–9.
42 A. Booth, *Postcards From the Trenches. Negotiation the Space between Modernism and the First World War* (Oxford: Oxford University Press, 1995), p. 31.
43 On Australia see J. Damousi, *The Labour of Loss. Mourning, Memory and Wartime Bereavement in Australia* (Cambridge: Cambridge University Press, 1999), esp. ch. 2.
44 C. Hämmerle, '"You Let a Weeping Woman Call you Home?" Private Correspondences During the First World War in Austria and Germany', in R. Earle (ed.), *Epistolary Selves. Letters and Letter-Writers, 1600–1945* (Aldershot: Ashgate, 1999), pp. 154–5.
45 Hämmerle, '"You Let a Weeping Woman Call you Home?"', p. 157.
46 M. Hanna, 'A Republic of Letters: The Epistolary Tradition in France during World War I', *The American Historical Review*, Vol. 108, No. 5 (2003), http://www.historycooperative.org/journals/ahr/108.5/hanna.html, para. 40.
47 Audoin-Rouzeau, *Men at War*, p. 128.

48 Audoin-Rouzeau and Becker, *1914–1918*, p. 36.

49 J. Bourke, *Dismembering the Male. Men's Bodies and the Great War* (London: Reaktion Books, 1996), p. 21; I. Bet-El, *Conscripts. Forgotten Men of the Great War* (Stroud: Sutton Publishing, 2003), p. 131, p. 143.

50 E. B. Proud, *History of the British Army Postal Service. Volume II, 1903–1927* (Dereham: Proud–Bailey, 1982), p. 13.

51 P. B. Boyden, *Tommy Atkins' Letters. The History of the British Army Postal Service From 1795* (London: National Army Museum, 1990), p. 28.

52 R. Bickersteth to mother, The Bickersteth War Diaries and the Papers of John Burgon Bickersteth, Churchill Archives Centre, GBR/0014/BICK, Vol. 2, 3 May 1915, p. 560. The moment reminded the middle-class officer Captain Reggie Trench of boarding school, when they would gather around in excited huddles as mail from home was handed out. R. Trench to mother, 31 March 1917, private collection.

53 E. Marchant to mother, 11 July 1915, IWM DS/MISC/26. The sense of anticipation was probably even greater when in trenches, as the post usually arrived with the rations. J. Ellis, *Eye Deep in Hell. Trench Warfare in World War I* (Baltimore: Johns Hopkins University Press, 1976), p. 138.

54 W. Owen to mother, 6 April 1917, in J. Bell (ed.), *Wilfred Owen. Selected Letters* (Oxford: Oxford University Press, 1985), p. 236.

55 M. Webb to mother, 11 August 1915, IWM 90/28/1.

56 E. F. Chapman to mother, 5 February 1917, IWM Con Shelf.

57 R. Foulkes to mother, 18 October 1915, IWM 82/4/1.

58 C. Ramsdale to mother and Mary, 17 August 1918, IWM Con Shelf.

59 N. Ferguson, *The Pity of War* (London: Penguin, 1998), pp. 350–7.

60 K. Grieves, *Sussex in the First World War* (Lewes: Sussex Record Society, 2004), p. xxiii.

61 Owen to mother, 4 February 1917, in Bell (ed.), *Wilfred Owen. Selected Letters*, p. 216; also Dominic Hibberd, *Wilfred Owen. A New Biography* (London: Weidenfeld & Nicolson, 2002), p. 218.

62 Mrs S. J. Dawson to Sam Dawson, private collection, 3 August, 11 August, 23 August 1919.

63 Bourke, *Dismembering the Male*, p. 170.

64 S. Grayzel, *Women's Identities at War. Gender, Motherhood and Politics in Britain and France during the First World War* (Chapel Hill, NC: University of North Carolina Press, 1999), p. 49. There are similar problems with the analysis by Karen Hagermann in which she argues that a gender perspective 'clearly marks the erasure of the lines separating the military and civilian realms.' What interests me here, focusing on emotional experience, is how those lines were constantly being communicated across and yet re-asserted. 'Home/Front: The Military, Violence and Gender Relations in the Age of the World Wars', in K. Hagermann, and S. Schüler-Springorum (eds), *Home/Front. The Military, War and Gender in Twentieth-Century Germany* (Oxford: Berg, 2002), p. 6.

65 Bourke, *Dismembering the Male*, p. 168.
66 McCartney, *Citizen Soldiers*, p. 257.
67 D. Englander, 'Soldiering and Identity: Reflections on the Great War', *War in History*, Vol. 1, No. 3, p. 318. As Audoin-Rouzeau and Becker recognise, 'the joy of returning home alive could not have erased all the heartbreak and pain', and they conclude that the longer-term psychological effects of traumas on the battlefield need further study. *1914–18*, pp. 166–7.
68 Harry Patch interview; Coppard, *With A Machine Gun*, p. 26.
69 Greenwell, *An Infant in Arms*, p. xxii.
70 Coppard, *With A Machine Gun*, p. 134.
71 Leed, *No Man's Land*, p. 189.
72 Mosse, *Fallen Soldiers*, pp. 169–81. Weisbrod, 'Military Violence and Male Fundamentalism', p. 81. Though for an interesting revision of the 'dehumanisation' perspective, which argues that the war in Germany could also be felt as a positive development in gender relations, see Birthe Kundrus, 'Gender Wars: The First World War and the Construction of Gender Relations in the Weimar Republic', in Hagermann and Schüler-Springorum, *Home/Front*, pp. 159–79.
73 Leed, *No Man's Land*, p. 167.
74 Susan Grayzel, for example, writes of how, in *Glory of Women*, Sassoon 'attacked all women'. *Women's Identities*, p. 18. See Nosheen Khan on Owen and Sassoon's hostility towards women. *Women's Poetry of the First World War* (Hemel Hempstead: Harvester-Wheatsheaf, 1988), p. 103.
75 J. Stallworthy (ed.), *The Poems of Wilfred Owen* (London: Chatto & Windus, 1990), p. 138.
76 *Siegfried Sassoon. The War Poems* (London: Faber & Faber, 1983), p. 100.
77 *Sassoon. The War Poems*, p. 101.
78 W. Owen to mother, 4 October 1918, in Bell (ed.), *Wilfred Owen. Selected Letters*, p. 351.
79 F. Manning, *Her Privates We* (London: Serpent's Tail, 1999), p. 215.
80 Bion, *War Memoirs*, p. 122. Bion's daughter, Parthenope Bion, points out her father's experience of being regressed in the war, 'Aftermath', *War Memoirs*, p. 310.
81 B. Bond, *The Unquiet Western Front. Britain's Role in Literature and History* (Cambridge: Cambridge University Press, 2002); D. Todman, *The Great War. Myth and Memory* (London: Hambledon, 2005), esp. ch. 1.
82 In some cases the stint was much longer than four days. Gladden recorded being twenty-six days in the front line without a break during the battle of the Somme, *Ypres*, p. 16.
83 Ellis, *Eye Deep in Hell*, p. 28.
84 C. Edmonds (C. E. Carrington), *A Subaltern's War* (London: Anthony Mott, 1984), pp. 95–6.
85 Edmonds, *A Subaltern's War*, p. 96.

86 D. Hibberd, *Wilfred Owen*, p. xvii, pp. 212–15.
87 F. E. Noakes, *The Distant Drum. The Personal History of a Guardsman in the Great War* (Tunbridge Wells: npub, 1952), p. 53.
88 Cited in D. Winter, *Death's Men*, p. 118.
89 R. Mountfort to mother, 7 November 1915, IWM Con Shelf.
90 S. Das, *Touch and Intimacy in First World War Literature* (Cambridge: Cambridsge University Press, 2005), p. 79; Graves quoted in Das, p. 79.
91 Greenwell, *Infant in Arms*, p. 63. The Medical Officer Charles Moran made a similar association between the sound of a breeze and the anticipation of shelling. The battle of the Somme, where his battalion experienced 403 casualties, would not leave his thoughts: 'I was to go through it many times in my sleep and then the mind was no longer doped, it hurt. Even when the war had begun to fade out of men's minds I used to hear all at once without warning the sound of a shell coming. Perhaps it was only the wind in the trees to remind me that war had exacted its tribute and that my little capital was less than it had been.' C. Moran, *The Anatomy of Courage* (London: Constable, 1945), p. 69. On fear see M. Roper, 'Between Manliness and Masculinity: The "War Generation" and the Psychology of Fear in Britain, 1914–1970', *Journal of British Studies*, Vol. 44, No. 2 (2005), pp. 343–63.
92 Bishop and Bostridge, *Letters From a Lost Generation*, p. 271. On 'crump' see Oxford English Dictionary online.
93 The central character in Frederic Manning's autobiographical novel *Her Privates We*, would not forget the shell which fell among men in the middle of parade, in a village behind the lines and hitherto largely unscathed (p. 54).
94 The account is from Charles Moran, and is cited by Denis Winter. Winter goes on to remark on the personal stress caused by the fact that the recruit was 'hardly ever out of danger', *Death's Men*, p. 131.
95 D. Winter, *Death's Men*, p. 31.
96 Cited in D. Winter, *Death's Men*, p. 248.
97 Manning, *Her Privates We*, p. 11. Manning evokes the men's state with a quote from Shakespeare's *The Life of King Henry the Fifth*: 'But I had not so much of man in me,/And all my mother came into mine eyes/And gave me up to tears.' (p. 12).
98 Edwin Vaughan thought that his laughter was actually a sign of mental fragility: 'my nerves had been giving way under the strain until I was reduced to the childishness of laughing at another man's fear'. *Some Desperate Glory. The Diary of a Young Officer, 1917* (London: Leo Cooper, 1987), p. 212.
99 On the 'subtle thrill' of killing, see N. Taylor to father 18 May 1916, IWM 90/28/1; on 'exaltation' at survival, G. Chapman, *A Passionate Prodigality. Fragments of Autobiography* (New York: Holt, Rinehart and Winston, 1966); p. 204; on 'elation', Vaughan, *Some Desperate Glory*, p. 192.

100 Quoted in Weisbrod, 'Military Violence and Male Fundamentalism', pp. 77–8.
101 The dead in war, says the veteran and cultural historian of the war, Samuel Hynes, are 'grotesque and astonishing'. *The Soldier's Tale. Bearing Witness to Modern War* (London: Pimlico, 1998), p. 20.
102 W. H. R. Rivers, *Instinct and the Unconscious. A Contribution to a Biological Theory of the Psycho-Neuroses* (Cambridge: Cambridge University Press, 1920), p. 226.
103 Herbert, *The Secret Battle*, p. 26.
104 W. Hate, diary 10 March 1915, IWM 86/51/1
105 Edmonds, *Subaltern's War*, pp. 46–9.
106 C. Carrington, *Soldier From the Wars Returning* (London: Arrow Books, 1965), p. 293; Edmonds, *A Subaltern's War*, p. 14.
107 Carrington, *Soldier From the Wars*, p. 221.
108 Nightingale wrote to his sister Meta about one of the new volunteer officers who was hit during dinner, and 'fell into the soup, upsetting the whole table, and bled into the tea-pot making an awful mess of everything'. G. W. Nightingale to Meta, 4 June 1915, IWM P216. See also Michele Barrett, 'Shell-Shocked', *The Guardian*, Review Section, 19 April 2003, p. 36.
109 Bond, *The Unquiet Western Front*, p. 27.
110 G. Chapman, *A Passionate Prodigality*, pp. 5–6.
111 W. R. Bion, *Learning From Experience* (London: H. Karnac, 1991), pp. 6–7. Bion coined the term 'alpha functioning' to describe the capacity of the mind to translate emotional experiences into thoughts; 'beta elements', by contrast were 'undigested facts', which were dealt with by more primitive psychic mechanisms such as splitting and projection.
112 W. R. Bion, 'Notes on the Theory of Schizophrenia', in W. R. Bion, *Second Thoughts. Selected Papers on Psychoanalysis* (London: H. Karnac, 1987), p. 31.
113 R. Holmes, *Tommy. The British Soldier on the Western Front 1914–1918* (London: Harper Perennial, 2005), p. xxiii.
114 Holmes, *Tommy*, p. xxiv.
115 H. J. C. Leland to wife, 4 October 1917, IWM 96/51/1.
116 Santanu Das makes a similar point about the difference between poetry and prose. Prose became possible only when the mind was able to 'heal the breach in time caused by the war and organise the war years into a coherent prose narrative.' *Touch and Intimacy*, p. 63.
117 On the emotional importance of food for the trench soldier see R. Duffett, 'A War Unimagined: Food and the Rank and File Soldier of the First World War', in J. Meyer (ed.), *Popular Culture and the First World War* (Leiden: Brill, 2007), pp. 47–70; R. Duffett, '"I believe 'e'd sell 'imself for a tin o' toffee": The Significance of Food in the Memoirs of the Rank and File Soldiers of the First World War', unpublished MA dissertation, Department of History, University of Essex, 2005.

118 Owen to mother, 9 January 1917, in Bell (ed.), *Wilfred Owen. Selected Letters*, p. 209.
119 Mother to A. H. Swettenham, nd, IWM 83/31/1.
120 S. E. Brown to mother, date illegible, IWM 89/7/1.
121 David Vincent, in his study of nineteenth-century working-class autobiography, makes a similar point about the resort to stereotypes. Self-educated writers borrowed clichés, he remarks, 'to give expression to their deeper feelings.' *Bread, Knowledge and Freedom: A Study of Nineteenth-Century Working Class Autobiography* (London: Europa, 1981), p. 41.
122 B. Chapman to mother, 19 June 1918, IWM 98/17/1.
123 Bond, *The Unquiet Western Front*, p. 31.
124 S. Freud, 'Thoughts for the Times on War and Death', *The Standard Edition of the Complete Psychological Works of Sigmund Freud*, tr. J. Strachey, Vol. 14 (London: Vintage, 2001), p. 284; Daniel Pick, *War Machine. The Rationalisation of Slaughter in the Modern Age* (New Haven: Yale University Press, 1993), pp. 218–20. Niall Ferguson argues that one of the reasons why men kept fighting was because they wanted to: the reassertion of primitive instincts proved seductive. *The Pity of War*, pp. 357–66. For an interesting application of Freud's ideas about life and death instincts to gunners and snipers, see Chris Corr, 'Killing and Dying: The Experience of Shell and Sniper-Fire in the First World War', unpublished MA dissertation, Department of Sociology, University of Essex, 2004.
125 S. Freud, 'Mourning and Melancholia', *The Standard Edition of the Complete Psychological Works of Sigmund Freud*, tr. J. Strachey, Vol. 14 (London: Vintage, 2001) pp. 243–59; J. M. Winter, *Sites of Memory, Sites of Mourning. The Great War in European Cultural History* (Cambridge: Cambridge University Press, 1995), esp. ch. 4, pp. 78–117.
126 S. Freud, 'Beyond the Pleasure Principle', *The Standard Edition of the Complete Psychological Works of Sigmund Freud*, tr. J. Strachey, Vol. 18 (London: Vintage, 2001), pp. 7–64. See also Dominick LaCapra, *Writing History, Writing Trauma* (Baltimore: Johns Hopkins University Press, 2001), e.g. p. 144; and Robert J. Lifton, *The Broken Connection. On Death and the Continuity of Life* (New York: Simon & Schuster, 1979), pp. 163–7.
127 Bion, *Learning From Experience*, p. 42.
128 Bion, *Learning From Experience*, pp. 36–7.
129 H. Hague to mother, 1 June 1918, IWM 98/33/1.
130 F. Wollocombe to mother and father, 22 November 1915, IWM 95/33/1. That writing home could make the writer appear to himself as more down than he actually felt, is also observed by Jennifer Hartley. See '"Letters are Everything These Days": Mothers and Letters in the Second World War', in R. Earle (ed.), *Epistolary Selves. Letters and Letter-Writers, 1600–1945* (Aldershot: Ashgate, 1999), p. 191.

131 Quoted in M. Tonnessman, 'Transference and Countertransference: An Historical Approach', in S. Budd and R. Rushbridger (eds.), *Introducing Psychoanalysis. Essential Themes and Topics* (London: Routledge, 2005), p. 192.
132 P. Roth, 'Projective Identification', in Budd and Rushbridger, *Introducing Psychoanalysis*, p. 51.
133 See Carol Acton, *Grief in Wartime. Private Pain, Public Discourse* (Basingstoke: Palgrave, 2007).
134 Acton, *Grief in Wartime*, p. 5. For a further commentary on discourse-based approaches see M. Roper, 'Slipping Out of View: Subjectivity and Emotion in Gender History', *History Workshop Journal*, Vol. 59 (Spring 2005), pp. 57–73.
135 Thompson, P. and T. Lummis, 'Family Life and Work Experience Before 1918, 1870–1973' [computer file], 5th edition. Colchester: UK Data Archive [distributor], April 2005. SN: 2000.
136 P. Fussell (ed.), *The Ordeal of Alfred M. Hale. The Memoirs of a Soldier Servant* (London: Leo Cooper, 1975).
137 J. Bourne, 'The British Working Man in Arms', in H. Cecil and P. Liddle, *Facing Armageddon. The First World War Experienced* (London: Pen & Sword, 1996), pp. 336–52; Bet-El, *Conscripts.*
138 Quoted in Grieves, *Sussex in the First World War*, p. xiii.
139 S. Rogerson quoted in Winter, *Death's Men*, p. 55.
140 J. Watson, *Fighting Different Wars. Experience, Memory and the First World War in Britain* (Cambridge: Cambridge University Press, 2004), p. 13.
141 Grieves, *Sussex in the First World War*, p. ix.
142 Grieves, *Sussex in the First World War*, p. xxv. The phrase about 'ridiculous' propinquity is Fussell's.
143 J. Horne, 'Soldiers, Civilians and the Warfare of Attrition: Representations of Combat in France, 1914–1918', in F. Coetzee and M. Shevin-Coetzee (eds.), *Authority, Identity and the Social History of the Great War* (Oxford: Berghahn Books, 1995), p. 223.
144 Bet-El, *Conscripts*, p. 143; McCartney, *Citizen Soldiers*, p. 140, p. 155.
145 A. Young, 'W. H. R. Rivers and the War Neuroses', *Journal of the History of the Behavioural Sciences*, Vol. 35, No. 4 (Fall 1999), pp. 364–8; Rivers, *Instinct and the Unconscious*, p. 206.
146 Quoted in Young, 'W. H. R. Rivers', p. 368.
147 Rivers, *Instinct and the Unconscious*, p. 209.
148 Young, 'W. H. R. Rivers', p. 368.
149 J. G. Fuller, *Troop Morale and Popular Culture in the British and Dominion Armies* (Oxford: Clarendon Press, 1991), p. 54.
150 Chapman, *A Passionate Prodigality*, p. 57.
151 On the envy of rankers towards their officers see Coppard, *With A Machine Gun*, p. 77.

152 See on the upper middle class, P. Thompson, *The Edwardians. The Remaking of British Society* (London: Routledge, 1992); on the lower middle class, G. Crossick, 'The Emergence of the Lower Middle Class in Britain: A Discussion', in G. Crossick (ed.), *The Lower Middle Class in Britain, 1870–1914* (London: Croom Helm, 1977), pp. 11–60; J. Hammerton, 'Pooterism or Partnership? Marriage and Masculine Identity in the Lower Middle Class, 1870–1920', *Journal of British Studies*, Vol. 38, No. 3 (July 1999), pp. 291–321.

153 E. F. Chapman to Miss Hare, 5 August 1916, IWM Con Shelf.

154 Rivers, *Instinct and the Unconscious*, p. 210.

155 J. M. Strange, '"She Cried a Very Little": Death, Grief and Mourning in Working-Class Culture C. 1880–1914', *Social History* Vol. 27, No. 2 (May 2002), p. 161.

156 Herbert's biographer Reginald Pound is in 'no doubt that *The Secret Battle* was being compulsively written under the duress of frightful memories.' Pound, *A. P. Herbert*, p. 55.

157 Pound, *A. P. Herbert*, p. 52.

158 Rosa Maria Bracco makes precisely this point about R. C. Sherriff's immensely successful 1928 play *Journey's End*. Through the neurasthenic officer Hibberd, she thinks, Sherriff may have been trying 'to explain the genuineness of his plight without exposing his own story.' R. M. Bracco, *Merchants of Hope. British Middlebrow Writers and the First World War* (Oxford: Berg, 1993), p. 162. See also M. Roper, 'Between Manliness and Masculinity', pp. 353–7.

# PART I

# Mothers and sons

# 1

# Keeping in touch

On 8 August 1914, three days after war was declared, Annis and Henry Urwick started out for Tidmouth barracks to pay their son Lyndall, a Special Reservist and Second Lieutenant in the 3rd Worcestershire Regiment, a final visit before he left for France. Lyndall had mixed feelings about the visit. He told his mother not to waste money on the journey but left the final decision up to her: 'You say that it shall be as I wish. But really we men do not understand these things. If, as I say, you feel that to see me will help you, come.'[1] His mother's needs, not his own, should dictate the decision.

Annis and Henry had to wait around at the barracks the following day for Lyndall to come off duty, but Henry, a partner in the long-established glove making firm of Fownes Brothers, found the movement of stores quite interesting. They finally met up with Lyndall and, as Henry reported in his diary, Annis was 'very much pleased to have seen him + was considerably cheered.' Her good spirits did not last long, however. Lyndall was her only son and as they waited back in Malvern over the next three days for news of his movements she became 'very much depressed'. Henry 'tried to cheer her up'.[2] As was often the case, Lyndall's mother was the emotional barometer for the family, and father and son kept close watch on her reactions.

On 13 August Lyndall sent his parents a telegram saying 'condition quite satisfactory no cause for alarm letter follows', from which they deduced that he was about to embark. He followed it up with a letter which asked his mother to keep his correspondence, as 'we are not allowed to make a war diary & a somewhat vague account of my movements may yet prove an assistance to memory.'[3] It would be Annis' job to preserve her son's record of his war, in letters addressed to her but with half an eye on posterity.

A long silence followed. On 26 August they received a letter from Lyndall but it was a week old, and they were learning of the first casualties among the 3rd Worcestershire men, including Lyndall's own commanding officer. Annis was 'much cheered' by a letter from Lyndall on 11 September reporting that he was all right.[4] On 18 September they received another letter saying he was well, but Lyndall had sent it on 4 September, and the Urwicks knew from the newspapers that there had been fighting around the Aisne since 15 September. The next they heard was that two of Urwick's fellow officers had been casualties in the recent fighting; they received a 'Very nice long letter from Lyn' but it was now 22 September and it was dated 11 September, so despite its comforting length, the letter gave them no idea how their son had fared at the Aisne.[5]

Annis wrote to Lyndall every day throughout this difficult time. She hoped that the strength of her love might protect him: 'I pray that what has now sustained you, may never fail you in your hour of need – I do not think it will, since you are a son of deep love + you must always feel that love stretching out to you, across the barriers of time + distance.' On 23 September she packed up some vests, drawers, half a pound of tobacco, quinine tablets and his old Jaeger coat, together with a volume of verse which was 'especially understanding, as to the women's portion of suffering in such times – since no horror is as hard as the waiting – waiting for you know what!' The news from the Western Front was still worrying her: 'I hear it said that the Boer war was child's play to what [*sic*] you are now living through.' It saddened her, she wrote the next day, 'how little I can do to show my Mother-love, but you know it follows you in all your marchings, rejoices in your happier hours + would fair comfort you in the sudden sterner side of life of which you must have had a terrible experience.'[6]

Henry and Annis would have read newspaper reports of the 150 or so casualties among the Battalion during fighting on 20 September, but they did not hear from Lyndall until 26 September, when he wired them to say that he was 'laid up' at a hospital in Versailles but that his condition was 'not serious'. The following day they received a War Office telegram which informed them that Lyndall had been slightly wounded, but then he telegraphed them himself to say he was suffering from colic.[7]

Henry and Annis Urwick were unable to ascertain for sure whether or not Lyndall was wounded until his letter arrived on 30 September, almost a week after he was admitted to hospital. Dated 25 September, it explained that he had found himself 'curled up with a stomach ache' around the fifth day of the battle of the Aisne, and had 'crawled down to the first field hospital' with the help of a stretcher bearer before being put on a hospital train to Versailles. On reading this and a subsequent letter, Henry concluded that Lyndall was 'not feeling very fit'.[8]

Annis was also feeling unwell. Throughout Lyndall's time in hospital she seemed to Henry to be 'very depressed + nervy', and 'very much worried'. Even when good news arrived on 10 October, 'though relieved about Lyn', she was 'not very fit.'[9] In fact, this last phrase was almost the very same one that Henry had used to describe Lyn's own state: the mental strain of this worried mother was felt by Henry as commensurate with the illness of his son, suffering from violent diarrhoea.

Henry Urwick's diary and his wife's daily letters to her son show the confusion and uncertainty which often dogged families as they tried to keep track of their loved ones, and the cumulative emotional toll of waiting. They show too how much store families set by any communication, no matter how contradictory, out of date, or seemingly impersonal. Over the top of Lyndall's enigmatic telegram from Tidmouth Annis wrote: 'Received by me Aug 13th 1914 from my beloved son – I <u>think</u> a signal of departure.'[10] This telegram would mark Lyndall's entry to the war.

Letters were, by comparison with official communiqués, especially evocative of the loved one, and families like the Urwicks lived in constant hope of their arrival. Wallie Goodwin's father liked to pen pithy little phrases urging his son to keep up correspondence. 'Write soon/write long/write often/+ then the distance + time will seem shorter', he signed off his letter on one occasion.[11] Even the writing on the envelope moved them, and in holding the letter, they were not only 'in touch' in the sense of being brought up to date with events, but touched the very paper that a loved one had held.[12] 'I am ever thinking of you', wrote Louisa Hooper to her son Kenneth, 'and fold and embrace you in imagination continually. Your letters are always kissed before I place them in the Box'.[13] The very paper that he wrote on, sometimes so thin that the writing stood out on the reverse side, and only partly protected from the elements in his greatcoat or tunic pocket, suggested how fragile a son's existence was. Harold Anderton's mother would have been brought close up against the rain, mud and cold of the trenches well before reading his apology for 'the filthy state of this paper', which had been stored in the pocket of his soaked overcoat.[14]

For the soldier, the letter from home provided an equally vivid sign of loved ones, and he too hungered for mail. Lieutenant Howard Bowser, stationed in Cairo, told his father he had received 'the very best mail I've ever had from England I think. It took us nearly an hour to read, gloat over and digest.'[15] On Christmas Eve 1915, Leonard Timpson recorded, 'A record, Mail arrives. My share of the spoils, 12 letters 4 parcels + two papers.'[16] Hedley Payne felt he was actually 'hearing Dad's voice again' when he read his letter, and many men kept their most cherished letters close to the heart in a breast pocket.[17] Amongst the photographs of lady friends and risqué postcards returned to A. G. Baker's parents after his death on the Somme in September 1916 was the 1914 Christmas card they had sent him almost two years earlier. It reads 'A link to bind where duty bids us part/A chain of thought stretches forth from heart to heart'.[18]

It was not only the news from home, but the writing of letters which drew these soldiers back into the lives they had left behind. Through his letters, Matt Webb explained to his parents, he was able to create a 'mind picture' of home.[19] The connection sometimes felt so vivid that awareness of the difference between the real and the imaginary was suspended. As he settled down in a French café to compose a letter home, Anderton observed the 'beatific smiles' of the men around him as they wrote to their sweethearts.[20] 'He has gone home', Henri Barbusse commented of a man lost in thought as he wrote a letter.[21]

Some historians have argued that the British soldier wrote home less often and with more 'emotional reserve' than his German or French equivalent.[22] Many sons, however, were avid letter-writers. The volume of mail sent home by the British Army on the Western Front kept increasing during the war and by 1917 over eight million letters were being sent each week, an average of nearly one a day for each soldier based in France.[23] The Army recognised the importance for morale of an efficient mail service and after 1914, letters home weighing less than 4 oz were free of charge.[24] Subalterns were often amazed at the amount the men wrote. The platoon commander Wilfred Owen, newly arrived at the front, censored 'hundreds of letters' on 3 January 1917 and three days later he was still censoring 'by the hundred'. 'Censoring letters all afternoon', he reported on 10 January, concluding that 'The men do practically nothing all day but write letters'.[25] The sheer bulk of their correspondence ensured that the officer's censorship was bound to be patchy.

It was not only the new recruit in France, the memory of home fresh in his mind, who was the avid letter-writer; many a seasoned soldier was equally conscientious. During his eighteen months' service in France, Milton Robinson wrote 490 letters to relations and friends and received 457 letters and parcels, recording each one as it was sent or arrived.

Another soldier reported receiving 167 letters and writing 242 letters during a twelve-month period.[26] Far from being reluctant correspondents, these men were actually writing more letters than they received, and the very fact that they counted their correspondence shows how important it was to them. Conditions were rarely conducive to writing, and men huddled in corners or on beds, scrawling in poor light on notepads balanced on their knees. Having come out of trenches, Hedley Payne found himself 'with half a dozen letters to answer in about five minutes, seated on the straw with twenty people shouting + jumping all over me + my only light – a candle at sufficient distant [sic] away to be well nigh useless'.[27]

While writing home enabled the soldier to revive his personal memory of home, it was also felt to be a duty, something that was *owed* to loved ones. Will Hate wrote to his mother although he felt 'more like sleeping than writing at present for I was up three parts of the night', and when Charles Ramsdale's mother suggested sending him some books, he replied 'I think I had better say "no", as I am hopelessly in arrears with letters now'.[28] Returning from leave, Tom Thorpe found a backlog of mail awaiting him. He explained to his sister that since his return 'I have done nothing much else but write letters. When I got back here I think I owed <u>15</u> from all over England, Wales + France but now the total has gone down to 2'.[29] Though it might feel onerous to keep up this amount of correspondence, Thorpe was proud of the geographical range across which his correspondents were spread.

Families also had to fit letter-writing into days that were, because of war work, lack of domestic help or voluntary work, busier than in peacetime. Mothers sometimes fell asleep over their letters.[30] Because letter-writing was a way of mothering at a distance, however, most put great energy into it, almost as if it was their equivalent to military service.[31] Louisa Hooper's letters to Kenneth, who was a POW, were printed in a minute and beautifully clear hand, which she cultivated after the German censor deemed illegible her initial letters. She soon adopted this hand for her other son Arnold, then serving in India, who wrote effusively about her 'Dear little writing, and that magnificent writing on the envelope', and whose friends were by also, according to Arnold, impressed with how 'beautiful' her script was.[32]

As mothers grew used to writing and cultivated the art, it developed its own attractions. Sarah Jane Dawson wrote to her sons Billy and Sam three times a week throughout the war, being careful always to warn them if a holiday or other excursion might break the routine, for 'one cannot write so well when away from home'. As Sam's de-mobilisation approached, she wished for his swift return, but she thought she would 'miss the writing when you are home for good'. [33]

Annis and Henry Urwick may have felt frustrated by the difficulty in getting accurate news of their son, but in fact, because of the Western Front's proximity to Britain, the ties between loved ones could be sustained in ways that were impossible for families further afield. The key factor was the time gap between sending and receiving mail. In the early weeks of the war it could take up to ten days for a letter to arrive at the front, and the post was also likely to be disrupted when a man was on the move or fighting, when of course families were especially anxious for news. The normal delivery time, however, was around two to three days. Mail from the front was a little slower due to censorship, typically taking around six days.[34] The time gaps for Colonial troops serving on the Western Front, or British troops serving in more distant theatres of war, were much greater. The journey time for mail from Australia to the Western Front, for example, was at least fifty days.[35] The effects of distance on the wartime relationships between Australian soldiers and their families are disputed. J. G. Fuller concludes that it reduced the importance of home ties, quoting a veteran's comment that 'Long separation from Australia had seemed to cut us completely away from the land of our birth. The longer a man served, the fewer letters he got, the more he was forgotten. Our only home was our unit.'[36] Joy Damousi, by contrast, argues that letters were treasured by Australian families and men serving abroad, being 'precious, even sacred'.[37]

Distance may not have diluted the emotional reaction to letters, but it did limit the ability of families to provide practical support. The mail to British troops stationed in Mesopotamia, Salonica or Gallipoli could take months to arrive and was often out of sequence. Goodwin's family were desperate for news of their son, who they knew was *en route* for Gallipoli after the heavy fighting of mid-1915. When his first letter was received – auspiciously, on the day of his birthday – his mother's relief was palpable: 'I cannot tell you how delighted and relieved we were, to get a letter from you. I had almost given up hope being over 5 weeks since we had the last card. Your dad had been, and written everywhere but no one would, or could not tell us any thing'.[38] The difficulties experienced by Captain Harold Standrick and his mother also illustrate how communication could become impoverished in more remote theatres of the war. He was serving in Palestine, from where his letters arrived out of order. As his mother's contradictory remarks and crossings out show, she tried unsuccessfully to place Harold's letters in a chronological sequence; she did not even know whether her mail was reaching him:

> Many thanks for all your interesting letters, we received one last Monday dated Dec 1st, bearing on the envelope post date Dec 31st, we received one of ~~an~~ a later earlier date before that one [*sic*]We are quite in despair about sending any more parcels, as we cannot hear that you have received anything we have sent dearest. I do hope they haven't all been stolen from you.[39]

So as to help sort out this kind of confusion, and gauge how much mail was going missing, Lieutenant A. G. Steavenson's mother numbered her letters to her son in Mesopotamia, the last surviving example from 1919 is numbered 123.[40] Though Mrs Steavenson wrote regularly, time differences made it hard for correspondents like her to stay in touch, for readers learned not of an almost contemporaneous situation but of one long past. Struggling to empathise, writers fell back on generalised statements of support and affection.

The comparatively fast post between Britain and the Western Front allowed correspondents to establish reliable routines for keeping in contact and similar time zones, weather and seasons intensified the feeling of proximity. Each could imagine what the other was doing in the very instant of writing. As Annis Urwick strolled about her garden in Malvern after breakfast in late September 1914, the heavy dew on her slippers led her to reflect that Lyndall's night under canvas must have been a cold one, although by then he was actually in hospital.[41] British soldiers – their awareness of weather and the seasons heightened by life outdoors – did the same. Writing in Autumn 1916 from a dug-out whose walls were decorated with drawings by his twelve-year-old sister Hilda, Edward Chapman's mind was fixed on his family: 'I think consistently of home, and know exactly what everything will be looking like, and the smell about the damp garden. I always wish I could pop in to tea, and find you all sitting round the table, and Hilda in the act of committing a bad manner!'[42] Home scenes relieved the stresses of the present. So as to ward off the gloom and solitude of night watch Jim Tomlinson rehearsed his family's preparations for bed: 'I think of home . . . + imagine just what is going on there you all waking up or about 10o/c Pa toddling off with his "good night Ma" You still to come in Ma reading the paper in front of the fire Hilda just getting ready to go. then at say 2 or 3 o/c I fancy you all fast asleep + there am I leaning against something struggling to keep my eyes open.'[43] Home had an immediacy for the

British soldier on the Western Front that it could not for those further afield, though this could also intensify the longing to get back. A man might almost be able to smell his Sunday dinner as he reminisced about home, but he still had to manage on the thin gravy and vegetables of his Maconochie stew.[44]

## Learning the art of letter-writing

The men who made up the wartime Army were on the whole better educated than soldiers of the Edwardian Army, 70 per cent of whom, between 1907 and 1913, had been unable to pass the educational standards normally set for eleven-year-old children.[45] Soldiering in Edwardian Britain had been an option mainly for the poorest and least secure. The volunteer George Fortune recalled his father's adage, whose occupation as a diver at the port of Dover put him among the respectable working class: 'a man who goes in the army is not fit for anything else. Once a soldier, never a man.'[46] Kitchener's Army changed that, and although around 56 per cent of the volunteers who served in the wartime Army were from industrial occupations, non-manual and professional workers were over-represented.[47] The latter signed up in droves early in the war, over half a million from the financial and commercial sectors between August 1914 and the introduction of conscription, forming the mainstay of many Pals' battalions of volunteers.[48] Contrary to Fortune's belief, the respectable were attracted to Army life precisely because of its physical challenges. Military service promised a way out of increasingly feminised office work. In J. B. Priestley's words, they wanted a 'challenge to what we felt was our untested manhood', to demonstrate that they too could 'leave home and soft beds' and drill, march and bear arms just like men from less comfortable backgrounds.[49]

Of these Army recruits – the 25 per cent who were drawn from central or local government, the professions, or finance and commerce – many were writers by trade, and would become prolific letter-writers during the war.[50] 'The more these wretched clerks write to their wives the less I can write to mine', wrote an exasperated subaltern, 'I have such a lot to censor'.[51] It is the letters of black-coated workers which tend to predominate in archival collections of the rank-and-file soldier, but, coming as they did from indoor occupations and comfortable homes, the shock of life in the ranks was undoubtedly greater for them than it was for some. Much as they wished to show that they could stick Army life, their letters were animated by the contrasts, as they found themselves eating and sleeping with men from whom, in civilian life, they had been anxious to mark themselves off.[52] For many of the agricultural workers who made up around 8.4 per cent of the volunteer Army, letter-writing would not have been as familiar as it was to the clerk, but at the same time, the physical conditions of Army life may not have felt quite so alien, as they were used to labouring in all weathers, a poor diet and paternalistic authority.

The traffic in mail across Britain expanded rapidly during the late nineteenth and early twentieth centuries but, as David Vincent shows, much of this was due to cards and especially picture postcards, which required only rudimentary writing skills.[53] Elementary school students were given little in the way of instruction in composition. They could probably copy a standard letter, but they had been neither taught nor encouraged to communicate their own thoughts and experiences in writing.[54]

Many rankers had probably never even written a letter to a parent before joining the Army. Reading through collections of letters, one can often observe men gaining confidence with practice. Not infrequently – drawing no doubt on examples remembered from their schooling – they opened with the formal salutations mocked by many a middle-class officer, such as 'hoping to find you in the best of health as it leaves me quite well at present', or 'Just a line to let you know that I am still in the pink'.[55] However, their letters contained much more besides, because convention was inadequate for the intimacy and individual requests that writers wished to communicate.[56] Most writers succeeded in making the form their own. Charles Ramsdale, born in 1898, left school at thirteen to work in a York miller's firm. He wrote long letters to his mother and sister, and was proud of how his travels had improved his facility with language. On one occasion he referred to his sister Mary's 'coiffeur' ('French for hairdressing if you don't know') and he liked to show off his facility with written English: 'You ask for my "candied" opinion. Well now, I thought it was peel, not opinions, that was candied!'[57] Ramsdale might have taken Mary to task for her spelling, but his own turns of phrase suggest that his prose style was based as much on the spoken vernacular as on the standard rules of written grammar.[58] Stephen Brown did not pretend to Ramsdale's facility with English but his concern for his family comes across powerfully enough in the last letter he wrote before leaving for France:

> dear mother do not worry about me for by God [*sic*] help I shall come home well Give my love to Lillie, Kitty and Freddie and tell him I will come and see him by and by you will receive 3/0 shilling from me and the same from the war office which will make six altogether give my love to all there is know [*sic*] need to put stamp on the letter you send put OHMS on it and it will come for nothing.[59]

Literacy was also a matter of generation, because compulsory education had been introduced during the 1870s when some of the war generation's parents were already past school leaving age.[60] The switch from face-to-face contact to letters was hard for those with a rudimentary education, especially when sons and even daughters were frequently away working and on military service, and could not be relied on to act as scribes. Many struggled with the difference between conversation and the formality which a letter seemed to require. John Carter signed himself 'Dadd' in his first letter to his son Harry, and then crossed it out and wrote 'father'. His next letter was yet more formal, signed this time 'Your affectionate father and mother John & E. Carter', although softened by the profuse crosses he added underneath.[61]

For some it was not just the writing of the letter itself, but the procedure for getting it to the recipient that had to be learned. A novice might address his or her letter using the nick-name of a Battalion and one correspondent, hoping to make sure the letter she had written would reach her loved one, put his age and date of birth on the envelope.[62] In response to such problems, sons gave precise instructions to parents about how to address their letters. Learning the art of personal correspondence was part of a larger shift in literacy on the home front, as people encountered a range of new official forms, from the ubiquitous field-service postcard or ration book, to claims for the Separation Allowance.

The need to keep in touch sparked new efforts in self-education. The teenager Robert Roberts observed the change from the vantage point of his parents' grocers' shop in Salford:

> Thousands of adults who perhaps had never before penned a single letter now felt the strongest desire to put words on paper. Then began the run in army canteens and every corner shop in the country for 'equipment': threepence bought the lot – a bottle of Stephens' ink, a packet of writing paper and envelopes and a pen. One cleared a space, sat four-square before the menacing blank page and began![63]

Some parents were inspired by having a son away at the war to not only take up a pen, but to try and master the art of letter-writing. Mrs Arnold compared her efforts with the 'lovly letters' written by her son Alfie: 'as you know I do not know how to place the brackets and so forth I hope that you did not have to leave my long one for three days before you could make it out.' Nevertheless, she continued, 'I believe if I had time and practiced a bit I could beat a good many . . . I am scribbling this on my lap.'[64]

The letters of lower-middle- and middle-class sons tended to adopt a less standardised form and were more playful with language than those of poorer rankers. This reflected their greater familiarity with letter-writing and with travel, while the formality of the urban working-class or rural labourer's letter, conversely, reflected the novelty of being away from his family and local community.[65] Arthur Gaunt's journey from his local recruiting office in Rochdale to the regimental depot was his 'first time away from home, rather strange but not bad'.[66] In the aftermath of an attack on German trenches in mid-March 1915 that was 'hell', Harold Anderton reflected ruefully to his mother that 'I don't think I have ever before spent Easter away from home'.[67] Men whose pre-war lives were strongly rooted in family, neighbourhood and the immediate locality were especially likely to miss the day-to-day contact with loved ones.

These pre-war differences in writing habits were exacerbated by the conditions under which men on the Western Front wrote home. Officers, even when in trenches, could generally write at tables, lit by candlelight, their paper kept dry by a dug-out roof. Privates in the line were less well protected from the rain and cold. They lacked light and their conditions were more cramped. One man described 'four of us squatting on the floor of a tiny dug-out, elbow to elbow, so that it is more than difficult to write'.[68] The comparatively expansive style of officers' letters was not due only to their superior education and familiarity with letter-writing, but to their more comfortable conditions.

Censorship also impacted strongly on the rank-and-file soldier, whose own platoon commander signed and stamped his every letter.[69] Although the actual standard of inspection was uneven,[70] men were discouraged from discussing the war or personal matters by the feeling that their commanding officer was looking over their shoulder.[71] On disembarking at Le Havre, Harold Anderton wrote 'There's not much news, and I doubt if the censor people will allow me to impart what little there is'. In his letter the following day he was 'almost at a loss to know what to say'. The past few days had been 'by no means uneventful' but he would have to exclude so many details of his actions that his letter would 'not only prove uninteresting but puzzling' to all at home.[72] Frustration was common: Charles Ramsdale complained about the deletions in an earlier letter, knowing full well that his message would be read by the very platoon officer responsible for the excisions.[73] The fear that a letter containing too much prohibited information might be destroyed was a strong disincentive to break regulations.[74]

Officers, able to censor their own letters, enjoyed a significant privilege. Their mail might be opened by the Base Censor but this rarely happened and many used the privilege to discuss topics that were technically out of bounds. Second Lieutenant Frank Wollocombe would refer to 'Lord C' when he was about to attack and he, like many others, used family names and other agreed codes as a means to convey information that would otherwise be censored.[75] Wilfred Owen told his mother that if she received a Field Service postcard with a double line through the sentence 'I am being sent down to the base', this meant he was actually at the Front.[76] That cipher like this was expressly prohibited by the Censorship and Publicity Section of the General Staff suggests it was prevalent.[77] Officers thus operated something of a double standard, censoring their men's letters whilst describing military action in detail in their own. A 1918 lecture on postal censorship pointed out this hypocritical behaviour, and appealed to gentlemanly honour to remedy it:

> many cases have been found which give the impression that some officers consider their letters to be above all censorship rules. What is sauce for the goose is sauce for the gander, and an officer who cuts information out of his men's letters and then writes it in his own is not playing the game to say the least of it. Remember that your signature on your own letters should be regarded as a guarantee of the contents as it is on the men's letters.[78]

## Who wrote to whom?

Much was demanded of mothers as correspondents, for it was felt to be their task to keep sons connected to home. After his first gruelling experience of trench warfare, Wilfred Owen set out his expectations: 'nothing but a daily one from you will keep me up. I think Colin [his brother] might try a weekly letter. And Father?'[79] Mothers in turn were keen to assure sons they were reliable. Helen Mercer, replying to her nineteen-year-old son's first letters from France, in which he reported that he had not heard from her, was quick to reassure. He ought not to worry, since 'you would know darling, that I should be writing often.' 'You are never out of my thoughts', she continued.[80]

The subjective impression that mothers formed a key link between young men and their families is supported by the larger patterns of correspondence. Amongst over 5,000 letters written by unmarried men to their families and now held at the IWM, almost half (47.5 per cent) were addressed to the mother. [81] Letters from sons to their mothers outnumber those to any other family member or any combination of family members; there are more than twice as many letters addressed to mothers as there are letters addressed to both parents or the whole family combined.[82]

A letter addressed to a mother was usually not meant exclusively for her, as sons expected her to relay news on to everyone in the family. Some men addressed their letters to 'mother and all', assuming that they would be read aloud or passed on. 'I'm flattered to know that my letters are so often read', Anderton commented to his mother.[83] At the same time, though sons assumed that their news would be shared with fathers, sisters and brothers, it still mattered that it was their *mother* who formed the mainstay. Edward Chapman also wrote to his sisters but as he explained to his mother, 'when I only have time to write one letter, I like it to go to you.'[84]

Although mothers predominate in the surviving correspondence there are striking variations, and these hint at the range of emotional relationships that could exist within families. At one extreme is Wilfred Owen, whose published collection contains 300 letters during his military service, only two of which are addressed to his father. His comment above, 'And father?', does more than express the ill-defined nature of epistolary expectations; it relegates his father to the emotional background. Alf Swettenham's letters to his mother and brother contain only one reference to his father: 'is Dad still working', he asks.[85] More commonly, collections contain letters to both parents or to the whole family, but favour the mother. Of the surviving letters written by Captain Arthur Gibbs in the twelve-month period after his arrival in France in December 1915, 120 were written to his mother and eleven to his 'dada'. Second Lieutenant Ernest Smith's collection contains fifty-one letters to his mother, five to his father, and five to his sister Ruth.

But not all writers were as focused on their mothers as these men seem to have been. In almost a quarter of the collections studied, letters addressed either to both parents or to all the family outnumbered other correspondence. Unmarried men also corresponded frequently with their brothers and sisters and letters addressed to siblings make up around 16 per cent of the total sample. Sisters were particularly close correspondents and in seven of the eighty-one collections considered here, letters to sisters outnumber those to any other family member.[86]

Other relatives outside the immediate family, particularly aunts, could also be significant. Captain B. G. Buxton kept regular contact with all his family, but his aunt seems to have been his most important correspondent, having the position normally occupied by a mother.[87] Twenty-one-year-old Tom Corless, whose mother had died in childbirth, did not stay in touch with his step-mother. She 'never wrote, but I put it down to the fact that Ma was never really keen on me.'[88] His aunt and 'wonderful grandmother' in Oldham were his principal correspondents. They sent him parcels, he stayed with them when on leave, and he returned to their home after the war.[89] A man's closest affections were not always reserved for his mother.

The figure who appears least often in family correspondence is the father. Around half the IWM collections surveyed in this study do not contain a single letter to a father, while letters to fathers constitute around 8 per cent of the sample overall. There are more than twice as many extant letters to sisters, and five times as many extant letters to mothers. This probably reflects the behaviour of fathers as correspondents. Lyndall Urwick's parents were not unusual: Henry wrote to his son two or three times in the first month of Lyndall's overseas service, while Annis wrote nearly every day. Fathers were widely believed to dislike letter-writing or to be too busy for it.[90] Yet this did not necessarily indicate a distant relationship. The letter was a feminine form, and because of its potential introspection and emotionality, for many mothers it felt a natural means of staying in touch.[91] Fathers and sons were likely to be intimate in different ways, through their shared participation in sports, hobbies or work, which were hard to sustain by letter. Lyndall Urwick, for example, had recently begun working for Fownes Brothers shortly before the war, and when father and son wrote to each other it tended to be about the family business.

These men certainly missed their fathers. Ernest Smith was delighted to hear from his father but, as an adult son with responsibilities of his own, was keen to acknowledge the reasons why his father could not write more often: 'I was so glad to get a letter from you as I quite appreciate the difficulty you have in writing. Even if it were not for this press of work which I am delighted to hear about.'[92] Second Lieutenant Arnold Hooper was prompted to put in a request for a letter from his dad via his mother: 'Father seems to have given all his time to other things. His hand-writing has not arrived with the Mail lately. Please call his attention to this fact. His second son admires and loves him to such an extent that he longs for him and his advice.'[93] Arnold's relationship with his father was based more on their common interests than on the expression of sentiment. His father was in the Kent Volunteer Corps and Arnold was following his father's profession as an architect. *The Architect* magazines that his father sent him in Mesopotamia were probably a more poignant reminder of paternal love than his letters. Though Arnold described his mother as his 'first friend', it was his father who, communicating by letter, he particularly missed.[94]

Not only the frequency but the tone and content of letters to fathers differed from those to mothers. Arnold Hooper summed it up when he signed off his letter to his mother with the following comment: 'I shall write a practical letter to the Father. I know you like the loving ones.'[95] Sons wrote to their fathers about the conduct of the war on the international stage, the military skills they were acquiring and the daily routines of Army life.[96] An officer might ask his father to 'pull strings' when he wanted a transfer or promotion, or ask for help to finance and purchase items of uniform and other kit. [97] Yet even requests were sometimes routed through mothers: Cecil Christopher wrote to his mother when he decided to invest in Exchequer bonds, explaining that 'I expect father to do the necessary business for me.'[98]

Sons were more likely to describe violent events to fathers than to mothers. John Middlebrook was vague about fighting in letters to his mother, but had no compunction in telling his father about the 'heavies' that hit a nearby dug-out. Two men had been 'killed outright and were more than that, they were unrecognisable and only to be identified by their discs.'[99] Captain Norman Taylor wrote to his sisters (his mother was dead) about domestic matters like his billets and dug-outs, but to his father he described in graphic detail his part in an attack on German soldiers who were sheltering in a crater:

> I reached the outer lip and went up to post sentries. Looking out, I saw a Bosch not more than 5 yards away with others behind. He threw a bomb plumb at me. I dodged and it rolled to the bottom of the crater. We opened sacks of bombs and started throwing. And so it went on for most of the night, intermittently . . .
>
> You have no idea what a subtle thrill there is in seeing on a good moonlight night, a Hun working party perhaps faintly silhouetted and opening a sudden burst of fire with a gun on them.

> I am sorry to say I had a gun knocked out the other day – a shell burst and blew it to bits. It took us half an hour to find and collect the unfortunate sentry.[100]

Though it was more acceptable for a son to present himself in a letter to his mother as a victim rather than a killer, the truth contained in Taylor's letter to his father was just as partial as any contained in a letter to a mother, for it hid his vulnerability.

There were exceptions. Some sons wrote just as often to fathers as to mothers. Frank Wollocombe appears to have been remarkably even-handed, and Eric Marchant wrote more often to his father than to his mother or sisters. But in only two of the eighty-one collections surveyed was the father the principal recipient. These patterns reflect what we know of the diversity of emotional relations in Edwardian families. It is often assumed that relationships between parents (especially fathers) and children were typically remote within the upper middle class and the most prosperous sections of the middle class.[101] Yet, as Elizabeth Buettner shows in her study of Empire families, some upper-middle-class parents deeply lamented their separation from children and wrote passionately of their love.[102] John Tosh has argued that there was not one but a variety of models of fatherhood in the late nineteenth-century middle class, ranging from the emotionally absent to the intimate.[103] The close involvement of men in the home is sometimes seen as distinctively lower middle class; yet there were also lower-middle-class sons – such as Wilfred Owen – who almost never wrote to their fathers. While working-class families were often very mother-focused, observers like the district nurse M. Loane noted the strong desire of fathers in South London for the company of their families.[104] Wartime correspondence highlights the different roles which fathers of this period could occupy, from being an equal domestic partner with the mother, through being the one who supported the mother, to being largely aloof from the emotional dramas of family life.

Sons may have counted their mothers among their most steadfast correspondents, but while they keenly anticipated their letters, they did not keep them long. Letters from wives and sweethearts, as Jenny Hartley notes in her study of Second World War correspondence, were 'more carefully tended than those from mothers' and hence are more likely to survive today.[105] When Vera Brittain found herself falling more deeply in love with Roland Leighton, it was not through face-to-face contact but through the exchange of *letters*. 'How I love writing to him!' she declared a week after receiving his first letter from the front.[106] Whereas letters between sweethearts had to nurture the fledgling relationship, the letters that mothers sent their sons harked back to a lifetime of shared experience. Their very ubiquity, and the fact that mothers wrote about everyday matters, made them dispensable. All the excitement of new love went into letters between sweethearts, whereas, though a son might expect a constant supply from his mother, the proof of her love did not lie in the letter itself.

## Confession and concealment

Historians of the First World War, though they often use letters home to build up a picture of life in the trenches, are frequently sceptical about their usefulness. Ilana Bet-El suggests that conscripts, 'prohibited from sharing the immediacy of their military experiences with their civilian contacts', were reduced to intimating 'a vague existence of eating in various climactic conditions.'[107] John Ellis describes the letter home as 'at best a prosaic document', with an 'enormous disparity between what men were going through and what they were able, or willing to communicate.'[108] By contrast, Gary Sheffield and Helen McCartney have argued that censorship did not stop rankers from giving intimate details of their war experience, and John Horne has described letters as part of a 'private information network' that conveyed the realities of life in trenches.[109]

Both those who emphasise the richness of accounts produced in letters, and those who question it, are partially correct. Sheffield and others are right that these letters do not just tell sanitised tales of war, but nor are they like the bloody and harrowing accounts that the war generation would produce in memoirs from the 1920s up to the 1970s.[110] When writing home sons were highly attuned to how their mothers would react, and the likely impact of their news on family members arguably formed just as strong a constraint on them as formal censorship. Everyone knew that mothers would be anxious. 'You who remain at home and worry about us here', wrote Edward Chapman, 'have far the worst of it'.[111] It was partly in response to this perceived anxiety that sons wrote home before going into the front line or into battle, as they knew the break in correspondence might be interpreted as a sign that they had come to harm.[112] They often tried to conceal the worst aspects of trench warfare. Frederick Noakes, looking back during the 1950s on the letters his mother had kept, was struck by 'the memories which they revive of the things I did *not* say'.[113] Indeed, the ability to protect a mother in this way was itself thought to be a sign of manliness. Howard Bowser 'concealed from my family not only our movements – this was strictly and wisely forbidden by order – but the mental ands physical ardours we endured – no man worth his salt would do less'.[114]

Despite their attempts at concealment, we can learn to read the emotions of sons between the lines of letters home, if we consider what it was about their situation that they were trying to protect their mothers from, and if we reflect on how mothers would have read these letters. Most sons, in trying to compose an account suitable for a mother's eye, conveyed feelings of which they were unaware. They dropped clues in their omissions, abrupt changes of topic, things alluded to but ultimately left unsaid, and contradictory comments about their spirits. The more stressful the circumstance, the stronger was the pressure *both* to want to confide in loved ones, *and* to resist confiding. The result was a characteristically oblique style of communication which can nevertheless reveal much about the emotional experience of Army life.

Edward Chapman was probably so concerned about his mother because of her situation, widowed eighteen months earlier and in her late fifties, with a twelve-year-old daughter Hilda and a twenty-seven-year-old daughter Constance still living in the Rectory in Freshford near Bath. A science graduate from Cambridge, aged twenty-three, who had been studying in Germany just before the war, Edward was a thoughtful correspondent, though rather hamstrung by his new responsibilities as head of the family. The first time he saw German shelling at close-hand was August 1916, when two shells fell on a bivouac close to his own. He told his mother, but stopped himself midway through, his train of thought broken by a sudden awareness of how she might react:

> I don't know whether I ought to tell you these incidents, for I'm afraid they make you feel anxious about me. I am really perfectly safe for this place is not shelled systematically at all. They pt one over every day or so just to keep up appearances. The danger is about equal to that in London from Zepps – certainly no greater![115]

On the night of 21 April 1916 he went into the front line for the first time, at Mametz Wood. The balancing act between confession and concealment was almost impossible to sustain in the letter he wrote from support trenches on 27 August, a day after leaving the front line. Though they were only holding the trench, not attacking, they were heavily shelled and 'lost a good many men.' On their first night a shell burst above them, wounding two or three men and killing Lieutenant Walker, who had been standing right beside Chapman at the time. Chapman himself got away with only a scratch on the neck and arm. His name would be in the casualty lists but it was 'absurd that I am put down as wounded, as I have often cut myself worse when shaving!' The remark was intended to make light of the wound, but in fact, underlined what a very close shave it had been. He lost everything in his pockets – including the little prayer book his mother had given him – when a flare went up during a digging party and he went to ground. The 'fearless' Lieutenant Humphreys, who had been with Edward in Ireland, was shot dead.

The countryside around them was a 'desolate waste', the forward areas littered with bodies from a failed attack by the battalion they had relieved. The blood and stench seemed to have got right into him:

> Dead bodies were lying out in front, and the trenches themselves were littered with old jam tins, equipment, bloodstained clothing etc. Naturally they were swarming with flies. By the end of the time half the company, including myself, were suffering from a mild sort of dysentery. I am better now, but don't yet feel very grand.

The contradictions abounded: he had dysentery but it was only mild, he was feeling better but was not 'yet very grand.' Chapman kept returning to the dead, and then invoking home as an abstract principle, a hallowed retreat rather than an actual place:

> All this area is one vast cemetery. Dead bodies taint the air wherever you go. It has robbed thousands and thousands of men of life, and thousands more of the things that made life seem worth living. I have come to look upon peace and quiet and home life as the Summum bonum. I feel now that all I want is to be able to live quietly, and tend a garden, and study a bit.
>
> I am sorry to be writing such a dismal letter, but I cannot always look at the war from the Bairnsfather point of view. Thank heaven so many people can. But of course the whole reason for feeling dismal is that I am a bit out of sorts. When I am fit again you will not find me depressing you with letters like this.

In the closing paragraphs he summoned a last effort to brighten up: 'Now for a piece of good news', he announced, and went on to explain how his friend Edwards, feared dead, had been made a POW. 'Isn't that splendid?' Chapman was searching for anything that might keep up his mother's spirits and his own.[116]

Chapman kept returning to the events at Mametz Wood in the weeks and months afterwards. The details emerged little by little throughout

September in letters to his younger sister and mother which were dotted about with exclamation marks and jovial comments, as if the very punctuation might lift his spirits. 'I am a pessimist no longer!' he announced.[117] Mametz Wood was clearly seared into memory, however, for in mid-February 1917, six months afterwards, he returned to it again. Having admitted how vulnerable he had felt, he quickly asserted his toughness: 'The first few weeks out here nearly broke me. Instead of breaking me it broke me in.'[118] Like many young temporary officers he was excited by the camaraderie, the experience of command, and the manly outdoors life, and did not want to appear a failure in this venture into military life.

Men circled around violent and disturbing events in letters home partly because writing itself unsettled them. 'Perhaps you will excuse my writing more at the present time + our present surroundings + possibly also the after feeling are not conducive to good writing', wrote Lieutenant Alick Knight after coming out of battle at the Somme with only a third of his Battalion unscathed. Three days later he was still 'so tired + lazy that even writing is an effort.'[119]

The problem with writing was that it encouraged introspection, while the ability *not* to dwell on disturbing events showed that they were in control. Ernest Smith wrote in his letter after battle that 'The taking over of that line seemed an unreal sort of dream to me, I am not going into details.'[120] Wilfred Owen wrote to his mother, after returning to the Western Front from Craiglockhart hospital for neurasthenic soldiers, that 'If I started into detail of our engagement I should disturb the censor and my own Rest.'[121] Once drawn into telling there could be no holding back. This fear led some to try and slow memory down. Like Chapman, they would reveal their experiences little by little over days, weeks, months and perhaps even years.

As well as circling around painful memories, men dropped clues about their feelings in errors and slips of the pencil. The letter that the seventeen-year-old subaltern Wilbert Spencer wrote just after coming out of trenches hinted at a gruelling time. In his 'first doze [*sic*] of shrapnel and shell', he had seen one of his men killed and another four wounded, a shell having '~~first~~ burst right on our trench'. Spencer's automatic repetition of the word 'first' intimated how much this violent introduction to modern warfare had upset him. Further down the page he returned to the incident, explaining that 'One of the worst ~~sights~~ parts of war is the sights one has to endure'. The word 'sights' is crossed out, and 'parts' added instead. It was the sights that filled his mind, the memory of them running ahead of his ability to put them into words.[122]

A man might skirt around the gruesome sights when corresponding with his mother, but relate graphic details to a sister or brother. Younger sisters in particular were sometimes told things that parents were not.[123] Edward Chapman's letter to his mother after Mametz Wood left many of the bloody details to her imagination, but he told Hilda that Lieutenant Walker, standing beside him that first day, was killed by a shell, 'a great fragment entering his head'.[124] Hardened soldiers found head wounds disturbing, so it was all the more shocking that Chapman wrote about them to a twelve-year-old girl. A letter to a sister might actually be aimed – deliberately or unwittingly – at a mother. Children then did not have the privacy accorded to teenagers today and in many families, younger sisters would have been expected to share the contents of their letters with their parents. Wilfred Owen would probably have assumed this when he wrote to his sister Mary, then aged twenty, from a Casualty Clearing Station in May 1917, shortly after he was diagnosed with neurasthenia. He explained to Mary that his condition had been brought on by lying opposite a dead subaltern officer, also from the Manchesters. Second Lieutenant Gaukroger was 'not only near by, but in various places around and about, if you understand. I hope you don't!'[125] Owen had intimated in a previous letter to his mother that Gaukroger was dead, but until this letter he had not mentioned that the body was dismembered.

Owen's comment that he hoped Mary would not understand was tendentious: she had been working as a voluntary nurse and doubtless knew well enough the damage that High Explosives could inflict. His account actually conveyed the very opposite of its apparent meaning, and drew attention to the horrific state of Gaukroger's body. Owen might assume that his mother would learn of the details, as Mary, quiet and frail by nature, was very much under her mother's thumb.[126] Such letters conformed to the notion that mothers must not be made anxious, but were equally motivated by the opposite impulse.

Men also dropped unconscious clues when discussing seemingly humdrum matters like washing, food, clothing and shelter. Domestic things conveyed the grotesque differences between home and trench. Roland Mountfort, who was fastidious in his personal habits, wrote pages and pages about the antics of the rats in 'Chateau des rat', the three months he had gone without a bath, drinking tea in which a slug had been found floating, drying off his clothes by sleeping in them, and 'the luxury of having sufficient clean space on your sleeve to rub your nose on!' Hoping to help him keep clean, his father sent him some soap. Mountfort's reply pressed home his misery. He was not in need of soap but water, which was so scarce that soap 'lasts a long time'. He used the same water to shave and wash his body and teeth: 'I suppose to you it hardly seems possible', he concluded.[127] Eric Marchant's description of home seems at first sight a fond memory, but it had a sharper point. He could 'imagine you all just now setting down to dinner and should like you to see us', covered in dirt, feeling 'a bit chilly', and living on nothing more substantial than tinned beef and biscuits,[128] The scenes from home that men conjured were not just wistful, but sometimes conveyed their fear, anger and disenchantment.

Sons also caught their mothers' attention in the descriptions they gave of their state of health. Since they almost always reported being in good spirits, any hint to the contrary would be seized upon. His stomach was a particularly sensitive indicator of a man's emotional state. The first time Charles Ramsdale got diarrhoea he wrote: 'I hope you are both quite well, as I am pleased to say I am, except for a touch of diarrhoea (not much)'. The second time he was 'quite well, hoping you are the same'. However, twice during the note he apologised for not writing more. He wasn't 'in the humour for letter-writing'; he couldn't say much because of the censor; and he had already caught himself almost falling asleep over his letter. Only in the final sentence did he offer an explanation, but immediately afterwards he reverted to his usual tone: 'Oh, I said I was quite well; really I've a touch of diarrhoea but am otherwise in the pink.'[129] On each occasion he left his ailment to the closing sentence, ensuring that all at home would be left pondering what was wrong. Stomach problems could register with mothers in a way that other ailments might not, connected as they were to deep concerns about nurturing, and the infant's need to hold down its food if it was to thrive.

The psychological dynamics of these letters were not just ones of confession and concealment, for the writers was not always fully aware of the emotional impulses that animated them. Mindful of the need to protect mothers from worry, they also experienced a powerful unconscious need to get rid of disturbing feelings and even to punish mothers because they were remote and could not help.[130] Reassurance could tip over into descriptions that were unwittingly aimed to make loved ones feel worried and guilty.

## Imagining home

Arthur Hubbard had an unusually gentle preparation for France. An office worker and member of a Territorial unit, the 1st London Scottish, he had trained with friends, and from his barracks in Roehampton it was possible to visit home in Streatham Vale.[131] On hearing in early May 1916 that he would be bound for France with the next draft, he dropped off a load of washing and looked forward to one last Sunday with his family. No doubt dinner was to be a high point, for in the barracks 'everybody is grumbling it is alright no doubt before it is cooked but rotten after and not sufficient by along [*sic*] way.'[132] Such comparisons with his family's Sunday meals would re-appear once Hubbard reached the Western Front.

By 22 May Hubbard was in France and organising his circle of correspondents. His letters were usually addressed to 'mother and all', and included married siblings as well as his sisters Nellie and Ivy, and brothers Will and Wal. His mother may have been surprised to learn that he had been 'keeping company' with a Miss Elson in Fulham; and that he had given Miss Elson his mother's address in case any of his letters home failed to arrive.[133]

It was not long before Hubbard had his first experience of the trenches, a six-day stint during a wet patch in early June that left him with a cold due to constantly wet feet and raw skin 'owing to keep on rubbing myself'. The lice in his unwashed shirt were probably the culprit. Hubbard was then sent away on a bombing course and when he returned to the battalion on 17 June it had been through a tough second tour in the front line. His friend Isaacs 'looks like an old man since I have been away' and as a soldier had become something of a liability. He was 'nervous, and seems to tumble down all the holes in the dark', and was prone to talking too loudly near the Germans.

Hubbard's mind was fixed on the big attack to come. He had broken the glass and hands of his much-loved watch, and had sent it back by registered post, but did not want it returned just yet. He would not tell them why, but the remainder of his letter more than hinted at the reason. He said nothing about fighting, but imagined what it would be like if they were successful and could 'pack up to return for good' in August.

Writing on a Saturday night, he was 'full of thoughts' of Sundays at home, but these only served to make him feel more homesick and envious: 'I can picture you all sitting around the table about 8.30 enjoying a good breakfast and me miles away in this miserable place which is being and has been blown to hell by the Huns who are at present as far away from us as you are from Mr Snelling's house'. His reference to their neighbour was not just a fond memory, but conveyed, in a manner they could not fail to understand, how close he was to the enemy. It was just as well, he continued, that his brothers Will and Wal were not out here, for they 'wouldn't stand the sights that I have seen since my short stay here, and the battle is not started yet.' Hubbard had a particular fear that he would have to fight hand-to-hand with the Germans; he only hoped that none would 'stay behind to tackle us.' On the final page of his letter he returned to the things he was missing most. He would like some of 'your jam if you have any, as it makes those hard biscuits eat better especially on Sundays', and he wanted 'to be able to see the garden before this season is over.'[134] This parting comment was more than a generalised wish that it would all be over by autumn. It voiced deep anxiety about whether he would get through the battle.

Hubbard's last letter home before he went over the top at Gommecourt was written on 30 June, the eve of the attack, in reply to letters from Nellie and Ivy. As he explained to his sisters what he was about to do, the mention of home served principally to shock: 'hope we shall be successful on Saturday morning July 1 at dawn when you are all fast asleep in driving the Huns out of their present position, and without any bad luck to myself. I have got to go over with the first batch'. He had had a pretty gruelling time since his last letter. Their tents were leaking and the floor was too wet to lie on, so they had stood up all night on 24 and 25 June, 'drenched through to our skins'. They were hungry. Hubbard was not so much stoic as aggrieved: 'they expect you to do your very best on the top of it, and short rations as well.' Now the Germans had started 'doing great damage' with their shells. He had been 20 yards away from a fellow London Regiment man who had 'shot himself through the foot just to get back to England out of it.' Hubbard, hoping to stop him from harming himself further, called for help and took away his rifle. Hubbard wondered how the man would live down his wound, knowing 'he done it himself', but he was not censorious, as he was 'not the only one that as [*sic*] done likewise.'[135]

The man's plight caused Hubbard to ponder his own future, and once again he turned to the memory of home. He thought of the garden, which 'as you say must be almost at its best', and wondered if they were having beans from it yet. But try as he might to picture a domestic haven, the hell of the trenches kept breaking through: 'I shall imagine I am in heaven when I get home, what a treat it will be to feel nice and clean, at present it is up to your neck in mud which all helps to make you feel miserable . . . I think Fred [a relative] will have a good time where he is going, no bayonet work I hope.'[136] Hubbard scrawled a final few lines before setting off for a church service, after which they would go into trenches 'ready for the attack in the morning.' He hoped he would get through alright, and closed with his 'best love to you all at home.'[137]

Hubbard's experience of battle on 1 July was as shocking as anything he had imagined, though Gommecourt was only a side-show, planned by General Haig to draw attention from the main attack.[138] After going over the top, cutting through the wire and crossing three lines of German trenches, Hubbard came across three soldiers emerging from their deep dug-out, crying for mercy and 'bleeding badly.' Ordered by his officers not to take prisoners, Hubbard had to 'empty my his magazine' on the wounded man.[139] His nightmare of having to engage German soldiers close-up had come true. Soon afterwards a shell landed nearby, smashing his rifle, knocking his helmet off and burying him in dirt. Major Lindsay came over to ask him what was wrong and at that instant was shot through the throat by a sniper. Hubbard was forced to retreat under heavy machine gun fire, leaving the Major's body for the Germans to bury.

Gruelling though these experiences were, in some ways Hubbard was a lucky man. Casualties among the London Scottish men stood at 40 per cent within an hour and three-quarters of the attack, and after ten hours in the German trenches this had risen to nearly 80 per cent. 'A' Company had been nearly wiped out.[140] His friend Isaacs was probably dead. Hubbard's only injuries were a cut knee from the German wire and a weakness in his back. His mind was another matter. In a letter written on 5 July he told 'mother and all' in a characteristically tortuous formulation that he was 'quite alright suffering from slight Shell Shock.' He was sure to 'be quite myself in a week or two, as you will notice by my writing only my nerves are shook up, severe headaches now and again when my mind is on the affair.'[141] Much as Hubbard tried to play down his condition, writing home put his mind 'on the affair'. He attempted another letter two days later, but writing made his hand shake. He did not wish to write any more 'as it makes my head jump to think about it'.[142] Hubbard seems never to have recovered from this experience: he committed suicide in the late 1920s and the official verdict was that his death was due to shell-shock.[143]

* * *

Men did not conjure the same images when they imagined home. For the lower-middle-class recruit Hubbard, home meant a house, garden, neighbours and Sunday meals. Wilfred Owen also thought of bricks and mortar, and though the house in Shrewsbury to which Susan and Tom Owen moved in 1910 was semi-detached and the bedroom that Wilfred occupied in the attic was tiny, he followed the upper-class habit of referring to it by name, 'Mahim'.[144] For Edward Chapman, brought up in the village rectory, home meant tea in the garden and his sister's table antics. A ranker from a rural background might be as likely to recall a particular landscape or the house of the local gentry. Private George Farndell, stationed in Le Havre but hailing from Chichester, wrote of how 'a nearby house reminds me very much of Goodwood.'[145] Given the rudimentary nature of his pre-war accommodation, the agricultural labourer or the poorest urban dweller was probably less prone to become nostalgic about the family home than his better-off comrades, but the surrounding streets or landscape might be the more fondly remembered, and so too might his Sunday dinner, one of the few times in the week when meat and other luxuries were sure to be on the table.[146]

Whatever home meant, and however different it was from Army life, men imagined it in their dreams, on sentry duty and at mealtimes, not just when writing home. In *No Man's Land*, Eric Leed concludes that these imaginings were nothing more than a kind of false consciousness, a 'defense against the realities of war and the sense of inferiority, degradation, and impotence imposed by these realities', which the battle-hardened recruit would eventually reject for the comradeship of other soldiers.[147] Hubbard and Chapman's accounts suggest that the more stressful the situation, the greater was the urge to construct home as a haven, yet the more the war intruded. Home became, not a parallel existence, but another world, beyond the reach of the trenches. These dreams of home, however, were neither naive nor dysfunctional, but essential to their survival. Despite all the pressures to keep a stiff upper lip, families were made to feel their pain, and this shows how strong the ties to home remained.

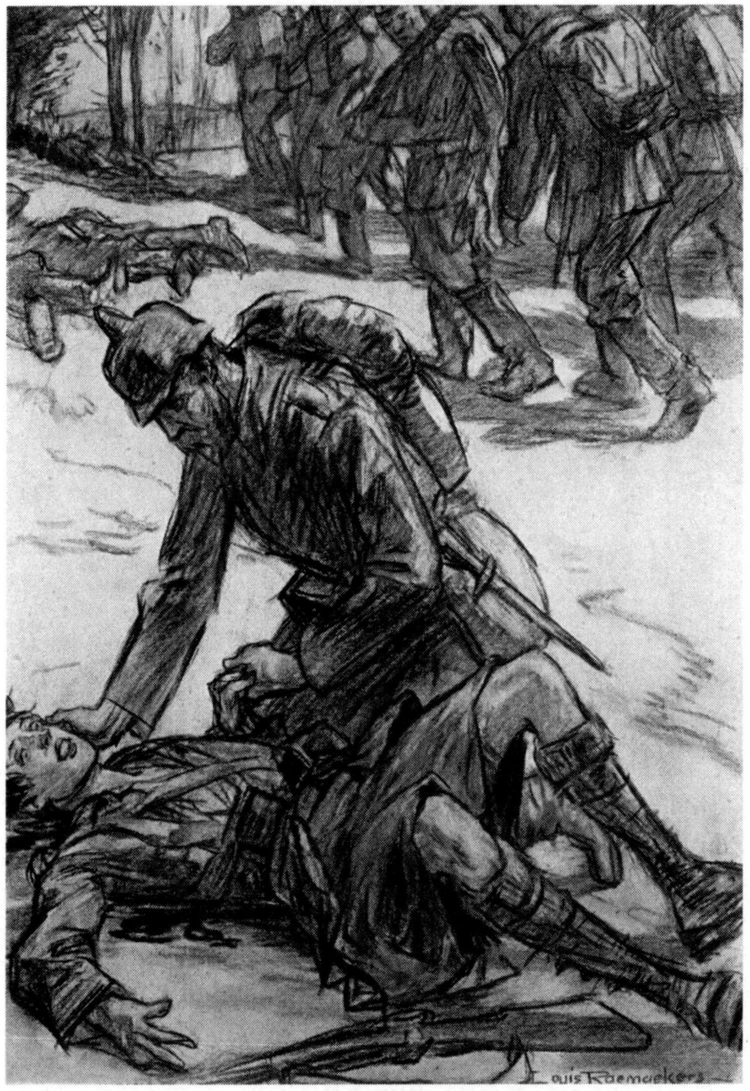


*1* 'Is it you, mother?', Louis Raemaekers

TO MY
SON
SERVING KING
AND COUNTRY
Though parted by duty
I trust this will cheer
'Tis a greeting from Home
To my Son, who's so dear;
May the smile of Good Fortune
beam down on your way,
Soon Peace to unite us –
GOD speed on that day.
POST CARD
FOR ADDRESS ONLY
With much
love from
Mother

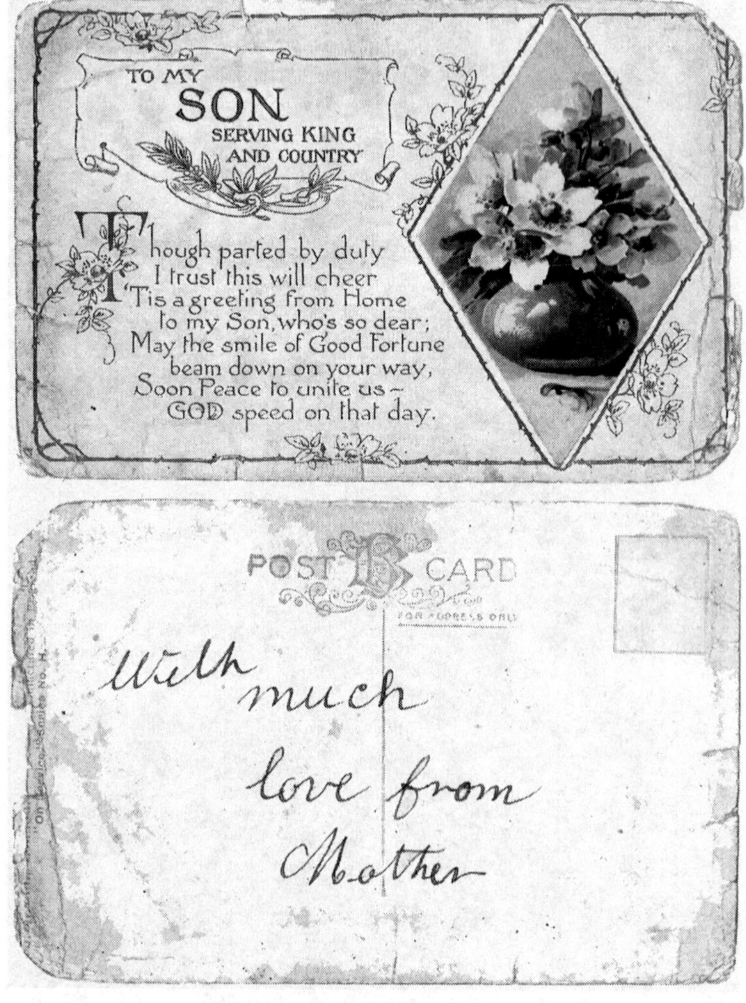

*2* 'To my son serving King and Country'. The message on the back of the postcard from Alf Swettenham's mother is brief; she lets the poem communicate her feelings

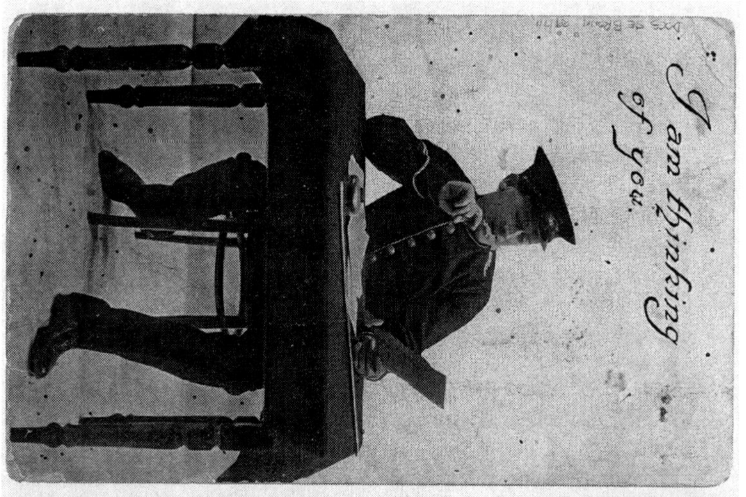


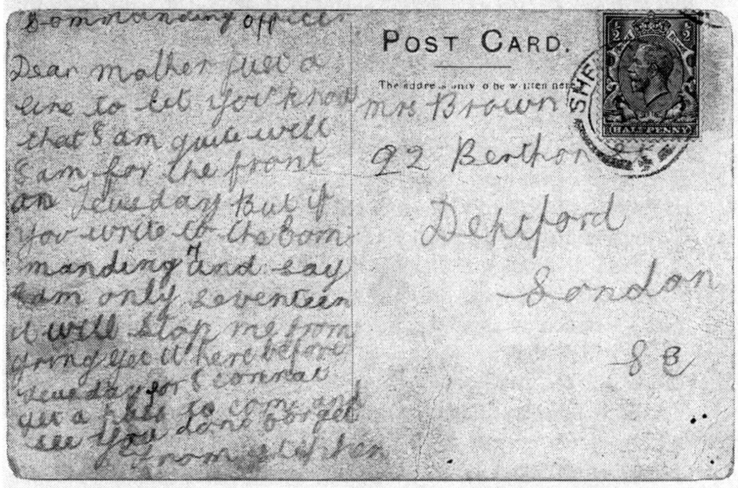

Commanding office[r]

Dear mother just a line to let you know that I am quite well I am for the front on Tuesday But if you write to the Commanding and say I am only seventeen it will stop me from going [illegible] here before Tuesday for I cannot get a pass to come and see you dont forget from [illegible]

POST CARD.

The address only to be written here

Mrs Brown
92 Berthon [illegible]
Deptford
London
S E

3 'I am thinking of you', Stephen Brown sent this postcard to his mother from Sheerness as he was about to embark for France. Brown was killed at Ypres in May 1915

## Notes

1 Lyndall Urwick to mother, 7 August 1914, private collection.
2 Henry Urwick diary, 9 August; 12 August 1914.
3 Lyndall Urwick to mother, 13 August 1914.
4 Henry Urwick diary, 12 September 1914.
5 Henry Urwick diary, 22 September 1914.
6 Annis Urwick to Lyndall Urwick, 22 September, 23 September, 24 September 1914.
7 H. Stacke, *The Worcestershire Regiment in the Great War* (Kidderminster: G. T. Cheshire & Sons Ltd, 1928), p. 20; Henry Urwick diary, 26 September, 27 September 1914.
8 Lyndall Urwick to mother, 25 September, 26 September 1914.
9 Henry Urwick diary, 30 September, 8 October, 9 October, 10 October 1914.
10 Telegram from Lyndall Urwick, 13 August 1914.
11 'Dadd' to W. A. Goodwin, 7 November 1915, IWM Con Shelf.
12 On the importance of letters as touched objects, see Santanu Das, *Touch and Intimacy in First World War Literature* (Cambridge: Cambridge University Press, 2005), p. 13. In holding their letter the recipient felt physically and emotionally connected to the writer. Likewise the historian, holding the fragile evidence of a life often lost shortly after the letter was written, becomes absorbed in that person's emotional experience.
13 L. Hooper to K. Hooper, 15 July 1915, LC DF066.
14 E. H. Anderton to mother, 26 February 1915, IWM 88/20/1.
15 H. F. Bowser to father, 7 November 1915, IWM 88/56/1.
16 L. Timpson diary, 24 December 1915, IWM 92/3/1.
17 H. S. Payne to mother, 23 October 1916, IWM 90/1/1. On receiving a letter from his father, Private E. Marchant was 'delighted to see your hand-writing. It isn't so much the news that makes letters so welcome but just the connection with home'. Marchant to father, 12 April 1915, IWM DS/MISC/26.
18 A. G. Baker, nd, IWM 01/6/1.
19 M. Webb to mother and father, 12 June 1915, IWM 90/28/1.
20 E. H. Anderton to mother, 12 April 1915, IWM 88/20/1.
21 Quoted in S. Grayzel, *Women's Identities at War. Gender, Motherhood and Politics in Britain and France during the First World War* (Chapel Hill. NC: University of North Carolina Press, 1999), p. 14.
22 M. Hanna, 'A Republic of Letters: The Epistolary Tradition in France during World War I', *The American Historical Review*, Vol. 108, No. 5 (2003), http://www.historycooperative.org/journals/ahr/108.5/hanna.html. Accessed 25 May 2007, para. 42.
23 P. B. Boyden, *Tommy Atkins' Letters. The History of the British Army Postal Service From 1795* (London: National Army Museum, 1990), p. 28. Statistics on manpower are from 'The Long, Long Trail. The British Army in the Great War of 1914–18', http://www.1914-1918.net/dukes.htm. Accessed 3 July 2007.

24 Boyden, *Tommy Atkins' Letters*, p. 30; D. Englander, 'Soldiering and Identity: Reflections on the Great War', *War in History*, Vol. 1, No. 3, p. 305.

25 W. Owen to mother, 4 January, 7 January, 9 January, 10 January 1917, in J. Bell (ed.), *Wilfred Owen. Selected Letters* (Oxford: Oxford University Press, 1985), p. 208, p. 210, p. 211.

26 Cited in Carol Acton, 'Writing and Waiting: First World War Correspondence between Vera Brittain and Roland Leighton', *Gender and History*, Vol. 11, No. 1 (April 1999), p. 61.

27 H. Payne to mother, 29 August 1916, IWM 90/1/1.

28 W. Hate to mother, 9 October 1915, IWM 86/51/1; C. Ramsdale to mother, 11 March 1917, IWM Con Shelf.

29 T. Thorpe to Nellie, 28 June 1917, IWM Con Shelf.

30 E. K. Smith to mother, 3 March 1915, *Letters Sent From France. Service with the Artists' Rifles and the Buffs, December 1914–December 1915* (London: J. Cobb, 1994), p. 29.

31 The importance of mothering as an 'alternative' to military service for women is pointed out by Nicole Gullace, *The Blood of Our Sons. Men, Women and the Renegotiation of British Citizenship in the Great War* (Basingstoke: Palgrave, 2002), p. 62.

32 A. Hooper to L. Hooper, quoted in L. Hooper to K. Hooper, 6 August 1915; A. Hooper to L. Hooper, quoted in L. Hooper to K. Hooper, 15 November 1915.

33 S. J. Dawson to S. B. Dawson, 16 July, 26 August 1919, private collection.

34 Ilana Bet-El, *Conscripts. Forgotten Men of the Great War* (Stroud: Sutton Publishing, 2003), p. 133.

35 J. Damousi, *The Labour of Loss. Mourning, Memory and Wartime Bereavement in Australia* (Cambridge: Cambridge University Press, 1999), p. 19. On the effect of time-gaps in the correspondence between Irish immigrants to Australia and their families, see D. Fitzpatrick, *Oceans of Consolation. Personal Accounts of Irish Migration to Australia* (Cork: Cork University Press, 1994), pp. 493–5.

36 From G.D. Mitchell, *Backs to the Wall* (1937), quoted in J. G. Fuller, *Troop Morale and Popular Culture in the British and Dominion Armies* (Oxford: Clarendon Press, 1991), p. 23.

37 Damousi, *TheLabour of Loss*, p. 19.

38 'Ma' to W. A. Goodwin, 4 November 1915.

39 Mother to J. H. Standrick 28 January 1918, IWM 96/23/1.

40 A. G. Steavenson collection, IWM 86/77/1. Damousi notes the numbering of letters by Australian families as a means of overcoming the confusion created by distance, and as helping to 'contain and structure the emotions'. *The Labour of Loss*, p. 24.

41 Annis Urwick to Lyndall Urwick, 24 September 1914.

42 E. F. Chapman to mother, 15 September 1916, IWM Con Shelf and 92/3/1.

43 J. D. Tomlinson to mother, 26 April 1915, IWM 87/51/1.

44 Machonochie was a tinned stew of vegetables and meat widely used as rations by the British Army. Bet-El quotes a conscript: 'queerest Sunday I have ever spent. 1.30pm thingking [*sic*] of Sunday dinner at home. We have midday dinner as a special treat – the old bully'. *Conscripts*, p. 72.

45 Fuller, *Troop Morale*, p. 47; P. Simkins, *Kitchener's Army. The Raising of the New Armies, 1914–16* (Manchester: Manchester University Press, 1988), p. 227.

46 G. Fortune, unpublished memoir, p. 1, IWM 04/5/1.

47 The enlistment rate for industrial workers was around 28 per cent compared with around 40 per cent for non-manual workers. J. M. Winter, *The Great War and the British People* (Basingstoke: Macmillan, 1985), p. 34. See also Ian Beckett, 'The British Army 1914–18: The Illusion of Change', in J. Turner, *Britain and the First World War* (London: Unwin Hyman, 1988), p. 105.

48 Jonathan Wild, 'A Merciful, Heaven-Sent Release?: The Clerk and the First World War in British Literary Culture', *Cultural and Social History* Vol. 4, No. 1 (March 2007), p. 75. On the Liverpool Pals' units, see Helen McCartney, *Citizen Soldiers. The Liverpool Territorials in the First World War* (Cambridge: Cambridge University Press, 2005).

49 Quoted in Wild, 'A Merciful, Heaven-Sent Release?', p. 75.

50 Winter, *The Great War*, p. 34; McCartney, *Citizen Soldiers*, p. 5, p. 36.

51 Quoted in Englander, 'Soldiering and Identity', p. 304.

52 This can be seen in accounts of the first night in barracks, which frequently mention the foul language and crude eating habits of fellow rankers, and the strangeness of sleeping together. Simkins, *Kitchener's Army*, pp. 195–8. On the importance of symbolic markers of separation from the working class, and especially the 'aggressive rejection' of manual work among the lower middle class, see G. Crossick, 'The Emergence of the Lower Middle Class in Britain': a Discussion', in G. Crossick (ed.), *The Lower Middle Class in Britain, 1870–1914* (London: Croom Helm, 1977), p. 49.

53 D. Vincent, *Literacy and Popular Culture. England 1750–1914* (Cambridge: Cambridge University Press, 1989), pp. 44–6.

54 One school inspector commented that schoolchildren 'have but little power of expressing in language or on paper what they actually know. They have words without ideas, and ideas without words.' Vincent, *Literacy and Popular Culture*, p. 43, pp. 90–3.

55 E.g. S. E. Brown to mother, 30 April 1915, IWM 89/7/1; Swettenham, nd, August 1918, IWM 83/3/1. Goodwin to father, 11 August 1915, IWM Con Shelf.

56 This is also pointed out by Fitzpatrick in his study of Irish immigrant correspondence, *Oceans of Consolation*, pp. 497–8.

57 Ramsdale to mother and Mary, 11 March 1917, IWM Con Shelf. The same pride in learning French comes through in Will Hate's letters. Thanking his

mother for her pies, he wrote 'I think as the French say they were 'Les Bon'. He then crossed out the 'Les' and inserted 'Trés' in its place; then crossed this out in favour of 'Très'. Hate to mother, 28 December 1914.

58 In reading and writing lessons, schools were encouraged to work on standard pronunciation because of concerns that, as David Vincent puts, children 'who merely reproduced the speech patterns of their parents would remain within the moral and intellectual environment of the family and the neighbourhood.' *The Rise of Mass Literacy. Reading and Writing in Modern Europe* (Cambridge: Polity, 2000), p. 139.

59 S. E. Brown to mother, Sheerness, nd.

60 Generational differences in literacy were observed by the district nurse M. Loane among working-class families in South London. *The Queen's Poor. Life as They Find it in Town and Country* (London: Middlesex University Press, 1998), p. 15. Vincent shows that in the period 1899–1914 there was still a sizeable gap between the generations in literacy. *Literacy and Popular Culture*, pp. 26–7.

61 Father and mother to H. Carter, 3 March 1915, IWM 86/8/1.

62 An article in the Post Office Magazine 'St Martin's Le Grand' was devoted to examples of badly addressed mail. E. B. Proud, *History of the British Army Postal Service. Volume II, 1903–1927* (Dereham: Proud–Bailey, 1982), p. 18.

63 Robert Roberts, *The Classic Slum. Salford Life in the First Quarter of the Century* (Harmondsworth: Penguin, 1971), p. 202.

64 Mother to A. J. Arnold, 28 August 1917, IWM Con Shelf.

65 On the novelty of leaving home, see Bet-El, *Conscripts*, p. 43; and Simkins, *Kitchener's Army*, pp. 207–9. David Vincent has shown that the *per capita* volume of post tended to be lowest in manufacturing towns and poorer neighbourhoods, where oral communication was strong and the need for alternatives less pressing. Vincent, *Literacy and Popular Culture*, p. 41, p. 43.

66 Quoted in Simkins, *Kitchener's Army*, p. 191.

67 Anderton to mother, 17 March, 4 April 1915.

68 Quoted in Bet-El, *Conscripts*, p. 102.

69 Soldiers were not supposed to write about impending movements or give their location. A pamphlet was circulated in late 1916 outlining the scope of military censorship, perhaps to try and ensure that conscripts would adopt good habits. Comments on defensive works, the effects of hostile fire, the physical and moral condition of troops and criticism of the Army itself were prohibited. In addition to their ordinary letters, men could write a limited number of 'green envelope' letters. These were exempt from censorship and operated on a system of trust which in which men agreed to write about 'nothing but personal and family matters'. The Base Post Office, however, might still open a green letter. Boyden, *Tommy Atkins' Letters*, p. 30; E. Wells, *Mailshot. A History of the Forces Postal Service*

(London: Defences Postal and Courier Service, Royal Engineers, 1987), p. 65; Bet-El, *Conscripts*, pp 132–3.

70 Some subalterns were known to pre-stamp empty envelopes, necessitating a warning against the practice. War Office, General Staff Censorship and Publicity Section, 'Lecture on the Postal Censorship Orders' (London: Censorship and Publicity Section, General Staff, 1918), p. 1.

71 'The C.O. enjoys reading all our letters' wrote one, in a teasing remark no doubt intended more for the censor more than the recipient. Quoted in J. C. Dunn, *The War the Infantry Knew. A Chronicle of Service in France and Belgium* (London: Abacus, 1994), p. 65.

72 H. Anderton to mother, 11 February, 12 February 1915.

73 C. Ramsdale to Mother and Mary, 10 March 1917.

74 Thorpe worried that if there was too much 'combatant news' in his letter, it would be destroyed, and 'you bet we don't care to risk that.' Thorpe to Nellie, 9 August 1917. As a result of such restrictions, men tried to bypass censorship, sending letters from hospital via the Red Cross, or getting friends on leave to post letters once they were back in Britain. The latter practice was prohibited, the suggested punishment being the sending back of the offender to his unit and the cancelling of leave. Percy Smith, determined that his parents should know the 'true state of us Tommies out here', sent a letter in September 1918 via a pal on leave which was highly critical of Army censorship. According to Smith, its purpose was less to stop the enemy gaining knowledge of Army movements, than to keep civilians ignorant, since if they knew what was actually going on, they would 'worry more'. Boyden, *Tommy Atkins' Letters*, p. 29; War Office, 'Lecture on Postal Censorship Orders', p. 17; P. Smith to mother and father, 18 September 1918, IWM 01/21/1.

75 F. Wollocombe diary, 9 October 1915, IWM 95/33/1.

76 W. Owen to mother, 1 January 1917, in Bell (ed.), *Wilfred Owen. Selected Letters*, p. 207.

77 War Office, General Staff Censorship and Publicity Section, 'Censorship Orders For Troops in the Field' (London: Censorship and Publicity Section, General Staff, 1918), p. 4.

78 War Office, 'Lecture on Postal Censorship Orders', p. 4.

79 Wilfred to Susan Owen, 19 January 1917, in Bell (ed.), *Wilfred Owen. Selected Letters*, pp. 214–15.

80 H. Mercer to E. C. Mercer, 28 September 1914, IWM 92/52/1.

81 This sample was constructed from eighty-one collections of letters listed in the on-line IWM catalogue and written by men on the Western Front to their families of origin. The sample was compiled by using the keyword search terms '1914–18', 'letter' and 'family', and included only those individuals who could be identified as family members. I am grateful to Ana Ljubinkovic for undertaking this research.

82 The IWM sample does not necessarily reflect the patterns of wartime correspondence, since mothers may have been more likely than fathers or siblings to hold onto war letters, and in fact, as Lyndall Urwick's instructions to his mother indicate, were sometimes explicitly requested to do so. Thus the bias towards mothers in the surviving collections might also be a function of their role as the keepers of family memory.

83 Anderton to mother, 12 April 1915. Similarly, among German and Austrian families, as Christa Hämmerle points out, letters from the front 'were not intended solely for the addressee and served to connect the lives of many people.' '"You Let a Weeping Woman Call you Home?" Private Correspondences during the First World War in Austria and Germany', in R. Earle (ed.), *Epistolary Selves. Letters and Letter-Writers, 1600–1945* (Aldershot: Ashgate, 1999), p. 162.

84 E. F. Chapman to mother, 31 October 1916. A mother might even have a claim on letters not addressed to her. David Fitzpatrick quotes an American commentary written in 1917, stating that 'no matter to whom it is addressed, it is always regarded as the property of the mother.' Fitzpatrick, *Oceans of Consolation*, p. 478.

85 A. Swettenham to mother, 3 October 1918.

86 On siblings, see Angela Woollacott, 'Sisters and Brothers in Arms: Family, Class and Gendering in World War I Britain, M. Cooke and A. Woollacott (eds.), *Gendering War Talk* (Princeton: Princeton University Press, 1993), pp. 128–47.

87 The Buxton collection contains 170 letters to his aunt, forty to his mother, forty-two to his father, and fifty-two to both parents. B. G. Buxton, IWM 78/60/3.

88 T. Corless to Grandma and Aunt, 3 November 1916, IWM 81/13/1. I am grateful to Mrs Sheila Roome for additional information about Tom's background.

89 Corless to Grandma and Aunt, 23 November 1916.

90 Captain Arthur Gibbs was particularly pleased to receive a letter from his 'dada', as 'I know you aren't fond of letter-writing'. A. Gibbs to father, 2 January 1916, IWM P317. Jenny Hartley remarks on the low expectations of men as letter-writers in the Second World War. '"Letters are Everything These Days": Mothers and Letters in the Second World War', in R. Earle (ed.), *Epistolary Selves. Letters and Letter-Writers, 1600–1945* (Aldershot: Ashgate, 1999), p. 185.

91 On the letter as a feminine form, see R. Earle, 'Introduction: Letters, Writers and the Historian', in R. Earle (ed.), *Epistolary Selves. Letters and Letter-Writers, 1600–1945* (Aldershot: Ashgate, 1999), pp. 6–7.

92 E. K. Smith to father, 26 March 1915, *Letters Sent From France*, p. 37.

93 A. Hooper to L. Hooper, quoted in L. Hooper to K. Hooper, 20 September 1915. A month later he wrote direct to his father asking for a letter: 'I believe

you are very busy, but try to find time to write to your old son. Mother is busy too.' A. Hooper to father, quoted in L. Hooper to K. Hooper, 25 October 1915. The problem of reluctant fathers was not restricted to the middle class, the printers' apprentice Bert Chapman, for example, passing the following message to his mother: 'Tell Dad I shall be very pleased for a line or two from him.' B. F. J. Chapman to mother, 17 June 1918, IWM 98/17/1.

94 A. Hooper to L. Hooper, quoted in L. Hooper to K. Hooper, 30 September 1915.

95 A. Hooper to L. Hooper, quoted in L. Hooper to K. Hooper, 30 September 1915.

96 For example F. Wollocombe to father, 2 January, 21 February 1916, IWM 95/33/1; E. J. Poole, 5 July, 18 July 1918, IWM 82/11/1.

97 Urwick to father 2 August, 12 August 1915; N. A. Taylor to father, 18 May 1916, IWM 90/28/1; E. R. Hutt to 'Dada', 18 January 1916, IWM 90/7/1; W. B. P. Spencer to father, 22 February 1915, IWM 87/56/1.

98 W. C. Christopher to mother, 18 April 1916, IWM 88/11/1.

99 J. B. Middlebrook to father, 21 July 1916, IWM Con Shelf.

100 Taylor to father, 18 May 1916.

101 Paul Thompson states that 'there can be little doubt that the most distant parents were to be found among the well-to-do'. *The Edwardians. The Remaking of British Society* (London: Routledge, 1992), p. 56.

102 E. Buettner, *Empire Families. Britons and Late Imperial India* (Oxford: Oxford University Press, 2004), esp. ch. 3.

103 J. Tosh, *A Man's Place. Masculinity and the Middle-Class Home in Victorian England* (New Haven: Yale University Press, 1999), pp. 90–101.

104 Loane, *The Queen's Poor*, p. 23, p. 26.

105 Hartley attributes this difference to the 'dailiness' of mothers' letters. '"Letters are Everything These Days"', p. 186.

106 A. Bishop, with T. Smart (eds.), *Vera Brittain. War Diary 1913–1917, Chronicle of Youth* (London: Victor Gollancz, 1981), p. 174.

107 Bet-El, *Conscripts*, p. 135, p. 137.

108 J. Ellis, *Eye Deep in Hell. Trench Warfare in World War I* (Baltimore: Johns Hopkins University Press, 1976), p. 139. Fuller believes that letters were not a reliable guide to morale, tending to either soften or exaggerate the truth. *Troop Morale*, pp. 2–3. An Australian collection of edited family letters goes so far as to say of a correspondent on the Somme during 1916 that 'there was really nothing he could write home about at all'. N. Carthew, *Voices from Trenches. Letters to Home* (Sydney: New Holland, 2002), p. 190.

109 J. Horne quoted in Hanna, 'A Republic of Letters', para. 6; G. Sheffield, *Leadership in the Trenches. Officer–Man Relations, Morale and Discipline in the British Army in the era of the First World War* (Basingstoke: Palgrave, 2000), p. 136; McCartney, *Citizen Soldiers*, p. 95. Hanna also argues that

French soldiers gave details of horror and hardship in letters home. 'A Republic of Letters', paras. 23–4.

110 On the incorporation of psychological ideas in veteran memoirs between the 1920s and 1970s see M. Roper, 'Between Manliness and Masculinity: The "War Generation" and the Psychology of Fear in Britain, 1914–1970', *Journal of British Studies*, Vol. 44, No. 2 (2005), pp. 343–63.

111 E. F. Chapman to mother, 14 February 1917. In a letter written in case of his death, Russell made a similar comment: 'The war is a terrible thing for all of us, but more especially for those who we leave behind to wait for the final issue.' N. R. Russell to mother, 6 July 1916, IWM 01/21/1.

112 See, for example, H. J. Savours to mother and father, 23 May 1917; Savours to mother and father and Madge, 30 July 1917, IWM PP/MCR/327.

113 F. E. Noakes, *The Distant Drum. The Personal History of a Guardsman in the Great War* (Tunbridge Wells: npub, 1952), p. 56.

114 H. F. Bowser memoir, np, IWM 88/56/1.

115 E. F. Chapman to mother, 7 August 1916.

116 E. F. Chapman to mother, 27 August 1916. Bruce Bairnsfather was a popular wartime cartoonist, whose character, 'Old Bill' was, as Bairnsfather put it, 'full of determination and Plum and Apple', the latter being a humorous reference to the ubiquitous ration jam. Bruce Bairnsfather, *Bullets and Billets*, Project Gotherburg, www.gutenberg.org/etext/11232. Accessed 18 July 2008.

117 E. F. Chapman to mother, 20 September 1916.

118 E. F. Chapman to mother, 14 February 1917.

119 A. Knight to mother, 6 July 1916; A. Knight to Peggy, 9 July 1916, IWM Con Shelf. After his close friend was killed, Marchant passed on the news in a short note to his mother: 'I feel greatly upset and do not feel up to writing a long letter yet'. Marchant to mother, 5 October 1915.

120 E. K. Smith to mother, 13 August 1915.

121 W. Owen to mother, 4 October 1918, in Bell (ed), *Wilfred Owen. Selected Letters*, p. 351.

122 W. Spencer to mother, 3 January 1915.

123 Janet Watson discusses two cases where men wrote about 'vivid and horrible' details to their sisters. *Fighting Different Wars. Experience, Memory and the First World War in Britain* (Cambridge: Cambridge University Press, 2004), p. 48, p. 50.

124 E. F. Chapman to Hilda, 28 June 1916.

125 W. Owen to Mary, 8 May 1917, in Bell (ed.), *Wilfred Owen. Selected Letters*, p. 242.

126 According to Owen's biographer, Dominic Hibberd, Mary 'sacrificed her adult life to her mother.' *Wilfred Owen. A New Biography* (London: Weidenfeld & Nicolson, 2002), p. 25.

127 R. D. Mountfort to mother, 11 October, 28 November 1915; 15 January 1916; Mountfort to father, 1 October 1915, IWM Con Shelf.

128 F. Marchant to mother and father, 28 March 1915.

129 C. Ramsdale to mother and Mary, 21 June 1917, 31 August 1918.

130 What Hartley observes of letters home in the Second World War could also apply to the First: there could be 'a need to punish the mother for failing to protect her child from these horrors.' '"Letters are Everything These Days'", p. 191.

131 The Territorial forces had been set up in 1908 by Lord Haldane, and were composed of civilians who trained one evening a week and one weekend every month. They were supposed to be given time off by employers to attend annual camps. R. Holmes, *Tommy. The British Soldier on the Western Front 1914–1918* (London: Harper Perennial, 2005), pp. 79–80.

132 A. H. Hubbard to mother and all, 4 June 1916, IWM Con Shelf.

133 Hubbard to mother and all, 22 June 1916.

134 Hubbard to mother and all, 17 June 1916.

135 Hubbard to Nellie and Ivy, 29 June 1916.

136 Hubbard to Nellie and Ivy, 29 June 1916.

137 Hubbard to Nellie and Ivy, 30 June 1916.

138 R. Prior and T. Wilson, *The Somme* (New Haven: Yale University Press, 2005), p. 71.

139 Hubbard to mother and all, 7 July 1916.

140 Pro Patria Mori: Gommecourt – The Battle, http://www.gommecourt.co.uk/battle.htm. Accessed 26 March 2007.

141 Hubbard to mother and all, 5 July 1916.

142 Hubbard to mother and all, 7 July 1916.

143 Malcolm Brown. *Tommy Goes to War* (Stroud: Tempus, 2005), p. 139; Helen Peters, '"Unmanned Men": In What Ways Did the Experience of Shell Shock Challenge Early Twentieth Century Notions of Masculinity?', unpublished MA Dissertation, Department of History, University of Essex, 2004.

144 Hibberd, *Wilfred Owen*, p. 51.

145 Quoted in K. Grieves (ed.), *Sussex in the First World War* (Lewes: Sussex Record Society, 2004), p. xxiii.

146 Seebohm Rowntree was told in 1914 by an Essex family of farm labourers that they were only ever 'completely satisfied' after Sunday dinner. This family 'was probably not untypical' comments Burnett. *Plenty and Want: A Social History of Diet in England from 1815 to the Present Day* (London: Scolar Press, 1979), p. 154. Chapter 4 of this study, 'Learning to care', discusses family backgrounds in more detail.

147 E. Leed, *No Man's Land. Combat and Identity in World War I* (Cambridge: Cambridge University Press, 1979), p. 189.

2

# Separation and support

On the evening of 3 February 1917, Alice Lubbock had a dream about her son Eric, a pilot in the Royal Flying Corps (RFC):

> I dreamt Eric and I were in a strange garden and we were watching a sort of big battering machine going over with guns and bombs coming from all parts. We both took it very calmly. Eric supposed it was a Hun and I wanted it to go as I had some interesting things to tell him. One seldom gets excited in dreams at the most thrilling or alarming events.[1]

The war in Alice Lubbock's dream certainly did not lack menace: it had armoury 'coming from all parts', and it was on home soil. Though this terrifying contraption had come closer to her than the war had ever done in reality, Alice, reflecting later on her dream, was struck by the fact that she and Eric had not felt anxious.

If, as Freud argued, dreams are a form of wish fulfilment, how might we understand Alice Lubbock's dream? Two weeks before she had written in her diary that her 'whole life is a big dread these days.' Alice had lost her husband in April 1913 and was still grieving when in August 1914 Eric joined the Army Service Corps as a driver, an option he took reluctantly as he wanted the opportunity to fight, but one which she must have hoped would give him some protection. Before being sworn in Eric telephoned his mother to ask for her permission, even though he was already twenty-one. His mother had told him that 'she would not stand in my way. It must have been a hard thing for a mother to say.' Alice Lubbock had felt unable to refuse him: 'Although I did mind most terribly, what could I do or say?'[2]

Her worries increased when, in July 1915, Eric finally received his much longed-for transfer to the RFC as an observer. He knew this would cause her pain: 'Mum bears it all so well but I cannot imagine what she suffers. She doesn't sleep well and somehow it is too awful to think of her suffering.' His mother, however, had concealed from him the true extent of her anxiety. She was convinced that Eric would not survive the war, but 'I did not tell him of my great dread.' '[F]rom now on', she recalled, 'the anxiety was terrible.'[3]

Eric's first flight was on 4 September 1915, his first crash just ten days later. Having watched it happen, the ground crew thought Eric and the pilot were bound to be injured, but they walked away. He crashed again on 18 September and gashed his leg on the machine gun. Eric himself had already come to accept he would probably die. He was in the air again by mid-October, taking photos on the Western Front and writing home about the deaths of fellow airmen. In November he was awarded the Military Cross, but his mother's letters to him still began 'MY LITTLE ONE'.[4]

The following year Eric began training as a pilot and by October 1916 he was in France. His letters were filled with descriptions of dog fights and Alice worried that he was taking unnecessary risks. He had got into trouble for going too far into the German lines and she thought his letters rather feverish. She was 'not at all happy about Eric. He seems to me to be living at very high pressure. It's only natural of course and he is in perpetual motion and excitement.' Reading his letters, we can see why she was concerned. In mid-November he sent his watch home because 'It is fast. I don't like fast people. It gains 2hrs in 24, ie 5 mins per hour. Not enough! I don't mind if time goes fast "pour le guerre" but this pseudo speed is a nuisance.' He wanted the watch 'slowed' and sent back to him; unconsciously perhaps, he was conveying the speeded-up state of his own mind.[5]

In Alice's dream a wish is certainly fulfilled. The war, though menacing, is in the background. Eric is not tempted to chase down the battering machine, but idly conjectures that it is probably German as the two of them stroll about the garden, caught up in conversation. Five weeks later, the threat that Alice Lubbock's dream had lifted momentarily would return: Eric died in France in a flying accident on the day her other son Harold left for the Dardanelles.[6]

## Waiting and worrying

With a son away at the front, life became a matter of waiting. Families settled into routines after the initial burst of activity, helping sons get their kit together for France and working out how to communicate with them, but it was difficult to keep their spirits up. Beatrice Pemberton wrote of how 'as the months drag by even the novelty of it all that buoyed us up at starting, wears off into a dull, enduring ache'.[7]

Unlike sons, who experienced bouts of intense anxiety in between longer periods of boredom, families were constantly worried. After her son left for France, Harry Carter's mother began attending special church services to pray for soldiers. 'Have you wrote to mother yet she is worrying over you', asked his sister, Lil.[8] Fathers were not immune to worry, as Goodwin's message to his son Wallie makes clear: 'your ma + myself . . . feel so helpless, on your account, + as soon as we hear that you are homeward bound + in good health a great load will be taken off our minds'.[9]

Anxious parents fixed on the inevitable gaps in correspondence.[10] Helen Mercer grew more frantic as she waited for her son's first letter to arrive from the front: 'I know you will try to send me a letter soon darling. It is the thing of all others, I long for, to know if you get any sleep, + have enough clothes.'[11] When the longed-for letter did arrive, even although families knew rationally that it could provide no guarantee of safety, they nevertheless felt it was proof of life. On receiving Second Lieutenant Reggie Hutt's first letter from front-line trenches, his mother immediately sent it to her husband, who was away from home. Her hurried note, scrawled on the envelope, betrays the tension of waiting, and how much importance parents attached to the most slender evidence: 'I am glad to say this came late last night – Thursday + I feel comforted + so will you dear – I am so glad it came in time for the mail.'[12] Whilst a parent might wish for a full account, ultimately what mattered was the simple fact of having the letter in their possession. After receiving two letters of little more than a sentence or two, scrawled on blotched paper as Joe Clarke was on the move, his mother was relieved, if a little disappointed: 'we are so glad to hear from you Although your notes contain so little news they convey to us what we chiefly want to know + that is that you are safe.'[13]

Mothers scrutinised every detail of their sons' letters for clues about their well-being. An unusually short letter or one that resorted to stock phrases might be seized on as a sign of poor health or spirits. Louisa Hooper became concerned when her son Arnold wrote her a 'very similar' letter to the one he had sent his father. As she reported to her other son Kenneth:

> one particular sentence [was] exactly the same; somehow that letter did not satisfy me like his dear letters generally do, I felt there was something between the lines, I am so glad that the dear Telegram, with the assuring words 'Very fit', was [composed] really some time after the letter. Those words "Very fit" have been constantly in my mind.[14]

Worry such as this about the health of sons made some mothers ill. When Cecil Christopher caught jaundice and was hospitalised, he wrote to his mother asking her to try and obtain a 'good blood tonic to pull me up a bit'. He later regretted having told her about his illness, for his sister replied telling him that their mother was sick with worry:

> I am sorry to see in both your letters, that Mother is so poorly. Really Val, there is absolutely no need for Mother to worry about me now. I have entirely got rid of the jaundice and I am still keeping fit. When I asked you to send me out a tonic I thought you would send Phosferine or something like that. It wasn't that I felt the after effects so badly, but I thought that a little pick-me-up would not do any harm. So you see Mother is only worrying herself needlessly.[15]

William Breakespeare thought his mother's death during the war was partly due to worry. Seven members of the family were in the Army and William had been reported missing; his mother was 'just a wreck'.[16] Henry Valentine also thought the war had claimed his mother, who had died of a stroke in 1916, 'worried 'cos she had four sons and a husband . . . at the war.'[17]

For mothers, war produced a split vision of sons. On the one hand they felt proud when they saw him in khaki. Families noted how the uniform and the rigours of training camps had filled out his frame. Seeing her brother Edward in uniform for the first time, Vera Brittain described how he 'seems so tall & absolutely grown up . . . He has never looked so well as he does in his military clothes.'[18] Geoffrey Bickersteth's three brothers 'all put on uniforms and made a great impression sitting together in the Vicarage pew at the Parish church with Mother and me.'[19] Mothers were impressed by this transformation from boy to soldier. When her son appeared at home for the first time in uniform Mary Charteris wrote in her diary, 'Yvo looked so nice in khaki to-day, he has a beautiful figure and his health has improved.'[20]

On the other hand, a son who was about to go on active service was vulnerable. British soldiers during the Great War had only a one in two chance of escaping death, wounding or being imprisoned.[21] Although nobody knew the statistical odds, the lists of casualties in newspapers and reports home from friends and relatives made them aware of the risks. They knew well enough, as Maggie Hobhouse wrote to her daughter after seeing her son Paul off at Waterloo station, that 'it might be for the last time.'[22] This vulnerability led families to imagine their sons as little more than children. Birthdays apart reminded them of the first moments of life. Goodwin wrote to his son Wallie of how 'Well I remember 23 years ago today, when your mother presented me with a red haired rascal'.[23] Louisa Hooper wrote effusively to her son Kenneth about the 'Glad day, when first I held your dear little form close to my heart.'[24]

Waiting re-kindled old anxieties. Infant mortality rates in the 1880s and 1890s, when the war generation were in their infancy, were comparatively high by today's standards, and did not begin to drop significantly until after 1900.[25] The poor were especially vulnerable but infancy was a risky phase of life for all classes. Though the chance of losing a child was greatest when it was very small, illnesses such as measles, scarlet fever and whooping cough also claimed the lives of older children.[26] Isabel Trench had a slightly drooping eyelid which her family put down to the fact that she had wept so much on the loss of her first daughter, Monica, who was less than a year old. We can only imagine the feelings that were re-awakened in her when all three sons enlisted in the First World War; when Herbert returned home in 1915 suffering from shell-shock, or when Reggie was killed on the first day of the German offensive in 1918.[27]

Most mothers of the war generation would have sat watching over sick children. As many working-class families would not have been able to afford a doctor, and medical care had little effect in cases of serious illnesses, a mother's nursing was, Ellen Ross observes, 'often the only hope for the seriously ill; a child's life was often literally in a mother's hands.'[28] Many mothers from lower-middle-class families would also have juggled their other work with the care of sick children.[29] It was only within the upper middle class that mother and child might be separated, children with infectious illnesses such as scarlet fever being quarantined, usually upstairs in the nursery. The memorial books produced by bereaved mothers sometimes recall the distress of looking on at a sick child through a nursery window but being unable to comfort them, or the loss of a child's companionship whilst it lay ill upstairs.[30] These mothers had been onlookers, prevented from touching their children, just as they would be again during the war.

The fact that they had risked their own lives in bearing sons, and nursed them through childhood illnesses, led Edwardian mothers to identify strongly with their sons' situations in the war. As Nicoletta Gullace argues, a mother regarded a son as a 'corporeal extension of herself'.[31] Public rhetoric reflected this and the enlistment of sons to the war was seen as a maternal sacrifice. But the association between mothers and care was as much practical as ideological, for they effectively underwrote the military effort through their nursing. Their ministrations became a national duty, making the mother part of the 'parallel army' on the home front.[32] Jack Kipling was looked after by his mother when he caught mild influenza during his officer training in early 1915 and was, Toni and Valmai Holt remark, frequently 'laid up at home'.[33] Men discharged from hospital but too badly injured to return to the front usually went back home.[34] For some mothers, it could be daunting to know they were responsible for caring for a disabled man. When John Middlebrook prepared to come home after having his arm amputated, his mother, who feared that John would be a complete invalid, organised the rest of the family to take over daily tasks like helping him dress and eat. Middlebrook's sister was given the job of dressing his infected stump. This mother seems to have reacted to her anxieties about the care of her son by delegating and trying to set up routines.[35]

Mothers were sometimes thought to have saved their son's lives through their nursing. When Edith Nugee learned on 31 July 1915 that her son Andy had been injured at Hooge she did not confide her feelings at length in her diary, but the depth of her distress is clear in her terse entry: 'Got telegram from War Office stating that Andy was seriously wounded. It is terrible'. For three days Edith waited for further information, tentatively going ahead with the preparations for her daughter Laura's wedding. 'Laura looks tired and worried', she reported, adding that she wished the 'news about Andy had not come till after her wedding'.[36]

On 3 August the family was told that one parent could visit Andy, news which they interpreted as meaning that he was not expected to live. Edith and her husband set out immediately for France, but the War Office insisted that only one parent could travel, so Edith took her son George with her, who was in any case returning from leave for the front. Edith must have been shocked the following day to see the extent of Andy's injuries – he had been hit by shrapnel – but what she noted was his fortitude. She describes her arrival at the hospital at Le Touquet: 'I then saw my darling Andy, oh how glad I was to be with him. He has lost his right eye, his other is impaired, his left leg is broken, + he has a wound in his right arm + shrapnel in his throat but he is quite brave and cheerful dear boy.'[37]

Edith Nugee visited her son every day for the next three-and-a-half weeks, sitting with him, writing his letters and reading the letters that arrived daily from his friends and fellow soldiers. Many of the diary entries during this time state simply that she 'was with Andy all day'. She was especially pleased to be able to feed him, holding out food to his mouth: 'I was allowed to give him his lunch, he has to be fed poor darling as he cannot see.' Laura's wedding went ahead on 7 August, and the next day, Edith received news that another son, Francis, had been injured in the shoulder. She wished to see him too but 'I do not want to leave Andy'.[38]

Edith Nugee's worries, with one son near death, another wounded, a third just returned to the Western Front, and a daughter having to manage her wedding without her mother, must have felt overwhelming at times. Yet her diary barely mentions her own feelings, concentrating instead on Andy's wounds and what she did to help him. She had seized on the chance to nurse him, and was 'sorry to go' when Andy was moved to another hospital at the end of August.[39] It was probably not the first time that Edith Nugee had seen her children through serious ill health. Much would then have depended on her ability to nurse, as it did during Andy's recovery in hospital at Le Touquet. Even the most professional nursing was thought no substitute for a mother's care: when George Nugee had visited his brother Andy on the day his mother arrived at the hospital, the doctors 'did not hold out much hope for him.' He recovered, and George believed that 'the quick arrival of mother may have helped to save Andy's life.'[40]

Some families were more used to being separated than others, and this influenced their feelings about the war. For men from working- and lower-middle- class backgrounds, the severing of ties to home could be a particularly disorientating feature of military service. The contrast with the public-school-educated officer could not have been greater. He typically entered the war with around a decade's experience of life away from home, having left his family at the age of around eight for preparatory school, boarded at public school and then perhaps gone on to university. He was also widely travelled: Lyndall Urwick and Gilbert Talbot followed in the footsteps of many a public schoolboy on their tours of Europe during summer 1914.[41]

The middle- and particularly the upper-class mother was used to supporting her son at arm's length. She knew what comforts he liked best.[42] At the same time, the longer history of separations in these families could mean that quite raw emotions were aroused when a son left for the front. Wilfred Bion kissed his mother a 'dry eyed goodbye' when she left him in the playground of his prep school for the first time. As she walked away he watched 'above the hedge which separated me from her and the road which was the boundary of the wide world itself, her hat go bobbing up and down'. He cried by night and suffered from repeated nightmares from which he awoke longing for his mother. On one of their days out together she bought him chocolates in his favourite tin, but although he said he wanted them, he would not take them back to the school.[43] During the war he fell into a similar pattern, barely corresponding with her and falling into irritable silence when on leave in London.[44] It felt easier to shut off contact with the world of home and mothers than to suffer the pain of separation.

While the wrench from home was probably particularly severe for Bion, who had spent his first eight years in India and was sent away to England to be schooled, the moment of leaving for public school constituted an epiphany for many middle-class sons.[45] After Eric Lubbock's first day at Eton, his housemaster wrote to his parents that 'it was very touching to see him struggling to check his feelings.' At the start of term in 1907, two years later, the housemaster wrote again to say that, although Eric was generally happy, 'he still looks rather sad at times at being away from home.' Eric's own diary, begun the following September when he was fourteen, described the first day back at Eton as a 'miserable day, especially when I woke up dreaming a High Elms dream.'[46] This was clearly not a one-off occurrence.

The pain felt by a mother when her son began preparatory school or embarked for France could be very deep. The first letter written by Theresa Cripps to her son when he left for boarding school began: 'Mother cried herself to sleep last night and perhaps you did too'. She proposed a way that they might stay in touch:

> Whenever you are unhappy, or in trouble, remember Mother's plan. Tell me at what time you are in bed, and that is when I will always think of you, and you must think of Father and me . . . The eight o'clock bell has just rung, and you are just sitting down to breakfast, feeling strange and shy, but soon you will know what a good thing it is to be at school, to learn to be courageous, to bear difficult things, and to go bravely through trials.[47]

Theresa Cripps' solution to the wrench of separation – to try and picture each other in synchrony – was one that many families would adopt during the war. Not all mothers grieved as openly as Theresa Cripps did when her son left for school and indeed, as Barbara Caine has shown,

Theresa was unusual among the nine Potter sisters in the degree of affection she showed her children. For some of Theresa's sisters, a son's departure for school provided relief from family problems; and some replied to their letters from boarding school, not with effusive expressions of love, but by correcting their grammar and spelling.[48]

Even those mothers who did not confide their feelings when a son began boarding school would have felt the moment as a turning point; for these mothers and for their sons, the experience could set the emotional terms of wartime separations. Bion was not unusual, as he prepared to embark for France, in being reluctant to have his mother see him off. Wanting perhaps to set an example to their comrades, and fearing that their resolve might be weakened, familiar ways of coping re-asserted themselves.[49] To the middle-class mother, the soldier–son remained a child. The Smiths described the younger of their dead sons, Arnold, who had been killed during his stint in the front line, as 'just a schoolboy and little more'.[50] Looking back in the early 1930s on her son Yvo's letters during the war (he had died at the age of nineteen), Mary Constance Charteris commented: 'He was so young when he went to the Front that he showed a childlike appreciation of the beauty of the "fireworks", and his imagination was impressed by the "sinister sound of the shells" which he described so vividly in his letters.'[51]

The fact that support for sons in wartime circled around basic bodily functions and needs encouraged mothers to see them as child-like. They worried about how their sons ate, the state of their stomachs, whether they were warm and dry and how often they washed. Although characteristic of mothering, this focus on bodily needs was a particular preoccupation in the early months of life, when a baby's inability to feed, or a stomach upset, might have fatal consequences. Once again, in trenches, a son's most basic needs were crucial and mothers responded just as they had earlier when care was a matter of life and death.

## The parcel

The main way in which families supported their sons in France was by sending parcels. And send parcels they did: 60,000 were handled by the Army every day, the highpoint being Christmas 1916, when over 4½ million parcels were despatched to the British Expeditionary Forces.[52] On the Western Front, where the British soldier's mail from home arrived in a matter of days, parcels could fulfil a wide range of needs. Minor ailments could be treated with home remedies and socks and underwear could be sent out on a regular basis. Fresh food from home could enrich monotonous army rations, whereas the soldier serving further afield had to put up with tinned or dried products.

In effect, families formed an adjunct to the army, helping to ensure that the soldier stayed clothed, well-fed and healthy.[53] Mrs Stephens began a comfort fund for the men in her husband's Battalion, the Second Rifle Brigade, in November 1914.[54] It was organised largely by the officers' wives and mothers, and financed by a combination of Battalion funds and donations from the Vickers Company, various magazines and daily newspapers and the Queen Mary's Needlework Guild.[55] In the first four-and-a-half months of its existence it sent 211 parcels weighing 11lb each, and 21 bales at 50lb each, along with cigarettes, and four cases of milk once a fortnight, in small tins that could be easily divided up among a section. Provisions on this scale required careful coordination, and Mrs Stephens corresponded with the Quartermaster, Major J. H. Alldridge, every couple of days. On 24 March 1915 he told her not to send any more mittens or comforters as the weather was getting warmer. The following articles 'would be useful', including socks, milk (small tins), sugar (moist), cocoa, pocket handkerchiefs, letter cards, black buttons small and large sizes, small towels and pocket books.[56] Curry powder was in big demand, perhaps because the Rifle Brigade had arrived on the Western Front direct from India.[57] So too, in November 1915, were safety pins 'large enough to fasten back the Great Coat', presumably to stop it dragging in flooded trenches.[58]

After Stephens was promoted to Brigadier, Mrs Nugent, the wife of the newly appointed Lieutenant-Colonel, was keen to do her bit too and at Christmas 1915 she collected £45.12.0. from the Ladies and Friends of the Regiment for the purchase and despatch of puddings, cakes, nuts and oranges. Her plum puddings alone weighed in at 504lb, and she was an equally energetic supplier of socks.[59] The Rifle Brigade Fund did more than top up army provisions. The 80lb of cocoa it sent each fortnight (Quartermaster Alldridge usually managed to get fresh milk to the men on the day it arrived), was probably enough to satisfy the Battalion's demand for hot chocolate.[60] By the end of the war the Fund had sent out nearly 1.75 million cigarettes, 10,226 socks, 2,901 gloves and mittens, and 240lbs of curry powder. It had become part of the machinery of the Battalion. Its contributions were circulated with the Battalion Orders each month, and its accounts were published.[61]

The scale and degree of coordination achieved by the Second Battalion Rifle Brigade comfort fund was exceptional, because this was a

Regular unit whose soldiers and womenfolk were used to supporting their men overseas. But women across Britain engaged in similar kinds of activities. Patriotism sprang from personal circumstances. When women knitted socks and mittens, sewed jute into sandbags, baked or collected blankets, they were driven by the same feelings as when making up parcels to their loved ones. Public provision was animated by the desire to keep loved ones warm, protected and nourished. At the very same time that Ella Bickersteth was helping her son Ralph, a Territorial soldier, to gather together his kit in preparation for overseas service, she was organising meetings of 'all the leading ladies of Leeds' to work together in the war effort.[62] Mrs Herbert Tritton, wife of the local squire in Great Leigh, Essex, managed to get the Mothers' Meeting to undertake an appeal for the men in her son Alan's regiment, the Coldstream Guards, even although most of the local men were joining the Essex Regiment. She judged from her son's letters home that what the men needed was mufflers and mittens: 'His last letter says the cold is intense at night in the trenches.'[63] Knowing about a son's situation gave mothers' voluntary efforts a practical direction.

War work allowed women to meet others in the same situation and helped take their minds off waiting.[64] Knitting, although sometimes criticised by men at the front (and by historians too) as a woefully inadequate response to the hardships they endured, could be therapeutic for the waiting mother or sister.[65] It 'was soothing to our nerves', wrote Mrs Peel, and 'comforting to think that the results of our labours might save some man something of hardship and misery.'[66] Knitting put to use the nervous energy that would otherwise dissipate in worry and could be fitted in amidst other tasks. Hetty Morris used to take her half-finished balaclava helmets, socks and mittens to church with her during the war, as the Minister 'agreed that we could knit as well as listen to what he was talking about.'[67] The homely quality of the finished article, its softness and even its imperfections, could be appreciated by the wearer: the Rifle Brigade Quartermaster thought 'any kind of socks useful but knitted best for marching', and he sent back consignments of them for repair, as 'the men like the knitted socks + don't mind the darning a bit.'[68]

Alongside these charitable activities were the equally time-consuming tasks of providing personal support for loved ones. It was the mother's job – often with the help of a daughter or servant – to chase up the order, no matter how arcane. Torches, for instance, were always in need of batteries but the range of makes frequently led to errors. Mothers read between the lines of letters, supplying what men needed for toothache, lice or constipation, sometimes when the son had not even asked directly. This required a certain practical imagination. Norman Taylor's mother had died in 1906 when he was eleven, and his sister Joyce, six years his senior, took joint responsibility for his parcels with their step-mother. When Joyce sent Norman a new tinder-lighter, she thoughtfully included a hair-pin so he could fray the wick.[69]

The parcel then had to be packed. Foodstuffs had to be well insulated from the rough handling that parcels received and it was not uncommon for men to write back with sorry tales of parcels whose contents were half spilt out or crushed, usually with a stern admonition to take more care in future. 'I think cake should really be sent in tins' stated Captain Reggie Trench after his cake arrived crushed.[70] Eric Marchant and his friends resorted to eating their cake with a spoon because it arrived 'all crumbs'. It was 'the second parcel running that has been smashed', so it was 'evident that stronger packaging is necessary'.[71] Once packed the parcel had to be taken to the post office, by mothers whose domestic routines were already stretched due to lack of help at home, shortages, housework and war work. Unlike more prosperous women, the mothers of most rankers were unused to, and could less readily afford, all this.

Families took the business of parcels very seriously. Herbert Best's mother kept a diary which recorded all the letters and parcels they had sent. In a single month in 1914, she wrote eight letters and made up six parcels.[72] On one occasion when paper was scarce, rather than write a letter home, Norman Taylor simply returned Joyce's letter with comments in the margin. Her letter is principally a list of queries about his wants, against which he stated preferences such as 'NO!', 'NOT YET', or 'VERY NICE'. One can see Joyce trying to imagine his situation, coming up with suggestions, sometimes off the mark, sometimes not. The letter included some sisterly advice for her young brother: 'I sent some sodomints in case of indigestion (VERY NICE). Very useful, I should carry several loose in my pocket not in glass bottle (YES VERY GOOD IDEA) in case of bullet hitting glass.'[73] When they stocked a parcel to a loved one at the front, families had to put themselves in his shoes.

Parcels from home were greeted with a degree of excitement that no gift from a comfort fund could match.[74] The twenty-one-year-old subaltern Arthur Gibbs wrote of how 'I love undoing them and it's just as much fun as opening a Christmas stocking.'[75] The home parcel typically contained a mixture of necessities and comforts. Necessities might include clothing, basic foodstuffs and remedies. Sarah Jane Dawson, noting that her son Sam's writing was faint, sent him a new pencil and kept him in a regular supply of notepaper.[76] Louisa Hooper proposed sending Kenneth some Berwick Coarse Oatmeal as a gentler alternative to the ubiquitous 'number nine pill' dispensed by the Medical Officer. The oatmeal would 'do you good, and help you in a particular way.'[77] Harold Hague asked his mother to send out a khaki shirt as 'the present one has a great tendency to walk off and leave me', and a tin of Boots vermin powder, which 'may persuade some of the animals to find a different home.'[78] Class distinctions were obvious even in the kinds of necessities that families supplied, some exuding more luxury than others. The subaltern's uniform would be sent back home by his batman with the change of seasons, and families would send out new or freshly laundered kit in its place, but rankers were prohibited from sending home items of personal clothing.[79] Lyndall Urwick asked his parents for silk underwear and tailor-made boots (his measurements were held in the boot-making department of the Savoy Tailors' Guild), whilst Reggie Hutt requested a new pyjama jacket after his other one tore when he turned over during his sleep.[80]

The greatest pleasure in a man's parcel was his 'comforts', and it was understood among families of all classes that a parcel must contain more than necessities. Wallie Goodwin could not conceal his disappointment when the first long-awaited parcel arrived for him at Gallipoli, though conscious that his reaction appeared ungenerous:

> I have just received the registered letter and parcel you sent me on the 30th Sept. and must confess being a little disappointed at the contents of parcel, finding only two tremendous writing pads, how I am going to carry them about I don't, know, I suppose I must give one away, however thanks all the same and don't think I am grumbling, but put yourself in my place, in bed in hospital the native postman coming in with a large parcel, registered too, and after signing papers, and laboriously undoing strings, I find two writing pads, after all this time too.[81]

Perhaps his parents had sent him writing materials hoping to hear more from their son; if so, they no doubt felt reproached but at least they had got a letter back. Parcels from home had to contain items that catered for the son's particular tastes. The element of individual pleasure was important.[82] This aspect of parcel-giving caused some difficulty for middle-class volunteers, used to the pre-war moral strictures governing charitable support. Having been taught that assistance must only ever extend to basic wants, anything more encouraging indolence, indulgence was now the order of the day. One volunteer, having thought that she should direct her efforts towards keeping the men warm, and not waste public money on tobacco or musical instruments, had to be educated into the new outlook. Beatrice Pemberton summed up the wartime spirit: 'In the main, women have a very generous and friendly idea of setting about this work of mothering. He is to have, so far as it is in their power to give it, whatever will help to make him happy and to keep him contented.'[83]

What a man received in his parcel by way of comforts depended greatly on his social background. Rankers were sometimes sent shop-bought foods such as chocolate or biscuits, though these were a rarity in many working-class households and such families would have made sacrifices to afford them.[84] Among the comforts received by Will Hate during his two years on the Western Front were peppermints, biscuits and nuts.[85] In addition to purchasing goods, less well-off families cooked pies and potted meats, baked cakes and biscuits, and sent fruit and vegetables from their gardens.[86] Charles Ramsdale thanked his mother and sister for a parcel containing tomatoes 'as fresh as if they'd just been pulled.'[87] Keeping up the supply of parcels put an extra burden on women who were already stretched, but they wanted to do it. A mother in the Essex village of Great Leighs took 'great comfort' from the fact that her son, who was training nearby, sent his washing home each week.[88]

At the other extreme of the traffic in comforts was Captain Arthur Gibbs, an old Etonian serving in the Prince of Wales Company of the Welsh Guards. He received twenty-two parcels from home in the five weeks following his arrival on the Western Front in December 1915, whose contents included pheasant, foie gras, fried fish and a regular supply of fruit. [89] Gibbs must have been popular in the officers' mess. There was little limit to what a better-off middle-class mother could provide in the early years of the war before shortages and rationing. She could send ready-made parcels through department stores like Fortnum and Mason's, or get her servants to do the shopping and cooking. Officers were allowed the additional luxury of alcohol as it was assumed that, being gentlemen, they would regulate their consumption responsibly. Making the most of this privilege, Gibbs requested 'an occasional bottle of Port and Champagne'. That the middle-class mother showed her love through the goods she selected rather than through her own labour was tacitly acknowledged by Gibbs when thanking his mother: 'Somebody at home showed great thoughtfulness when they made up the parcels.'[90]

The ranker was thus more likely than his officer to savour the taste of food cooked by a mother or sister, and by virtue of this his parcel possessed a particularly intimate connection with home. Thanking his mother for the parcel she had recently sent him and his brother, Cecil Christopher singled out the potted meat, for 'There was quite a bit of home about it.'[91] Matt Webb thanked his parents for 'a glorious home-made cake', and Bert Chapman commented, 'Gee, didn't we enjoy ourselves, eating cake like Mother makes it . . . Even the Sergt had a dip + said how nice the cake was.'[92] Home-made food was especially important at Christmas, the most family-centred festivity in the year. So as to make sure that he was not bereft, Wallie Goodwin, who was serving in Gallipoli, put in his order for 'a bit of "pudding"' in late October 1915.[93]

As the term 'comfort' itself suggests, there was something quite primitive about the soothing effect of such foods. The poet Katharine Tynan noticed this after bringing oranges, cakes and cigarettes to a hospital for wounded soldiers in Dublin, recording in her diary that 'These soldiers are babies in their enjoyment of sweet things.'[94] As the war continued the sugar and fat which went into most home-made comforts grew hard to come by, and before they were rationed nationally in mid-1918, many a mother would have spent hours waiting in queues to stock up, and paying exorbitant prices when they finally got hold of them.[95] Even the middle class had to cut down on personal consumption of butter and sugar, but for some poorer families the home-baked cake, let alone the shop-bought one, became unaffordable: the 'very nice parcel' that his 'Ma' triumphantly dispatched 'on speck' to Sid in late 1918 contained plenty of smokes and 'A fruit cake the first for nearly 2 years.'[96]

Sons wanted things that were sweet and which they could suck on; the gratification provided by smoking among men who were by turns anxious, bored and homesick, is probably one reason for the tremendous popularity of smoking among soldiers.[97] Wilbert Spencer requested a pipe-filling machine, as 'a pipe is lovely at times in the trenches', along with 'milk chocolate, condensed milk – ju jubes – lemon acid of some sort as well as biscuits and cake. You don't know how glad we are to get something luxurious to eat.'[98] Whilst on sentry duty, peering into the darkness for signs of enemy activity, Roland Mountfort 'simply craved for a bit of butterscotch or something to suck'. He arranged with his parents to send out chocolate, cake and butterscotch every four days, to coincide with his cycles in the front line, but comforts could also be consumed before going into the trenches, a last taste of home before the privations to come.[99]

The high expectations of sons raised the stakes for their mothers, who were constantly asking for guidance.[100] 'Tell us what you like best, it makes one feel happier if the things are what you want', wrote Wilfred Hoyle's mother, though she was pleased that her sausage rolls had gone down well as she was 'afraid if they would keep.'[101] Lieutenant 'Winkie' Steavenson's mother told him that she 'would like to know *exactly* what I am to send.'[102] A letter from his mother which listed things he might possibly want was jokingly called a 'catechism' by Arthur Gibbs. [103] The anxiety of mothers to get it right, and the cost of the goods themselves, discouraged them from the intuitive guesses that were a source of particular delight when they hit the mark.

Small lapses assumed momentous significance, being felt as a personal deprivation for which mothers were in some way responsible, even when reason told them otherwise. There is a tone of impatient recrimination in Reggie Hutt's letter home shortly after arriving at the front: 'I have written you lots of letters it seems to me, but I haven't had a single one from you, or the parcel I am expecting so much. I need some Gold Flake cigarettes badly'.[104] 'Dear Mother', wrote Ted Berryman, 'Can you please see about some cigarettes for me. Jim said he had fixed up a regular weekly or monthly supply, but since I came back from leave I haven't had any at all! Except what other fellows didn't want. *Please* don't think I'm complaining, only I can't help thinking there must be some mistake.'[105] Charles Ramsdale tried to put a brave face on it when his birthday passed without anything from home, but he could not conceal his disappointment:

> I was really pleased to get that letter from mother and the lovely birthday card. How nice it would have been if they could have really reached me on the proper day, when I was feeling ill and rather miserable. But I tried to comfort myself with the knowledge that there was something on the way; and your letters, dear Mother, never spoil with keeping however long they are in coming.[106]

Parcels and letters from home could bring to the surface quite childish feelings, not only of excitement, but also of being neglected and hard done by. Ramsdale's reaction was typical: his mother hadn't judged it right, he felt let down, but at the same time, he loved his mother and sister and did not want to seem ungrateful.

The reason why men felt easily disappointed was that in the end, apples from the garden or the home-baked cake, despite their wonderfully familiar taste, were little more than a sop. When the sweetness had gone from the mouth of the man on sentry duty, he was left staring out into the pitch black of night and feeling just as cold and miserable as he had minutes earlier. There was something manic about the efforts of mothers to get it just right, and their sons' need for them to do so. Unconsciously, each hoped that by itself, the parcel – if only its contents were selected and packaged carefully enough – could make good the separation.[107] But in the last instance, these men, no matter how well cosseted they were from the cold or how well they ate, were beyond their families' help. Home comforts, despite the heightened expectations that surrounded them, could not compensate for the terrors that, sooner or later, most sons would face.

## The cost of support

While officers and rankers alike waited expectantly for the parcel post to be given out, their parcels were funded in different ways, revealing in turn, the existence of distinct financial and emotional economies within families. The middle- or upper-middle-class mother whose son had attended a boarding school supported him in a similar way during the war. His parcels were gifts and she did not expect to be recompensed, although a son might remark on their cost as a way of expressing his gratitude. Reggie Hutt asked his mother to keep an account of the cost of the 100 Woodbines he issued the men in his platoon, but his correspondence contains no evidence that he paid her back. He certainly considered the personal items in his parcels to be gifts, giving extravagant praise to his mother for his 'most thrilling' parcels, which 'contained plenty of new ideas'.[108] Many subalterns had entered the army straight from school and although comparatively well-paid, they retained the attitude of dependants. Brigadier-General Frank Crozier lamented their extravagance: 'Mere boys of eighteen and upwards, who otherwise would have been at school or the university, or learning some profession or trade, were rushed into commissions, armed with stars, cheque books and authority, and often possessed of a quite erroneous knowledge of the value of money or the value of the things they imagined they had do to keep up an appearance.' They knew nothing about banking, and thought little of demanding 'rich and unwholesome foods' from home.[109]

This attitude towards parcels reflected the middle-class ethos of motherhood, which presumed it was the mother's role to intuit her child's wants, and devote herself to fulfilling them. Lyndall Urwick intimated this when thanking his mother for the parcel of Jaeger waistcoat, air pillow, knife and torch he received at Christmas 1914, which he valued because of their practical utility, but 'much more for the love which is so careful to supply all needs.'[110] Such ideals of maternal service often permeate the historical record. The evidence of mothers' *efforts* is everywhere; not least in the thousands of letters thanking them for parcels, though their own voices are hard to detect. When Ella Bickersteth took over the family diary that would reach eleven volumes and 7,000 pages, it was with barely a word of her own. She merely reported that as her second son Geoffrey 'is still at Heaning, I (Mother) am taking up the diary.'[111] The diary would allow her six sons, four of whom served in the war, to keep abreast of each other's news.

Louisa Hooper's letters to her son Kenneth, a POW, are equally short of news about her life at home. Instead, Louisa painstakingly copied out the letters of her other son, Arnold, for Kenneth. While this might appear an act of self-sacrifice, it was not entirely so, since Arnold's correspondence was full of declarations of devotion to Louisa, being aptly described by her as 'love-letters'. By conveying the effusive personal tributes of one son to the other, Louisa became (in Arnold's words) 'An Angel in our midst.'[112] Yet, honoured as she was by her own sons, Louisa sometimes felt a sense of frustration at her subsidiary role in the war effort. As she explained to Arnold, 'You by your cheerful bravery are placed in a higher plane than your poor old mother'.[113] Her sons reinforced this idea, as when Louisa thought of doing more war work, Arnold wrote:

> In the name of all that is good, do not do any more. If you love me don't. You do too much as it is . . . Your job is to keep in touch with your loving Sons, and to remain your dear self. Our most treasured part of our life. Our greatest Blessing. You have done your share. You have to put up with our absence.[114]

Though Arnold couched his comments as a compliment to Louisa, he clearly did not want his mother dividing her time between her sons and other soldiers, for it implied a diminution of maternal love. Yet for a mother it could feel claustrophobic to focus all her energy on her own sons, not only because, as Louisa Hooper implied, her private labours were invisible to others apart from her family, but because work outside the home could be a welcome distraction from worry.

Men from working-class families tended to have different expectations of their mothers. Unmarried sons usually lived at home, and even if they were earning their own wage, their mothers would buy their clothes and other personal articles.[115] This was a more reciprocal relationship than in the middle class, for a wage-earning son was likely to have been already giving over part of his wages when he joined up. In households which hovered precariously above subsistence levels, his contribution to family income was vital, for a son in full-time work was likely to be better paid than his sisters. His income could mean that mothers were able to afford small luxuries.[116]

Reflecting these pre-war responsibilities, many working-class recruits worried about their families' standard of living during the war. They found it difficult not to be able to help their mothers out, though some tried to where they could. Tom Thorpe, stationed in army camps in Britain for much of 1917 when food shortages were at their most severe, sent regular parcels of rabbits to his family, who were shop-keepers: 'I expect you will have a job to get them in the shops now but I can get you as many as you like; they only cost me 9d each + postage + I know that s [*sic*] cheaper than you can get them in the shops at Bournemouth.' On one of his home leaves he showed them how to skin the carcasses.[117]

Many worried about what it cost their families to keep up the supply of parcels. Thorpe was also more conscious of money than many subalterns. He viewed his parents' expenditure not as generosity, but as coming out of the family budget, with implications for everyone. When they sent him out a postal order he replied that although 'it is very good of you', he wished they 'wouldn't send me money as I can manage on what I get.' Thorpe's use of the plural reveals the sense of responsibility he felt for family finances: 'It would please me much better if you would put it by for a rainy day. Don't think I'm trying to throw dirty water but I have the feeling that I'm spending money needlessly that perhaps some day we'd be glad of.'[118] Will Hate instructed his mother that 'as things are so bad please do not worry about sending anything else. I can manage with the cigarettes.' Writing to thank his mother for the Christmas presents, he was 'only sorry I cannot send anything to you in return.'[119] The Christopher brothers asked their mother to send them the bill for their parcels so they could work out whether it was cheaper for them to buy items at the front.[120]

Hedley Payne, a ranker from a fairly prosperous family, epitomises the contrast between the well-heeled and the rest. After requesting new batteries for his torch, repairs to his watch and new socks, he wrote to his mother 'I feel quite ashamed of myself asking for things in all my letters but I am sure you will understand how things are.'[121] Payne was apologetic and thankful of his mother's help, but he did not see any reason to limit his requests.

Men from less prosperous families might be considerate when it came to money, but they did not want to miss out on their comforts either. At home they had often been shown favouritism by their mothers, for example enjoying larger portions of food, especially meat, than their sisters and younger brothers. This reflected the special bond between mothers and sons within working-class culture.[122] Arthur Hubbard was delighted to get 'mother's parcel with some eatables in', though he worried that the postage for his parcels would cost more than the goods:

> it comes very expensive to you all, going by what the very acceptable one cost I received last Sunday from you, times are getting very hard for you now, everything so dear. I wish I could send parcels back to you. There is no end of stuff wasted especially cheese and tobacco which would keep Dad going without buying at all.[123]

Hubbard had one eye on his family's hardships; he could even think of things in abundance on the Western Front that they would appreciate. But his other eye was on the 'very acceptable' parcel he had received, a further supply of which would not have been unwelcome. Hubbard clearly regarded his comforts as a right, and was a little resentful that, as the war went on and more women were drawn into paid work, they did not share the spoils with soldiers. He wrote a sharp note to a family friend telling her that, since 'the ladies were earning all the cash, while we are away . . . they were in a position to do a little for us every now and again.'[124]

Hardship sometimes made it impossible to keep up a supply of parcels. There is an occasional tone of irritation in Alf Swettenham's correspondence with his mother during 1918, though she had eleven children to look after, three of whom were on overseas military service.[125] Alf could not understand why he did not hear more often from her, for she knew how much he depended on letters from home: 'Bill told you what it is like being out here and not getting a letter. Now mother just see what you can do for me'. He wanted some treats : 'I hope you will write soon and please send something to smoke in the way of fags or some tobacco and fag papers as I was two days without a smoke and two days in the line at that, so just see what you can do for me.'[126]

Swettenham wrote again a month later, in the full swing of the Allied advance. The tone of his letter was urgent, his pangs of hunger appealing to the deepest maternal instincts:

> So if you will send out that little parcel as soon as possible I shall be very glad and my stomach will feel tight for once Well Mother as soon as I can get a registered envelope I will send you a few francs to help to pay for the cost of the parcel but for goodness sake sent [sic] it at once as I am always feeling half starved. Well what is a loaf between 3 men for a day's ration just see what you can do for me.[127]

Swettenham may have intended to pay his mother back, but he also expected her, despite rationing on the home front, to help him out. His phrase 'just see what you can do for me', repeated in each of these letters, was at once an invitation and a mild rebuke.

For many rankers, the problem of how to fund parcels reflected financial difficulties created by the war. A working-class mother with sons at the front might miss both his company and his income. The Reverend Andrew Clark reported that one of the reasons given for slow recruitment before conscription was the fear of mothers that if a son was wounded they would not receive an adequate pension.[128] Bereaved mothers often acknowledged the value of their sons' financial contributions. The mother who described her son as 'the kindest of all her family to her' was most likely referring to his financial help and not just his demeanour.[129]

The War Office responded to such concerns through a system of remittances which allowed soldiers to have a proportion of their pay sent directly to their families. The Christopher brothers, both clerical workers before the war, sent regular amounts of money to their mother.[130] Others sent irregular sums. Stephen Brown had borrowed money from his parents and was 'sorry for what I done when at home'; he hoped to join the Regular Army so he could pay them back with the 30/- bounty. When passes from his barracks were cancelled, he became anxious that his mother would miss out on her allowance, as he had intended to hand it over in person. In future she would get six shillings, 3/- in a remittance from him and 3/- from the War Office.[131]

When the wives and other dependants of wage-earners became entitled to a Separation Allowance in the summer of 1915, rankers were keen that their mothers should receive what was due to them. Joe Clarke gave his mother in Lewisham clear instructions on how to go about it. He had taken it upon himself to find out what monies should come her way, and wanted her to present the best case she could to the pension people:

> I made enquiries re. Separation Allowance this morning + I was informed that this was the procedure. Do not forget to tell them – should they ask

> you – that I contributed 16/- towards the home in civilian life. You will remember that this is what I told them at Camberwell + also tell them that I am making an allotment of 4d a day. You should receive altogether about 9/- per week since the Government make a grant of about 6/- per week. At Camberwell they told me you would receive 9/- per week.[132]

Will Hate was equally eager to see that his mother received the Separation Allowance. He too was well informed, knowing the value of the allowance and the information needed to complete the application forms. He had sent his details off to the Paymaster and felt she deserved support as 'You were pretty dependent on me before the War do not forget that.' He urged her to fill out the form as best she could: 'So you will see that you answer them properly for it.' His subsequent letters repeatedly ask if 'the grant' and his pay (which was presumably being remitted) have come through yet.[133]

The Separation Allowance was received by 1.5 million mothers in the war, equalling the number of wives who drew it. The extent of its take-up shows how widely it was felt that mothers were entitled to compensation for having a son away at the war.[134] Money loomed large in the affections of mothers and sons from poorer families. Sons showed their love by trying to make mothers more comfortable, and their efforts were as much a source of manly pleasure and pride as a burden.[135]

The history of wartime parcels and how they were paid for tells us a good deal about Edwardian cultures of parenting and the differences between the sons of poorer and more prosperous families. Second Lieutenant Lyndall Urwick, aged twenty-two, just out of university in 1919 and on an annual allowance of £140 in addition to a starting salary in the family firm of £100, could have enjoyed a lifestyle that was comfortable by any measure, but as was often the case in middle- and upper-middle-class families, his father kept the purse strings.[136] By contrast most of the men in Urwick's platoon of Reservists in the 3rd Worcesters in Autumn 1914 were probably drawing their own wages before they enlisted, while a ranker of Urwick's age could have had as much as seven years' work experience. Paradoxically, as Chapters 3 and 4 show, Army life reversed the pre-war statuses of middle- and working-class sons within the family. It was the economically dependent men of the middle and upper middle classes who would take on the functions of command during the war, and they frequently led men whose civilian status – as workers and economic contributors to the household – conformed more closely than their own to Edwardian ideals of manliness.

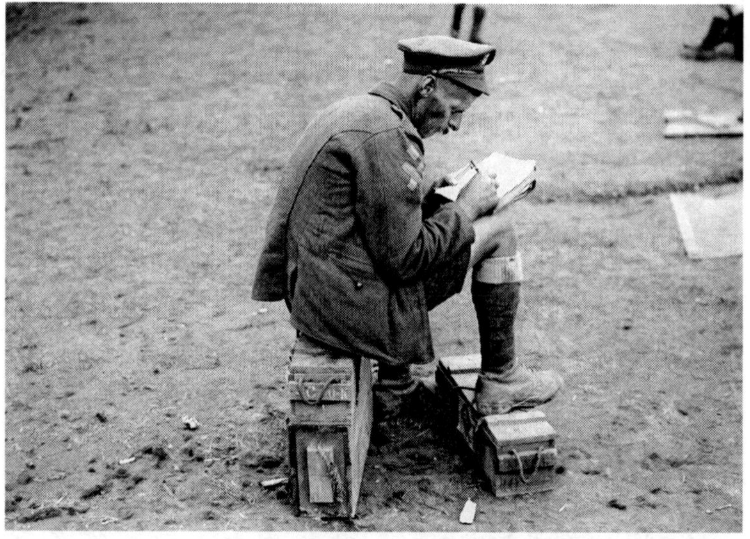

*4* Writing home. A soldier of the 2nd Leinsters at rest after the battle of Pilckem Ridge, 1917

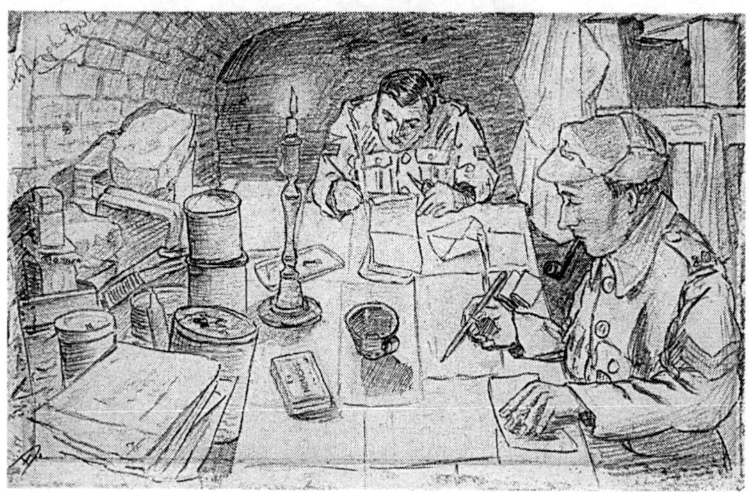

*5* ‘A slight idea of our cellar in Loos. We are here for four days. Sergt. Hicks is at the end; Corporal F. Carter on the right.’ Both men are deep in thought as they write home. E. L. Douglas-Fowles (1897–1952) produced many such sketches during his military service

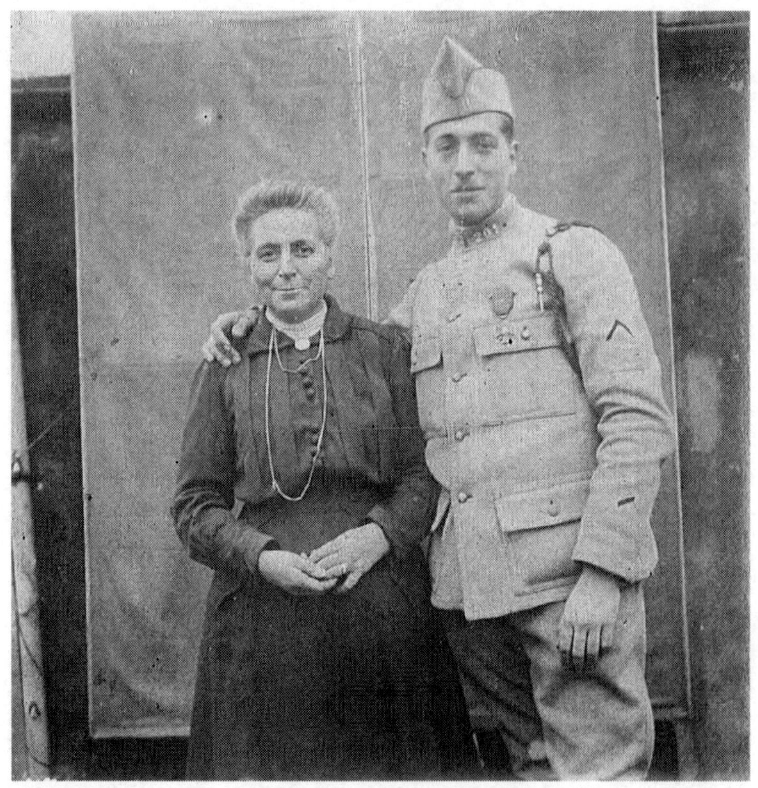

6 Joe Clarke with his mother. Clarke died from dysentery in 1918 while a POW in Germany

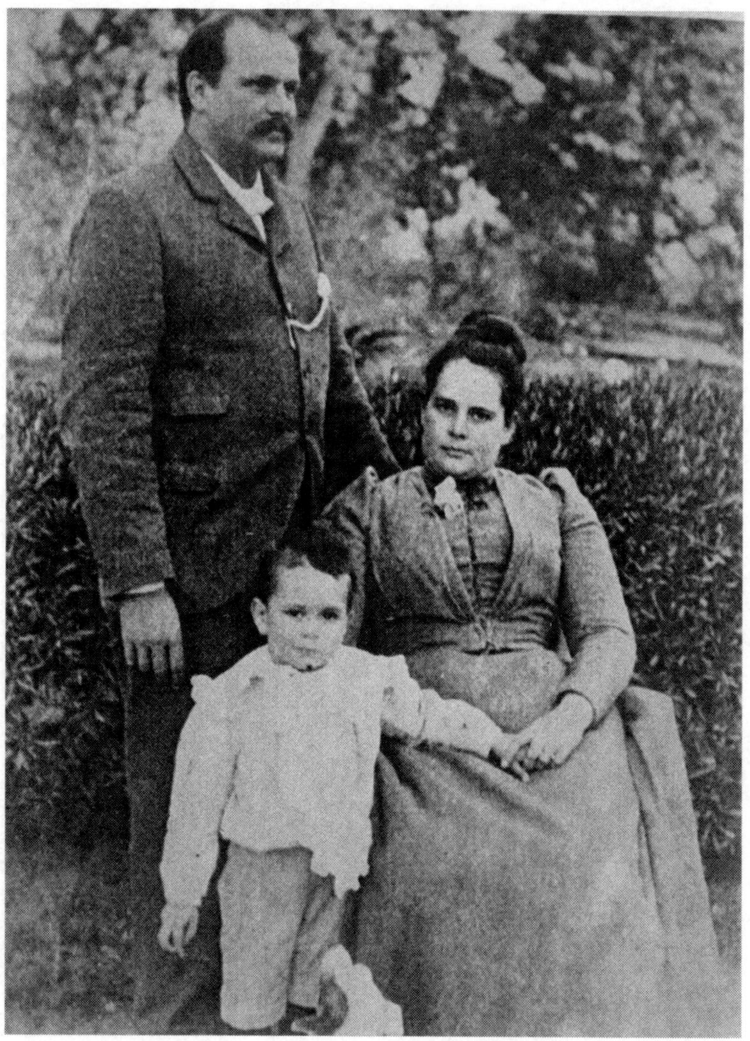

*7* Wilfred Bion with his parents at age three. Bion left India at the age of eight for a preparatory school in England

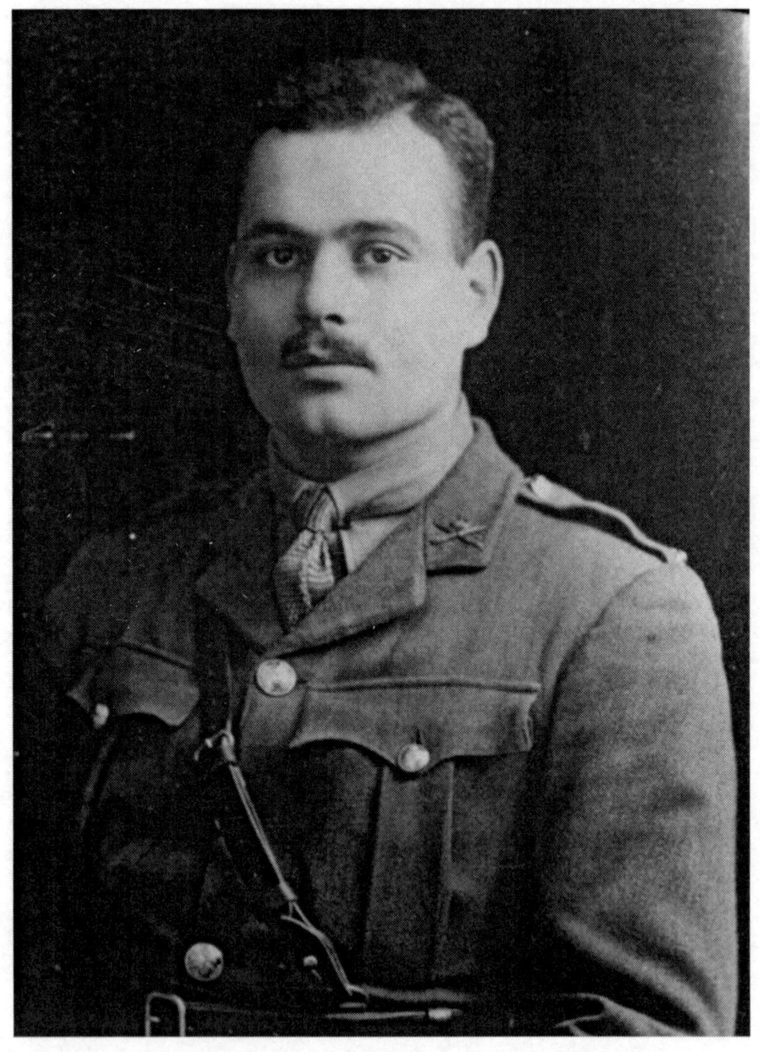

*8* Wilfred Bion in uniform, aged nineteen, 1916

## Notes

1 A. A. Lubbock, *Eric Fox Pitt Lubbock, born 16[th] May 1893. Killed in Aerial Fight Near Ypres, 11[th] March 1917. A Memoir by his Mother* (London: A. L. Humphries, 1918), p. 215.
2 Lubbock, *Eric Fox Pitt Lubbock*, p. 209, p. 24.
3 Lubbock, *Eric Fox Pitt Lubbock*, p. 68.
4 Lubbock, *Eric Fox Pitt Lubbock*, p. 82, p. 83, p. 173.
5 Lubbock, *Eric Fox Pitt Lubbock*, p. 208, p. 192.
6 Lubbock, *Eric Fox Pitt Lubbock*, p. 68.
7 B. Pemberton, 'Mothering the British Soldier', in Lady R. Churchill (ed.), *Women's War Work* (London: Arthur Pearson, 1916), pp. 82–3.
8 Gert and Lil to H. Carter, 13 March 1915, IWM 86/8/1.
9 Father to W. A. Goodwin, 7 November 1915, IWM Con Shelf.
10 M. Hanna, 'A Republic of Letters: The Epistolary Tradition in France during World War I', *The American Historical Review*, Vol. 108, No. 5 (2003), http://www.historycooperative.org/journals/ahr/108.5/hanna.html. Accessed 25 May 2007, para. 31. This dread was not unique to the war. Among Irish and Australian correspondents in the nineteenth century, comments Fitzpatrick, 'silence signified death'. D. Fitzpatrick, *Oceans of Consolation. Personal Accounts of Irish Migration to Australia*, (Cork: Cork University Press, 1994), p. 479.
11 H. Mercer to E. C. Mercer, 25 September, 28 September 1914, IWM 92/52/1.
12 E. R. Hutt to mother, note on envelope, 2 July 1915, IWM 90/7/1. Christa Hämmerle observes in her study of Austrian and German correspondence that 'every letter, every card was literally a "sign of life."' '"You Let a Weeping Woman Call you Home?": Private Correspondences during the First World War in Austria and Germany', in R. Earle (ed.), *Epistolary Selves. Letters and Letter-Writers, 1600–1945* (Aldershot: Ashgate, 1999), p. 159.
13 Mother to J. A. C. Clarke, 16 March 1918, IWM 96/57/1.
14 L. Hooper to K. Hooper, 28 February 1916, LC DF066.
15 C. Christopher to Val, 13 February 1916, IWM 88/11/1.
16 P. Thompson and T. Lummis, 'Family Life and Work Experience Before 1918, 1870–1973' [computer file], 5[th] edition. Colchester: UK Data Archive [distributor], April 2005. SN: 2000, interview 042, p. 3.
17 Thompson and Lummis, 'Family Life and Work', interview 419, p. 15. Milton Robinson returned from the front in early 1918 to be with his mother, who had influenza. 'To think that this had been caused by the war!', he exclaimed in his diary. M. Robinson diary, 12 February 1918, IWM 96/7/1.
18 A. Bishop, with T. Smart (eds.), *Vera Brittain. War Diary 1913–1917, Chronicle of Youth* (London: Victor Gollancz, 1981), pp. 132–3.

19 G. Bickersteth, 25 October 1914, The Bickersteth War Diaries and the Papers of John Burgon Bickersteth, Churchill Archives Centre, GBR/0014/BICK, Vol. 1, p. 169.
20 M. C. W. Charteris, *A Family Record* (London: Curwen Press, 1932), p. 258.
21 P. Jalland, *Death in the Victorian Family* (Oxford: Oxford University Press, 1996), p. 373.
22 Quoted in B. Caine, *Destined to be Wives. The Sisters of Beatrice Webb* (Oxford: Oxford University Press, 1988), p. 201.
23 Father to W. A. Goodwin, 4 November 1915, IWM Con Shelf.
24 L. Hooper to K. Hooper, 3 April 1917.
25 Jalland, *Death in the Victorian Family*, p. 120. David Cannadine takes a contrasting view, arguing that death rates fell in the last quarter of the nineteenth century and that consequently Edwardian parents were relatively unused to grieving for lost children. Infant mortality rates did not begin to fall dramatically until after 1900, when the war generation had already survived the crucial early years. 'War and Death, Grief and Mourning in Modern Britain', in J. Whaley (ed.), *Mirrors of Mortality. Studies in the Social History of Death* (London: Europa Publications, 1981), p. 193.
26 E. Ross, 'Labour and Love. Re-Discovering London's Working-Class Mothers, 1870–1918', in J. Lewis (ed.), *Labour and Love. Women's Experience of Home and Family 1850–1940* (Oxford: Blackwell, 1986), pp. 81–2; Jalland, *Death in the Victorian Family*, p. 120.
27 A. Fletcher, 'Richard Chenevix Trench and his Legacy: An Appreciation by Anthony Fletcher', unpublished essay, p. 25; D. Fletcher, 'Isabel Chenevix Trench: A Fond Memory from her Grand-Daughter', unpublished essay, p. 1.
28 E. Ross, *Love and Toil. Motherhood in Outcast London 1870–1918* (Oxford: Oxford University Press, 1993), p. 167.
29 D. Copelman, '"A New Comradeship Between Men and Women": Family, Marriage and London's Women Teachers 1870–1914', in J. Lewis (ed.), *Labour and Love. Women's Experience of Home and Family 1850–1940* (Oxford: Blackwell, 1986), p. 184.
30 Gilbert Talbot sent his mother a message via the nurse: 'It *is* hard that I should have measles and scarlet fever, when I am so happy downstairs!' G. Talbot, *Gilbert Walter Lyttleton Talbot. Born September 1 1891. Killed in Action at Hooge, July 30 1915* (London: Chiswick Press, 1916), p. 9.
31 N. Gullace, *The Blood of Our Sons: Men, Women and the Renegotiation of British Citizenship in the Great War* (Basingstoke: Palgrave, 2002), pp. 57–63.
32 The phrase is Gullace's, *Blood of our Sons*, pp. 56–7.
33 T. and V. Holt, *'My Boy Jack'. The Search for Kipling's Only Son* (London: Pen & Sword, 1998), p. 71.

34 See Deborah Cohen on the domestic care of disabled men, *The War Come Home: Disabled Veterans in Britain and Germany, 1914–1939* (Berkeley: University of California Press, 2001), esp. ch. 3.

35 J. B. Middlebrook memoirs, IWM Con Shelf, p. 137.

36 G. T. Nugee, diary of Edith Nugee, 31 July , 2 August 1915; IWM 77/102/1. I am grateful to Edward Nugee (nephew of Andrew Nugee) for further information about the events described here.

37 Nugee diary, 3 August, 4 August 1915.

38 Nugee diary , e.g. 12 August, 24 August 1915; 14 August 1915.

39 Nugee diary, 28 August 1915.

40 Memoirs of Brigadier G. T. Nugee, IWM 77/102/1, p. 170.

41 L. Urwick to mother, 13 July 1914, private collection; Talbot, *Gilbert Walter Lyttleton Talbot*, p. 40.

42 On the significance of parcels for Colonial officials whose children were schooled in Britain, see E. Buettner, *Empire Families. Britons and Late Imperial India* (Oxford: Oxford University Press, 2004), p. 135.

43 W. R. Bion, *The Long Weekend 1897–1919. Part of a Life* (London: Free Association Books, 1986), p. 33, p. 37, p. 42.

44 W. R. Bion, *War Memoirs 1917-19* (London: H. Karnac, 1997), p. 76.

45 See John Tosh on the transition from home to public school, *A Man's Place. Masculinity and the Middle-Class Home in Victorian England* (New Haven: Yale University Press, 1999), pp. 117–19.

46 Lubbock, *Eric Fox Pitt Lubbock*, p. 5, p. 6.

47 Quoted in Caine, *Destined to be Wives*, pp. 128–9.

48 Caine, *Destined to be Wives*, p. 124, p. 127.

49 For example, L. Urwick to mother, 7 August 1914. Ernest Smith hoped that his mother 'did not think me too selfish in not letting you see me off'. E. K. Smith to mother, 31 December 1914, *Letters Sent From France. Service with the Artists' Rifles and the Buffs, December 1914–December 1915* (London: J. Cobb, 1994), p. 3.

50 E. Smith and A. Smith, *Two Brothers. Eric and Arnold Miall Smith* (Edinburgh: Constable, 1918), p. 5.

51 Charteris, *A Family Record*, pp. 312–13.

52 D. Winter, *Death's Men. Soldiers of the Great War* (London: Penguin, 1979), p. 164; D. Englander, 'Soldiering and Identity: Reflections on the Great War', *War in History*, Vol. 1, No. 3, p. 304.

53 On the economic contribution made by Australian women in supplying comforts for soldiers, see Bruce Scates, 'The Unknown Sock Knitter: Voluntary Work, Emotional Labour, Bereavement and the Great War', *Labour History*, Vol. 81 (2001), esp. pp. 31–3. On Britain see Paul Ward, 'Women of Britain Say Go: Women's Patriotism in the First World War', *Twentieth Century British History*, Vol. 12, No. 1 (2001), pp. 23–46; and Paul Ward 'Empire and the Everyday: Britishness and Imperialism in

Women's Lives in the Great War', in P. Buckner and R. Douglas Francis, *Re-Discovering the British World* (Calgary: Calgary Press, 2005), pp. 267–83.

54 The Buffs also had a comfort fund, run by the Brigadier-General's wife 'unaided, except by her maid.' It despatched weekly bales of comforts. R. S. H. Moody, *Historical Records of the Buffs East Kent Regiment 1914–1919* (London: The Medici Society, 1922), p. 113. See also the interesting account of the 'Comforts For Soldiers' War Work Depot, which was set up four days after war was declared and continued to the end of the war. K. Grieves, (ed.), *Sussex in the First World War* (Lewes: Sussex Record Society, 2004), pp. 184–9.

55 Second Battalion The Rifle Brigade, Battalion Orders, 15 April 1915, 16 November 1915, National Army Museum Mrs E. D. Stephens, 8902–201–1043 to 1396.

56 J. H. Alldridge to Mrs E. D. Stephens, 24 March 1915.

57 *Report of the 2nd Battalion Brigade Comforts Fund*, 1919, p. 4.

58 Alldridge to Mrs Stephens, 18 November 1915.

59 Alldridge to Mrs Stephens, 16 December 1915; Battalion Orders, 20 July 1915.

60 Alldridge to Mrs Stephens, 22 March 1915.

61 Frank Nugent to Mrs Stephens, 30 January 1916 and *Report of the 2nd Battalion Comforts Fund*, 1919. The fund often targeted its parcels. NCOs were sent regular supplies of torch batteries, the battalion's eight runners were sent individual parcels, and the Aid Post was supplied with electric torches and batteries, hot water bottles, note-books, towels, soap, folding chairs and table, drugs and other supplies. Battalion runners to Mrs Stephens, 18 August 1915; Battalion Orders, 20 July 1915.

62 J. Bickersteth (ed.), *The Bickersteth Diaries 1914–1918* (London: Leo Cooper, 1995), pp. 12–13.

63 A. Clark, *Echoes of the Great War* (Oxford: Oxford University Press, 1985), p. 30.

64 On the solace provided by war work see C. S. Peel, *How We Lived Then. 1914–1918. A Sketch of Social and Domestic Life in England During the War* (London: Bodley Head, 1929), p. 71; Scates, 'The Unknown Sock Knitter', p. 36, p. 45. The public activities undertaken by Maggie Hobhouse, according to Barbara Caine, 'utilised her energy and filled her time – even if they did not still her anxieties.' *Destined to be Wives*, p. 201.

65 Ian Beckett describes how in the early months of the war, 'vast quantities of unwanted garments flooded the army.' *Home Front, 1914–1918: How Britain Survived the Great War* (Kew: The National Archives, 2006), p. 66. For a more positive assessment see Ward 'Empire and the Everyday', esp. pp. 275–7.

66 Peel, *How We Lived Then*, p. 61. In her poem 'Socks', the patriotic poet Jessie Pope imagines a woman knitting, and how it 'Checks the thoughts

that cluster thick'. C. Reilly (ed.), *Scars Upon My Heart. Women's Poetry & Verse of the First World War* (London: Virago, 1981), pp. 89–90. But worry could also get in the way of knitting, as the last line of Philadelphia Robertson's poem, 'A Woman's Prayer', suggests: 'Pray to God to see to it/ That I keep sane enough to knit.' Quoted in N. Khan, *Women's Poetry of the First World War* (Hemel Hempstead: Harvester–Wheatsheaf, 1988), pp. 76–7.

67 Thompson and Lummis, 'Family Life and Work', interview 065, p. 21.

68 Alldridge to Mrs Stephens, 11 May 1915. The knitted item was not always superior. Hilda Barker from Brighton made an honest appraisal of the sock she had just knitted: 'I don't think any soldier would be very comfortable wearing it.' Quoted in Grieves, *Sussex in the First World War*, p. 163. John Liddell wrote to his family in November 1914 that: 'some of the efforts that arrive are very thin and shoddy. Especially do I condemn the atrocity known as the heelless sock.' Quoted in Beckett, *Home Front*, p. 66.

69 J. Taylor to N. Taylor, 26 March 1915, IWM 90/28/1.

70 R. Trench to mother, 20 June 1917, private collection.

71 E. Marchant to mother, 11 July 1915, IWM DS/MISC/26.

72 O. H. Best, 'Letters + parcels for Herbert', IWM 87/56/1.

73 J. Taylor to N. Taylor, 26 March 1915.

74 Captain John Liddell blamed the traffic in comforts from support groups for holding up personal mail: 'The people who send them mean very well, but . . . these huge bales stop everything else coming through the post.' Quoted in Beckett, *The Home Front*, p. 66.

75 Gibbs to mother 2 January 1916, IWM P317.

76 S. J. Dawson to S. B. Dawson, 15 August, 23 August 1919, private collection.

77 L. Hooper to K. Hooper, 23 March 1917.

78 H. W. Hague to mother, 12 April 1918, IWM 98/33/1.

79 War Office, General Staff Censorship and Publicity Section. 'Censorship Orders For Troops in the Field' (London: Censorship and Publicity Section, General Staff, 1918), p. 10.

80 L. Urwick to mother, 23 March, 3 June 1915; E. R. Hutt to mother 20 September 1915, IWM 90/7/1. Frank Wollocombe ordered his military great-coat as Autumn drew on, and a new set of clothes in Spring 1916. F. Wollocombe to mother, 31 October 1915; 6 March 1916, IWM 95/33/1.

81 W. A. Goodwin to father, 17 November 1915, IWM Con Shelf.

82 The comforts in a man's parcel resembled the Christmas or birthday presents that became part of family rituals in the second half of the nineteenth century, and which symbolised the special affections of a parent, brother or sister. J. R. Gillis, *A World of Their Own Making. Myth, Ritual and the Quest for Family Values* (New York: Basic Books, 1996), p. 79.

83 Pemberton in Churchill (ed.), *Women's War Work*, p. 72.

84 Ross, *Love and Toil*, pp. 51–2.

85 Letters from W. T. Hate to mother, IWM 86/51/1.
86 C. Christopher to mother, 24 March 1916; Hubbard to mother, 17 June 1916; 'Ma to my dear Sid', 16 December 1918.
87 C. W. Ramsdale to Mother and Mary, 17 August 1918, IWM Con Shelf.
88 Clark, *Echoes of the Great War*, p. 17.
89 Gibbs to mother, 22 January 1915; 11 March 1916.
90 Gibbs to mother, 22 December 1915; 11 March 1916.
91 C. Christopher to mother, 24 March 1916.
92 M. Webb to mother and father, 12 June 1915, IWM 90/28/1; B. Chapman to mother, 21 June 1918 IWM 98/17/1.
93 Goodwin to father, 20 October 1915.
94 Katherine Tynan-Hinkson diary, nd, 1914, p. 51, Vol. A, Tynan/Hinkson Collection, John Rylands University Library of Manchester.
95 T. Wilson, *The Myriad Faces of War. Britain and the Great War, 1914–1918* (Cambridge: Polity, 1986), p. 513. A national rationing system for meat, butter, margarine, lard and sugar was in operation by July 1918. Wilson, pp. 648–9.
96 J. Burnett, *Plenty and Want. A Social History of Diet in England from 1815 to the Present Day* (London: Scolar Press, 1979), p. 249; 'Ma to my dear Sid', nd.
97 Niall Ferguson goes so far as to say that without tobacco and alcohol, 'the First World War could not have been fought.' *The Pity of War* (London: Penguin, 1998), p. 351.
98 W. B. P. Spencer to mother, 3 January, 2 February 1915, IWM 87/56/1.
99 R. D. Mountfort to mother, 16 September 1915; 2 February 1916, IWM Con Shelf. Arthur Hubbard had 'a good feast from your parcel on Friday evening before we went to the trenches.' Hubbard to mother, 5 July 1916, IWM Con Shelf.
100 Carter's father wrote saying 'Mother wishes to know do you want anything sending as we are not sure whether we can do so, whereas [*sic*] you are . . . Can we send a parcel of chocolates and do you want any papers to read, if so, say which you would like then we can send them.' Father to H. Carter, 3 March 1915, IWM 86/8/1.
101 Mother to W. Hoyle, 27 December 1914, IWM 85/22/1.
102 Mother to A. G. Steavenson, 19 March 1919, IWM 86/77/1.
103 Gibbs to mother, 2 January 1916.
104 Hutt to mother, 19 May 1915.
105 F. Nesham (ed.), *Socks, Cigarettes and Shipwrecks. A Family's War Letters 1914–1918* (Gloucester: Alan Sutton, 1987), p. 69.
106 Ramsdale to Mother and Mary, 17 August 1918.
107 On manic reparation see Melanie Klein, 'A Contribution to the Psychogenesis of Manic-Depressive States' in M. Klein, *Love, Guilt and Reparation and Other Works 1921–1945* (London: Virago, 1994), pp. 262–89.

108 Hutt to mother, 11 June, 14 July 1915.
109 F. P. Crozier, *A Brass Hat in No Man's Land* (London: Jonathan Cape, 1930), pp. 153–4.
110 L. Urwick to mother, 18 December 1914.
111 E. Bickersteth, 14 November 1914, 'The Bickersteth War Diaries', Vol. 1, p. 203.
112 L. Hooper to K. Hooper, 9 April 1916; A. Hooper to K. Hooper, quoted in L. Hooper to K. Hooper, 9 April 1916.
113 A. Hooper quoting L. Hooper, quoted in L. Hooper to K. Hooper, 3 July 1916.
114 A. Hooper to L. Hooper, quoted in L. Hooper to K. Hooper, 18 October 1915.
115 L. Jamieson, 'Limited Resources and Limiting Conventions: Working-Class Mothers and Daughters in Urban Scotland c. 1890–1918', in J. Lewis (ed.), *Labour and Love. Women's Experience of Home and Family 1850–1940* (Oxford: Blackwell, 1986), p. 59.
116 Ross, *Love and Toil*, pp. 159–60; Jamieson, 'Limited Resources', p. 67.
117 T. Thorpe, 'To Mama + Dada', Upwey camp, nd, IWM Con Shelf.
118 Thorpe to Mama, Dad and Nellie, 13 September 1917.
119 W. T. Hate to mother, 8 August 1915; 21 December 1914. Similar self-restraint among working-class children is noted by Ross. *Love and Toil*, p. 151.
120 C. Christopher to mother, 13 May 1916.
121 H. S. Payne to mother 13 December 1917, IWM 90/1/1.
122 See M. Tebbutt, *Women's Talk? A Social History of 'Gossip' in Working Class Neighbourhoods 1880–1960* (Aldershot: Scolar Press, 1995), pp. 102–16.
123 Hubbard to mother, 22 May, 9 June 1916.
124 Hubbard to mother and all, nd, 1918.
125 I am grateful to Swettenham's niece, Mrs Marriott, for information on his family background.
126 Swettenham to mother, 9 September 1918; nd but late December 1918.
127 Swettenham to mother, 12 October 1918. On the disruption of supply lines and shortage of food during the spring and summer of 1918, see I. Bet-El, *Conscripts. Forgotten Men of the Great War* (Stroud: Sutton Publishing, 2003), p. 115.
128 Clark, *Echoes of the Great War*, p. 76.
129 Clark, *Echoes of the Great War*, p. 42. See J.-M. Strange on the mourning of 'excellent' sons, whose financial contributions were also seen as a sign of their selflessness. '"She Cried a Very Little": Death, Grief and Mourning in Working-Class Culture c. 1880–1914', *Social History* Vol 27, No. 2 (May 2002), p. 150.
130 For example C. Christopher to mother, 24 January 1916.
131 S. E. Brown to mother, nd; Brown to mother, nd but postmarked Sheerness, IWM 89/7/1.

132 J. A. C. Clarke to mother, 11 April 1917, IWM 96/57/1.
133 Hate to mother, 1 August, 8 August, 4 October, 9 October 1915.
134 Uptake of the Separation Allowance among mothers was initially halting, but grew to equal or surpass uptake by wives, although the overall amount given to mothers was less. Given this, it is not clear why Susan Pederson concludes that wives were 'the most important recipients.' 'Gender, Welfare, and Citizenship in Britain during the Great War', *American Historical Review*, Vol. 95, No. 4 (1990), n. 4, p. 985.
135 Ross 'Labour and Love', p. 87; Ross, *Love and Toil*, p. 159.
136 H. Urwick diary, note on inside cover, private collection.

PART II

# Mothering men

# 3

# Staying alive

The days before Captain Reggie Trench's departure for France were spent in a flurry of activity. He had to organise the despatch of his collapsible bed, canvas bath and basin. He was also issuing the 250 men in the company with gas masks, steel helmets, satchels for use in the trenches, field dressings, clasp knives, and '400 pants, 300 pairs of socks, 200 pairs boots'. He had to make sure that he took back 'from every man' the kit that they had been using in Camp, including kit bags, hairbrushes (the men's hair had been clipped close to the scalp and a comb was considered sufficient), boot brushes, jackets, trousers and canvas shoes, as in theory he would have to pay for any missing articles. Along with a new wagon of Lewis guns and ammunition, he had charge of the Field Kitchen, which had to be carried in twenty-eight separate compartments.[1] This was domestic management on a grand scale.

Trench's duties became more onerous once they arrived in France. After a 14-mile march, the men weighed down by 83lb packs, he got his company settled into billets ten miles from the front line. They fed well, as the cook was fluent in French and could negotiate supplies, but after three days of marching and living amidst 'pretty awful mud', the men needed a wash. 'With great difficulty' Trench managed to rig up a bath. His letter to his mother ended on a proud note: 'The Town Mayor tells me that it is the only one in the whole Corps area!'[2]

Hygiene became even more of an issue once they moved into the trenches. His men were not even allowed to take their parcels into the trenches because of the mess they made with the paper. Creosol solution had to be scattered about. 'Sanitation is a great worry to me just at present', he explained.[3] He observed his surroundings with an eye trained in military efficiency, and this meant good house-keeping. In one delightful letter, he compiles a two-page list of the uses of the sandbag, which many men carried in their kit. It would not only stop bullets, but make hat covers, curtains, carpets, blankets, puttees, bed-socks and even pudding cloths. Trench was greatly impressed by this improvisation.[4]

Historical accounts of the Western Front sometimes assume that nothing could be more remote from the soldier's existence in the trenches than his past life at home. In *No Man's Land*, Eric Leed writes that 'the traditional figure of the veteran is derived from everything that is presumed to lie "outside" the boundaries of domestic existence.'[5] Leed picks up on a feeling, often voiced in letters, that the two worlds of home and the front were incommensurable. On returning from his first home leave, for example, Roland Mountfort wrote

> I discovered during the past two nights that my efforts to picture trenches in winter from an armchair at home were about as successful as a blind man's to imagine Niagara. At the same time I was disappointed to find on returning here how little (comparatively with what I had many a weary time imagined) I had appreciated the luxuries of pyjamas, clean sheets, good food, England, home + beauty; having taken it all as a most natural matter of course.[6]

Soldiers may have imagined home and trench as opposed worlds, but in fact on the Western Front they were more deeply involved in domestic work than they had ever been before the war. Water was unavailable in the line and had to be carried up the trenches in old petrol cans. Meals had to be conveyed in heavy dixies from the company cooker behind the lines through the maze of communication trenches. Sometimes it was too difficult or dangerous to get hot food up the line, so men carried cold rations with them, and small cookers.[7] The 'homely smell' of bacon in the trenches after morning stand-to momentarily overpowered the stench of chloride of lime, while the guns fell silent in a 'tacit truce' that allowed each side to enjoy breakfast.[8]

After a spell in the trenches the men would go back to billets. Clothes had to be cleaned and bodies washed, but this was no easy task. When Trench retired to billets after a gruelling stint in the front line, which claimed the lives of his commanding officer and five of his men, he found there was enough water only for cooking and drinking. Nevertheless he explained, 'I'm getting the men bathed in water of a sort by degrees and have had a fine bath myself'.[9] Hours 'at rest' were spent on the 'spit and polish' for which the British Army was famous, shining buttons and boots, brushing down the tunic and picking out the lice that infested the seams.[10]

These 'house-keeping' activities were not distractions from military routine but constituted its very basis. Ilana Bet-El estimates that military activities occupied only around a third of the conscripts' time, the rest being spent in 'very human survival activities' such as sleeping, eating and constructing shelter.[11] The primitive conditions of the trenches and exposure to the elements made domestic skills not only desirable but essential. In summer the trench soldier suffered from heat and dust, while in winter, unable to move about much, the cold and wet penetrated through his layers of clothing. Frostbite and trench foot, a condition caused by standing in wet trenches, claimed fingers and toes. The winter of 1916–17 was the coldest on record since 1894–95. Of men admitted to hospital in 1917 with conditions not related to enemy action, only VD outnumbered frostbite.[12]

When it was wet it was muddy, and since many of the British trenches in Northern France and Belgium were barely higher than the water table, they were in a semi-constant state of flooding. The 'porridgy mud' around Ypres was so bad that trenches often had to be built up with sandbags, rather than dug down. The trenches around the Somme were generally drier, but when wet the chalky ground turned to the consistency of half-wet cement.[13] Because the British Army preferred to concentrate its efforts on offensive action, its trenches tended to be more poorly constructed than those of the Germans, and were not only less well drained, but shallower and lacking deep dug-outs. Trench walls or dug-out roofs could cave in under heavy rainfall, suffocating those within.[14] It took effort and ingenuity to stay alive, let alone achieve a modicum of comfort.

In his remarkable book *The War the Infantry Knew*, which drew on the testimonies of over fifty men of the Second Battalion of the Welch Fusiliers, J. C. Dunn was determined that it should explain to the reader not only the events of battle, but what 'ordinary trench life' was like. In a departure from the traditions of military history, the book describes billeting, washing and bathing, rations, parcels, entertainments and delousing.[15] Siegfried Sassoon's contribution to the volume underlines the importance of day-to-day survival:

> The truth is that infantry soldiering in the battle-zone was an overwhelmingly physical experience. Such human elements as food, warmth and sleep were the living realities, and it may not have occurred to many a writer of military histories that the weather was a more effective General than Foch,

> Haig or Ludendorff. A bad blister on a man's heel might be the only thing he could clearly remember after a week of intense experience which added a battle honour to the colours of his regiment. For those whose active unit was company, platoon or section, physical sensations predominated. Mental activity (detached from feet and belly) was strictly limited by gross physical actualities.

The 'details of discomfort', Sassoon concluded, 'constituted the humanity of infantry soldiering'.[16]

Soldiers tried to ameliorate such hardships with homely touches. Mirrors, clocks and family portraits were not unknown in officers' dug-outs.[17] Reggie Trench's dug-out near Sanctuary Wood was about as long as a bus, its roof made of elephant iron, a door at one end and a canvas window at the other. Inside were a stove, two chairs, boards raised off the floor for beds and a table consisting of raised earth covered by boards. His fellow officers had added a couple of shelves and some boxes to hold their post. Trench had laid 'a blue and white little cloth that I got in Amiens' on the table, and there were 'many flowers in empty fruit jars!'[18] A divisional intelligence officer in the Ypres Salient was even reputed to have a dug-out lined with books on shelves, and a garden resplendent with flowers and vegetables with which he supplemented his rations.[19]

For the 'other ranks' it was a matter of securing the best shelter they could from the weather. If sleeping under canvas and their tent was full, they learned to turn over in unison. A billet in a barn, sleeping on straw, could give a good night's sleep as long as it was not infested. When Gilbert Talbot took over a billet from a Territorial Battalion he found it 'indescribably foul – filthy straw, old clothes, stale food, odd bits of equipment , etc, etc, etc, – all old and filthy and verminous.' As a result most of his men were forced to bivouac the first night, and 'pretty chilly they were.'[20] In trenches men slept in funk holes, shelves of around four feet wide which were scooped out of the trench wall and could accommodate three men. These gave slight protection from the weather but there was stiff competition for them and the legs of the man on the edge still poked into the trench. Many just huddled together on the duckboards wrapped in their groundsheets, their sleep disturbed every time a man stumbled up or down the line. Griffiths described the discomforts:

> To lie for two hours on a plank half sinking into a dream-ridden sleep, half hearing every noise within reach of audibility, there was little rest of body or mind. On such a bed, flesh was no protection to the bones; it was a

> small envelope containing a jumble of crossing nerves. Bone pressed down and wood pressed up until the sting changed slowly into a dragging pain. Getting up was a process of re-assembling the members.[21]

When they were totally exhausted most managed to get sleep despite the discomfort, but the officer's privilege they coveted most of all was his dug-out. He kept relatively warm and dry, and he had some protection from shelling. He could eat at a table and sleep lying down, and he had somewhere to stow his letters and pictures of loved ones. When George Coppard decided to become a batman, it was so that he too might enjoy '"a little bit of Heaven" . . . a refuge in between patrols.'[22]

## Food, comradeship and family networks

The question of where the next meal would come from, and what it might be, assumed great significance among soldiers. Some men kept daily diaries of what they were fed, their record of the war amounting to little more than a menu.[23] This concern, which at times amounted to an obsession, can partly be explained in terms of the privations of Army life. Days were long and often monotonous. Soldiers behind the lines spent much of their time doing 'bull', cleaning their kit, parading and doing fatigues. In the front line, 'stand-to' took place half an hour before dawn and again at dusk, and in the long hours in between, working parties would repair trenches or transport supplies to and from the front line. Hungry from their exertions, boredom also aroused their anticipation, even when standard rations were all they could expect.[24] When it arrived, Army food rarely failed to disappoint. It probably constituted an improvement in diet only for the very poorest recruits.[25] Some complained of hunger, and many more about the monotony of the diet: hard biscuits, apple and plum jam, bully beef and tinned Maconochie stew.[26] Percy Smith thought its unreliability was as great a problem as the lack of variety: 'bully beef & biscuits is the chief item on the menu, sometimes we get plenty, & other times very little, we have to take things as they come.'[27] Food supplies were especially unreliable when men were in trenches. Rations often arrived cold. Whilst in the Northumberland Fusiliers Norman Gladden claimed to have gone for twenty-six days in the forward trenches with 'practically no cooked food.'[28] Moreover, Coppard noted, 'irregular appropriations' could occur as food travelled up to the line.[29] Supplements to the Army rations were thus particularly welcome when men were in the line.

Informal food supplies were not only an individual pleasure, but provided one of the ways in which men made friends within their section or platoon. Fenton fished in the canal near his trenches, eking out his comrades' rations with bream and roach.[30] At Arras, Coppard provided for his mates in the roofless kitchen of 'Whizz-bang villa', right under the noses of the Germans:

> The lads gave me full marks when I produced three big rissoles per man, made of bully and potatoes fried in swimming bacon fat. Real good they were. Stewed fruit was on the menu every day. This domesticity and house-keeping lark was rudely shattered every now and again when machine-gun bullets struck the walls, making us scuttle into the cellar like rabbits.[31]

Men often regarded food as common to the group, just as it had been shared within their families. Two 'classic' accounts of life in the trenches illustrate the importance of food in comradeship. In the German writer Erich Maria Remarque's *All Quiet on the Western Front*, the narrator Paul Bäumer scrounges and steals, aided by a remarkable character, Kat, whose capacity to obtain food in the most unpromising situations assumes an almost magical quality. The culinary high-point of the novel is a clandestine meal of freshly caught turkey, cooked amidst a growing bombardment as the two men huddle together over a fire. As they eat their illicit catch together, they share a tender moment: 'we are brothers, pressing one another to take the best pieces.'[32] In his autobiographical novel *Her Privates We*, the Australian Frederic Manning also writes a good deal about food: where it came from, what it tasted like and how it was shared among friends.[33]

Food and comradeship did not always go together, however. Memoir writers sometimes recalled the unseemly scrambles they witnessed on their first meal in the camp canteen.[34] The unwritten rule was that looting was acceptable as long as it was supplying a basic need and not just for personal gain, but the line between looting to survive and theft was far from clear.[35] Captain Herbert Leland, who spent long periods away from divisional headquarters, looted fowls and ducks from surrounding farms and had his 'eye on a couple of "porkeens", but I don't think it will be wise to "pinch" them.'[36]

Grace and favour in the distribution of food could disadvantage the less gregarious, those who had little to put into the kitty, and those who for whatever reason were not liked within the section or platoon. The task of distributing rations within each section of around fifteen men commonly fell to the corporal, who was not always fair. Fifty years after being drafted into a Territorial unit of the Northumberland Fusiliers, Gladden's resentment at the NCOs who held back the best food for the old hands was still palpable.[37] Frank Richards thought 'there was always a bit of sharking' done with the bacon ration, 'the same as with the rum'.[38] Coppard reckoned that his senior NCOs drank far more than their ration of rum, and that supplies to his machine gun team were 'a hit or miss affair.' He recited a ditty that suggests the behaviour of these NCO's was not unusual:

> If the sergeant drinks your rum,
> Never mind!
> And your face has lost its smile,
> Never mind!
> He's entitled to a tot,
> But not the bleedin' lot,
> If the sergeant drinks your rum,
> Never mind![39]

Men could, by the same token, show great generosity. A private soldier in the Second Welch Fusiliers who had been given a job on the canteen staff because of his frailty, was reported to have walked seven miles up into 'noisy' trenches to bring cigarettes to his old comrades.[40]

Within these informal systems of pooling among friends, the food sent by families in parcels was not only appreciated for the personal comfort it provided, but because it could be offered to others. The artillery gunner Ray Christopher described how, with the help of parcels sent from home, their diet had improved:

> We are six in our dug-out, and when a parcel arrives for anyone, or anybody buys anything, we all share it. We have quite decent little suppers sometimes. When we get any surplus bread I make rissoles, out of bread crumbs, onions and bully-beef, and they are jolly fine when fried with a tin of tomatoes. Then perhaps another night we have fried sausages and onions, so we don't do so badly. Tonight we fried some tinned herrings and they were good. Talking about fish, we were wondering if a small crate of kippers would reach us in anything like condition; or failing kippers some haddock.[41]

On receiving a parcel from his mother containing apples, sweets, chocolate and cake, Charles Ramsdale reported 'I've not been able to acquaint those bad lads with my good fortune, but I know they (or such of them as share my abode tonight) will rejoice with me over the good things and will do their duty most manfully in assisting in the consumption thereof.'[42]

The expectation that food from home would be shared aroused mixed feelings. It could lead to generosity as men became aware of each other's domestic situation, and how well they were provided for by their families. In the run-up to Christmas 1915 the Christopher brothers asked for a parcel to be sent to a fellow soldier who 'hasn't a solitary relation in the world', noting that everyone else seemed to be 'getting parcels now except him'.[43] Yet parcels from home were jealously guarded among men who had not seen home for up to a year and who deeply missed their families. When Fenton returned from a grenade course he was not altogether pleased to find that his mates had consumed the five parcels that arrived in his absence, though it was common practice to share parcels when a man was away on leave or a course.[44] After returning from a particularly difficult stint in trenches at the Somme, Frank Richards found that the contents of his parcels had been consumed by his friend Paddy, who had heard that Frank was wounded: 'I almost smelled a rat. I was hard up for tobacco at the time and I thought my luck was dead out.'[45] In *The Secret Battle*, A. P. Herbert described how the problems of communal feeding created simmering resentment in the mess, particularly over parcels, because those who got the fewest parcels sometimes consumed the most.[46]

When a home parcel arrived, men were faced with a real dilemma: the sight of their favourite foods brought loved ones vividly to mind, yet they had to give some of it up for comrades. As Herbert noted:

> A man would willingly preserve its treasures for himself to gloat over alone, in no mere fleshly indulgence, but as a concrete expression of affection from the home for which he longs. This is not nonsense. He likes to undo the strings in the grubby hole which is his present home, and secretly become sentimental over the little fond packages and queer, loving thoughts which have composed it. And though in a generous impulse he may say to his companions 'Come and eat this cake', and see it in a moment disappear, it is hard for him not to think, 'My sister (or wife, or mother) made this for me; they thought it would give me pleasure for many days. Already it is gone – would they not be hurt if they knew?' He feels that he has betrayed the tenderness of his home.[47]

It was hard not to feel envious when the parcel post was handed out and the same men always garnered the biggest harvests.[48] Willis Brown suggested that his mother might get other people to send him parcels in Gallipoli; 'any one will do, as there is quite a lot of competition as to who gets most mails, some get ten or twelve things a week regularly.'[49] The prosperity of the volunteer reinforcements was a source of irritation among Regulars in the Royal Welch Fusiliers. When they were integrated with new recruits from the 20th Battalion of the Royal Fusiliers in November 1915, the old soldiers fumed at these University and Public School men, 'accustomed from infancy to be waited on, with not a soul to show them an active soldier's chief job – rough casual labour.'[50] The Royal Fusiliers became known as 'The Chocolate Soldiers' because of the size of their mail parcels, and because they 'spent so much on the costlier foodstuffs, sauces, and confectionery'. Stealing from them was considered almost fair game: when a parcel post arrived as the Royal Fusiliers were getting ready to go into the line and they began to grumble about the 'bore of carrying their parcels themselves', a few 'Old Sweats' lit a fire upwind of their billet and, as the men evacuated, ran off with their parcels.[51]

The arrangements between rankers tended to be ad hoc, but food from home contributed in a more routine way to the officer's social circle, and on a scale that the ranker could only envy. When out of the line officers ate in the mess, which had elaborate rules and rituals. New subalterns were told that 'Your mess is your home, and you should behave in it as if you were in your own home.'[52] This domestic ethos continued in the line, when dug-outs were typically occupied by the three or four subalterns that constituted a Company along with their batmen. Captain Arthur Gibbs explained that, in his dug-out, 'Food is shared among 3 of us'.[53] Subalterns usually had a mess president who was responsible for menus and for purchasing food that supplemented their rations. A mother's help was invaluable for the mess president. Greenwell was proud of the grand style in which the officers in his company were able to entertain as a result of his careful provision and he got his mother to supplement their diet with supplies from Harrods.[54] Richard Foulkes asked his mother to send out fried fish and a plum or ginger pudding, to be paid for out of the mess subscriptions.[55]

The food in Hall's mess was always common property among the nine officers, and Hall asked his parents to send a cake or anything home-made, as 'I should naturally like to supply my share.'[56] Like Hall, Arthur Gibbs generally referred to 'we' when mentioning his parcels. On Christmas Day 1915, he told his mother, 'We had the pheasant and the swiss roll up in the trenches: they were splendid. We have just had a halt for refreshment – Insole, Crawford, Wood and myself – we have had the 2 bottles of fizz, and now there isn't much left of the excellent hamper you made up for me.'[57] These parcels allowed the officer to reciprocate the hospitality offered by his fellow subalterns, and the fact that they came from his home added to their value. 'Clark has been talking about your rock cakes ever since your last parcel', wrote 2nd Lieutenant Edward Chapman to his mother.[58] One mother continued to bake cakes for the officers in her son's mess even after his death.[59]

## The subaltern's 'housewifery'

As Reggie Trench's animated descriptions to his mother show, the domestic duties of the officer on the Western Front were many and varied. In addition to the military tasks he carried out in the trenches, like supervising the repair of trenches, inspecting men on watch, preparing for and leading patrols or raiding parties and administering discipline, he was responsible for the general comfort and morale of his men. The job combined discipline and service, exercised in the most difficult emotional and physical circumstances.

After the war became bogged down in late 1914, outbreaks of trench foot, which was caused by standing in cold and damp conditions, began to occur. The condition was potentially very serious, the worst cases turning gangrenous.[60] It could seriously affect fighting strength: one Battalion in the wet December of 1916 was said to have lost 200 men through trench foot. Subaltern officers were detailed to carry out regular preventative measures. They had to ensure that the trenches were drained as far as was possible, conduct regular inspections of the men's feet and supervise the application of whale oil. Carrington recalled 'nursing' his men's blistered toes, ensuring that they had clean socks, and insisting on 'ritual washings'.[61] A conscientious subaltern would be constantly on the look-out for fresh socks. Reggie Trench was so pleased when he managed to secure a large shipment of fresh socks for his men that he wrote to his mother about it: 'I'm lucky in having 54 new pairs of socks to distribute, and, fancy, 12 pairs of good boots'. A couple of days later he felt himself even more 'lucky as regards socks as I have got 70 new pairs'.[62] Rifling through the packs of dead Germans looking for socks was one of the more bizarre acts of 'housewifery' recalled by Guy Chapman after they occupied a German trench in 1917.[63] A low incidence of trench foot was a matter of pride among subalterns.[64]

Officers also had to keep an eye on the general state of cleanliness of the men, making sure that they had baths as often as could be managed, that their uniforms were kept as clean as possible and that they were de-lousing regularly. As a result they gained close knowledge of their men's personal hygiene. The aptly named 'Piggott' was the 'prize filthy man' in Ernest Smith's company. He smelt so bad that 'there was not a man in the platoon who would consent to sleep with him in the same tent.' Neither Smith nor the other subalterns in the company found it easy to discipline Piggott, since in his personal manner he was 'so very civil'. In 'sheer despair', Smith passed the matter over to the Medical Officer, who, to Smith's great amusement, found a job for Piggott in the Division laundry.[65]

Rest and shelter preoccupied the subaltern. Though they did not sleep in the same shelters as the men, they were aware of the men's conditions and were often shocked by their hardships. 'The Tommy stands or sits down in a cramped position nearly all the time. He gets no shelter from the rain for 3 days', reported Wilbert Spencer to his mother.[66] Frank Maxwell stood up to his divisional commander over the matter of blankets, when, after a tour of the trenches he found 'only wretched shelters of corrugated iron, under which those not on the parapet sit freezing with cold. No blankets allowed.' His anger towards his superior officers was animated by empathy: what he had seen in the trenches 'made me very sorry for the poor men in it', and determined to improve their situation.[67] On one occasion the tank commander Wilfred Bion and his fellow officers got the men to dig hollows in the ground to sleep in, over which they parked their tanks so as to form a roof. 'The feeling of comfort and security' this provided, he explains, 'did much to improve their spirits'. Bion was distraught when the men were discovered insensible the next morning, temporarily poisoned by carbon monoxide gas.[68]

Subalterns also kept an eye on what the men were fed, since nothing was more likely to stir discontent than poor or insufficient meals.[69] Conscientious officers tried to vary the army rations. While Vernon Merivale, a temporary Captain in the Northumberland Fusiliers, was putting together hot food containers to get the tea up to the trenches in, his brother Frank, acting Quarter-Master in the same Battalion, wrote to his mother in December 1917 that:

> I am giving my men hot tea + rum before they get up for early morning stables, they appreciate it very much.
>
> I have also bought a 100 kilos of potatoes for Fr 20 (175lb) wonderfully cheap isn't it. I am going to mince up every oddment I can get add minced bully beaf [*sic*] + potatoes and make hot rissoles for the men's suppers.

> I think they want a lot of food this cold weather + especially fat, the rissoles are boiled in dripping.[70]

Meanwhile Vernon and Frank's cousin Herman, who was stationed in Gallipoli, had written to his family 'asking for recipes + simple explanations for cooking rations. His men have no notion how to set about it, + he is getting very tired of their efforts. So we are trying what variations can be made of bully beef, onions, rice + bacon – with (sometimes) oatmeal + flour; tinned milk + dried vegetables.'[71]

Reggie Trench observed his men's diet with a well-practised eye. Three months into his service in France, he reported to his mother that he was 'experimenting on the Company in the food line', cooking up a spinach made of nettles, and boiling up young hops with margarine, which 'taste and look very much like young asparagus'. On another occasion he listed every single item of food served up to his men that day, concluding proudly, 'Not a bad day's feed is it? And all for [*sic*] the rations issued to us made up with a little care & forethought.'[72]

Promotion to Major in August 1917 gave Trench more scope for improving the men's diet. He was charged with supervising the messing arrangements of the Battalion, a task which he found 'very interesting', and which he embarked upon with characteristic energy.[73] The Army had established this function earlier in 1917, in response to the rising price of commodities during the war, which had led to cuts in the ration. Trench would have attended a short course in cookery as part of his training.[74] He wanted to relieve the monotony of Army food, and set up a battalion canteen whose stock was designed to 'satisfy all tastes'.[75] Such arrangements were not uncommon, but Trench took the idea a step further than most, returning the profits to the men in the form of comforts. In February 1918 he reported proudly to his mother that 'today each man in the front line got either an apple or a piece of chocc: or a packet of cigarettes!! Also I have enough papers to distribute two to every 7 men in the front line. This helps them to get thro' the day when not on sentry without getting too bored.'[76]

No problem, no matter how apparently insignificant, seems to have escaped Trench's impulse for domestic innovation. He designed his own cooker for use in the trenches.[77] He was very pleased when he managed to secure a lorry with which to deliver vegetables to the men, who had not had fresh cabbage since they came out.[78] Convinced of the merits of sausages in providing a 'pleasant variety for the men' (one result of the cuts in rations had been the substitution of rabbit and sausage for meat[79]), he tried to obtain a range of sausage-making attachments for the battalion mincing machine. He even got his mother involved, repeatedly asking her to visit a local ironmonger and see if such an attachment could be bought.[80] When this failed, he got one of the handymen to improvise a device, only then to find that sausage skins had become scarce. Consequently, he wrote to his mother, 'we shall have to roll the sausage meat in flour to get it to bind.' Trench was undeterred even when this scheme foundered, and finally hit on a solution: 'I have procured bigger skins which I intend to fill with meat, minced herbs, fat, bread & biscuit crumbs etc: these boil and serve in slices. I think it should be rather good & very portable and if the men like them I shall arrange for some to be made for sending up to us when we are in the trenches.'[81] For Trench, the satisfaction of soldiering lay as much in working out how best to get the men fed, as in more obviously military responsibilities.

In taking care of the men, subalterns could draw on the often considerable resources of their families. It was not unusual for an officer to supply the men in his platoon with cigarettes, sweets and other comforts, especially in the early years of the war, when foodstuffs were more plentiful, and when the mainstay of volunteer officers, drawn from the public-school-educated elite, were well heeled.[82] Reggie Hutt distributed cigarettes from home 'as follows: 23 signallers get 230, officers' servants at Headquarters get 70 (there are 7 of them) and the 350 remaining cigarettes go to the old platoon No. 15.'[83] Urwick's mother sent out regular parcels of socks to his men, and he wrote to her about some 'lonely soldiers' who might appreciate parcels.[84] Edward Chapman asked his mother to send comforts to his men, as many of them 'are very poor, and from the poorer parts of London, And I want to do all I can for them'.[85] Officers, animated by the ideal of 'noblesse oblige', sometimes used their own money to supply goods.[86] In a scene reminiscent of the squire and his bailiff dispensing charity to the villagers, Sassoon, finding that his men were short of cigarettes, bought some and got his batman to dole them out.[87] Charity could extend to the men's families, particularly in Territorial and Pals' battalions where local and military networks frequently overlapped. Vernon Merivale asked his mother to see if she could find work for some of the families of men in his platoon.[88] One of the men's wives had requested his help directly:

> The wife of 3670 Pte Easton J of my company writes saying that she is in great trouble as her daughter has become insane etc. She wants her husband to come home which is impossible. She lives at 67 Rothsay Terrace Bedlington. Would you mind asking the local secretary of the Relief Fund (or whatever its called) to look her up.[89]

Vernon Merivale had no compunction in calling on his mother to assist in a situation where family troubles were affecting the morale of one of his men. This kind of help, extending from the subaltern via his own family to the families of his men, drew on established middle-class networks of charitable support, bringing the battle and home fronts into a close relation.

How typical were men such as Vernon Merivale and Reggie Trench, who were energetic and capable in caring for their men? Some of the measures undertaken by officers – such as establishing the Battalion canteens which allowed the men more ready access to comforts such as chocolate, sweets and cigarettes – were voluntary, though they also supplied the officers, who tended to get preferential treatment.[90]

The historian J. G. Fuller, though he doubts whether British officers were as well regarded as they liked to think they were, acknowledges their success in setting up entertainments such as sporting events and concert parties.[91] When Wollocombe's men came out of the trenches at Meaulte, he strove to make their rest as comfortable as possible. Although he had been suffering from violent sickness and had 'felt rotten' the previous day, he busied himself with 'getting things ready for the company which came in about 1pm. Our men had no furniture, but I borrowed some chairs and a table from the YMCA.'[92] In some Battalions, officers made special provision for the men at Christmas. The officers of the Royal Welch Fusiliers subscribed to funds to buy them extras. On Christmas Day 1916 they had roast meat with potato, carrot, turnip and onion, an apple or orange, and nuts for their Christmas lunch, followed by cake, candied fruit and sweets, and a half-pound of Christmas pudding sent by the Comforts Committee.[93] Well-organised celebrations were not universal however, and the Royal Welch Fusiliers were probably better organised because they had been a Regular unit. George Coppard, in the Queen's Royal West Surrey Regiment, recalled his Christmas in the trenches in 1915. Their officer, Mr Clark, was killed early on Christmas Day, no post or parcels arrived, and the 'soggy rations were of the meanest kind, the only pretence at Christmas being a few raisins covered with hairs and other foreign matter from the inside of a sandbag.'[94] Grace-and-favour probably declined as the war continued, as many of the officers who were promoted from the ranks later in the war did not have the largesse of wealthy families to fall back on. After 1917, shortages and rationing made it difficult even for the more prosperous officer to supply his platoon.

Standards, in any case, varied widely. Many officers stayed in their dug-outs and left the 'housewifery' to their NCOs. Gladden's experience may not have been atypical: he had a four-month spell back in England in 1916 after developing septic ulcers on both his feet, which he blamed on 'the lackadaisical conditions' within the Battalion, a Territorial division of the Northumberland Fusiliers. They had endured long spells in inadequately drained trenches in wet and dirty clothing, with little shelter, and their officers 'never appeared unless there was some mission to perform.'[95] When he returned to another battalion of the Northumberland Fusiliers in 1917, however, he found a different world. The trenches were well organised, the rations arrived warm in proper containers, and they were efficiently and fairly distributed. These were 'well-organised units under officers who bothered about the welfare of their men and took their responsibilities seriously.'[96]

Crucial to the subaltern's identity was the idea of sacrifice. A good officer, reported General Crozier's batman, was one whose men came 'first with him all the time'.[97] When Reggie Trench was killed in battle in March 1918, the Captain charged with discovering the circumstances of his death wrote to Trench's wife conveying exactly this sentiment. 'His first thoughts were always for his officers and men'.[98] There could of course be an element of self-interest in being seen to go out of their way to help the men and one officer admitted that he sometimes offered to carry the men's packs when marching because 'it makes them love me'.[99] Donald Hankey was unusually frank about the advantages to be gained by seeming to appear altruistic: 'if ever you have a chance of showing that you are willing to share the often hard and sometimes humiliating lot of the men it is that which above all things will give you power over them.'[100]

The officer's moral universe was divided between the selfless and the egotistical. Often there was a subaltern among the Company who, in the view of his fellow officers, failed in his responsibilities towards the men. The intensity of life in the front line, and the small groups of officers who occupied the dug-out, contributed to strong feelings and allegiances. Wilfred Spencer got on well with Captain Rowe but not with the other subaltern in his company, who was 'not at all nice. No-one in the battalion likes him.' The man had come from another regiment and 'thinks too much of himself, making himself generally unpopular.'[101] The single-minded pursuit of promotion in others was widely criticised, even although most were themselves anxious to get on. Bion's commanding officer, 'Aitches', was always trying to 'curry favour with everyone'. 'Aitches' kept well clear when attacks were imminent and it was even 'discovered that he wore body armour under his tunic when he was still forty miles from the line. What he did when he reached the line was never quite clear. But by 1918 his name was a legend in the battalion for everything contemptible.'[102]

Such descriptions, which harped on the conspicuous failures of others, made the teller appear conscientious by comparison and deflected self-scrutiny. Yet personal failures were unavoidable. Sooner or later the subaltern would have the death or wounding of men on his conscience, and he would wonder what he might have done to avoid it. Gilbert Talbot was deeply upset after one of his NCOs died trying to retrieve the body of a dead German from the parados (bank behind the trench), the stench of which had been upsetting the men. The night the NCO was killed, Talbot 'nearly cried, and reproached himself for letting Sergeant Dawson go out on such a dangerous undertaking.'[103]

Wilfred Owen also felt the strain of not being able to protect his men. During his first experience of battle near Beaumont Hamel in January 1917, his platoon crouched for fifty hours in a dug-out forward of the British lines, under constant bombardment from the Germans. One of the sentries, a man whom Owen had rejected as a servant, was killed, and another was blown down the entrance tunnel into the dug-out and blinded. In a letter to his mother written shortly afterwards, Owen blamed himself for the sentry's death. If he had not rejected him, Owen reflected, 'he would have lived, for servants don't do Sentry Duty'.[104]

The subaltern's ability to care for his men was conditioned by the fact that it was also his job to discipline them. At the sound of the whistle that announced battle, the officer had to make his men go over the top, and he had to prevent them, sometimes at gunpoint, from retreating. Field punishments were handled by the Commanding Officer of the Battalion, but the majority of offences, from overstaying leave or absence from parade to drunkenness or self-inflicted wounds caused by negligence, could be dealt with by the Company Commander.[105] He might also have to initiate proceedings for more serious offences. Private Fox was Court Martialled and shot for threatening his Company Commander during a kit inspection. When the officer had pulled Fox up for having a dirty rifle and boots, Fox had kicked him.[106]

Caring for the men was emotionally exhausting, and sometimes these young officers balked at the task. Gary Sheffield reports the case of an officer who, when censoring his men's letters, read that one was intending to approach him for advice about his family problems. The officer went into 'a most horrible funk' and tried to avoid the man.[107] Even an older and more experienced man might blanch at the painful tasks he had to undertake. After Reggie Trench received 'such a pathetic letter' from the mother of his dead friend Alliban, he agonised about how to respond. '[W]hat can I do', he appealed to his mother, 'I can't tell her any more than I have told her; that news is bad enough. I don't know what to do and his loss is very great to me.' In despair he asked his mother if she would write. Grieving himself over the loss of his good friend, and with no-one left in the Battalion 'to discuss things with now', he simply had no capacity for sympathy left. [108]

As Gladden's contrasting tales of the Northumberland Fusiliers suggest, officers' ability to care for their men varied widely. Regular battalions (in the early years of the war before they became diluted) and Territorial units certainly had greater experience and expertise in matters of day-to-day survival. At the same time many temporary officers were anxious to learn how to look after the men, and proud of what they achieved. Much depended on the lead given by the senior officers in the Battalion, the make-up of the particular company or platoon, and the individual characters of subaltern officers and NCOs. The memoirs of two rankers, Charles Taylor, Clerk of Works at the London Docks, and the railway worker George Fortune, point to the variations. The socialist Fortune thought his officers and NCOs were 'wonderful the way they used to do their duty. They were always watching over us and seeing we got a hot drink.'[109] The retired manager Taylor 'did not see much of our officers. They used to visit us in the front line while we were at work and where they went to after that we did not know.'[110] Try as the Army might to introduce uniform standards, the subaltern's 'housewifery' on the Western Front, like the management of domestic affairs within his family home, depended a lot on individual ability and the character of personal relationships.

## Looking after the officers

Underpinning the officer's care of his men was another kind of service whose anonymous drudgery contrasted with the officer's heightened moral purpose. Every regimental officer, from the Second Lieutenant to the General, had the right to a batman. Essentially he was a manservant, and in selecting possible recruits, the Army looked for previous experience of service. In practice however the job was more wide-ranging than most servants in a comfortable middle-class household would have been used to: the batman was valet, butler and cook rolled into one.

His regular tasks out of the line included waking his officer in the mornings or when he was due to go on duty, providing hot water to wash or bathe, making his bed and tidying up, keeping his uniform clean (ex-batmen particularly recall the polishing of buttons, belt and boots), packing his things when the Battalion was on the move and lugging them about, and dispatching unwanted items to the officer's family when the seasons changed. General Crozier's servant, David Starrett, spent his time 'getting his shaving water, cleaning belt and his boots, keeping room or tent or dug-out tidy, running his errands.'[111] George Hewins claimed to have been selected as a batman because he could shave and cut hair.[112]

The batman took on additional responsibilities in the line, securing billets or dug-outs for his officer, and preparing the officer's meals when it was impossible to get food up the line. It was hard work keeping the officer looking smart and more than a half century after the war, Coppard and Starrett recalled the effort involved in scraping the mud off their officers' uniforms.[113] In addition there were some military considerations, for the batman was meant to stay by his officer's side in battle. Owen remarked to his mother (perhaps rather devilishly) that his choice of batman had been dictated by the man's 'excellence in bayonet work'.[114]

Being a batman had some advantages. They were paid and were usually given tips. They learned new skills. Eric Marchant enjoyed being Captain Green's batman for, as he explained to his mother, 'I really think I have picked up a bit by taking on that job that I didn't know before, you wait till you've seen me wash up! Also make beds!'[115] They were exempt from many of the parades and drill that made the ranker's life out of the line a misery, and, perhaps the most important advantage, they had access to the officers' mess or dug-out, and thus to warmth, shelter from the rain, additional protection from shells and better food. 'I fancied the Officer's Mess', said George Hewins when explaining why he had opted to become a batman rather than be promoted to Corporal, which paid better.[116] The 'creature comforts' of the officers, and an income of at least half a crown a week, were the principal attractions for Coppard.[117] Arthur Hubbard looked forward to cigarettes, good food and tinned fruit, all of which would help save his mother money in parcels.[118]

At the same time the job was unremitting and physically taxing. Alfred Hale ended up working as a batman during 1917–18 and in 1922 he wrote a long memoir of his war. An ex-Uppingham boy and a musical composer, Hale was conscripted when the Military Service Act came into force in January 1916, along with other unmarried men between the ages of eighteen and forty-one. On joining the Royal Flying Corps he was classified as 'C2' – fit only for service in home camps – and most of his military service was spent within Britain.

A less suitable batman than Hale would be hard to imagine. He could barely carry his own kit bag, so the officer's hold-all, with its heavy roll-up bed and canvas basin, was 'too heavy by far for me or any other middle-aged category man.'[119] Hale struggled to make himself, let alone his officer, presentable. On the first occasion he used an Army razor he cut his face about so badly he was told to present himself to the Flight Sergeant every day for inspection.[120]

Hale was unusual in being able to see the relationship between batmen and officers from both sides. A man of independent means, he employed a housekeeper at his cottage in Hampshire. Though he gathered together his officer's washing to be sent to the camp laundry on a Monday morning, he sent his own washing – including his pillowcases – home to Mrs Ling each week. She would return it the following week with a parcel of his favourite foods, including eggs, 'tiny loaves cut in half ready spread with butter, some with jam, the two halves arriving sandwiched together' and fruit from his garden.[121]

Hale's working days in camp near Bedford were long. The batmen woke with the first whistle at 6.30. After rolling up and putting away their blankets and straw mattresses they dressed and washed in a tin basin in the kitchen yard. They would then creep quietly into the officers' tents and fetch their tunics, belts and boots, which had to be polished. Hot water would be begged from the kitchen so the officers could wash, but if the cook was in a bad mood they had to light the kitchen boiler themselves. The officers' slops had to be emptied out and their tents brushed out and tidied. Hale often felt hungry in the mornings, because the batmen had to serve the officers' breakfasts before they were permitted to eat their own, and the officers were often late risers. He sometimes managed to get an hour or so to read in the afternoon before tea, but the head batman worried that they might be spotted by an officer, so they were often put to trivial duties. Tea was the 'one bright spot' in the day, the cook's temper by then being mollified, and there was plenty of jam, bread, butter and tea. Hale's overriding memories were of lugging buckets of water around the camp, and lighting fires for the officers' stoves, baths and the camp kitchen.[122] His hands became cracked with the constant polishing and washing. Such was the life of a batman, 'the lowest and most despised being in the Royal Flying Corps.'[123]

Because of his age and privileged background, Hale suffered from bullying. Soon after his arrival in the training camp at Thetford most of his kit and personal effects were stolen.[124] From the start of his time at Bedford, 'nothing I could do was right'. The cook conspired with the head batman to short-ration him, and he was given the jobs they did not want. Early tea was poured for the other batmen but Hale had to wait until breakfast for his.[125] Later, his fellow batmen moved Hale's bed from the centre of the tent to the entrance, which caught the freezing wind and rain, and installed their beds where his had been. This, reported Hale, 'made me more miserable than I can put into words.'[126] For Hale the job of batman was a 'sore bondage', not only because he was a conscript but because he was always at others' beck and call. Some of his fellow rankers agreed: one, on hearing that he was destined to become a batman, remarked that he had tried it and found it a 'rotten business. "You're never off duty", he said.'[127]

Being party to the officer's privileges could make batmen resentful. Though on the whole Hale liked his officer, he wished he could enjoy the same facilities for washing and shaving, and the same food. Mr Cowper was able to lie in and take afternoon naps, but Hale was kept busy simply for the sake of it.[128] Hale's background probably made him more openly resentful of his officers than others, who were fascinated by the comparative luxury of the officers and hoped to enjoy some of it. Coppard, who joined the Royal West Surrey Regiment at sixteen and became a machine gunner, took on the job of batman in early 1916 because he was a 'domesticated person', and wanted the opportunity to see things from the officer's point of view. On his visits to the Company Headquarters he was amazed to see the life that the officers led, with proper bedding and 'room to stretch out to sleep.' Batmen were on hand to serve whatever they wanted and there were unlimited supplies of cigarettes, rum and Old Orkney whiskey, or, as the troops called it, 'Officers Only.'[129]

Though they shared the same spaces, batmen were rarely at ease in the company of their officers. Coppard was struck by the stark differences between the subalterns' 'creature comforts' and 'the almost complete absence of them for the men', and it was not long before he opted to go back to the ranks: 'Being a batman had its good points but somehow I felt less than a complete soldier, for though there was almost as much danger in the job there was certainly more personal comfort. I was glad to be back in the team. The little pin-pricks they had occasionally dished out about my having a cushy job ceased.'[130] Outnumbered in the mess or dug-out by his superiors, cut off from his comrades and sometimes resented by them for his easy conditions, the batman was neither one thing nor the other.

Officers sometimes had inflated expectations of their batman. Roland Leighton got his batman to write his letters out for him after he cut his finger slightly, while Will Hate was made to carry his officers' souvenirs after Neuve Chapelle.[131] The military guide *Straight Tips For 'Subs'* reminded the subaltern that his batman was 'a soldier more than a servant and should be treated as such . . . If you overwork him you should overpay him.' It issued a note of warning: the subaltern who over-taxed his batmen would give him cause for discontent and 'your back-slidings will be duly re-counted by him to the men of your company.'[132] Army officials worried that temporary officers lacked the paternalistic outlook of the Regular officer, and would fail to look after the batman's welfare.[133] A Regular officer in the Royal Welch Fusiliers noted a batman struggling up to the front line with his Company Commander's valise and bedding, muttering '"God strike me, and (obscene) the (obscenity) what's got this kit."'[134] The kit probably belonged to one of the pampered 'chocolate soldiers' of the old 20th Battalion.

Officers tended to commend their batmen only if they did something out of the ordinary to make them comfortable. Simply doing the domestic chores was not enough. H. A. Munro recorded the efforts of his batman: 'DANGER! THIS DUG-OUT IS MINED! So ran a notice carried by Graham and used by him on entering a trench to lay an early and permanent claim on a good dug-out for me.'[135] Owen reported to his mother how, after being on the march and reaching a village where no billets had been prepared, his new batman had managed to find a 'fine hut, with a little chair in it!' He 'keeps a jolly fire going', he later reported, thieving wood 'with much cunning'. Owen was irritated when his batman did 'nothing off his own bat', but praised him when he used his 'enterprise and initiative' to make him more comfortable.[136]

The job could be frustrating for the batman because his officer's individual likes and dislikes counted for so much. Small matters assumed inordinate importance. Did he like his porridge smooth or lumpy, his bacon lean or fatty? On one occasion when Hale had to rise at 4 a.m. to bring a cup of tea to Captain Ross' bedroom, he was bawled out because his Army boots made too much noise. The bawling out continued when Ross received his tea: 'You know I don't like milk. Take it back and bring another cup.'[137]

When men were on the move, or occupying muddy trenches, in leaky dug-outs and surviving wholly on rations, it was difficult to protect the officer entirely from discomfort. Rather than blame the conditions, however, officers were apt to blame the batman. Greenwell was annoyed that he was unable to shave during a heavy bombardment, as his batman 'can't get near me or doesn't' want to.'[138] Wilfred Owen's first batman managed to wipe mud all over his belongings; his successor, when Owen went on a Transport course, forgot to pack his photographs and poems, leading Owen to regret that, in taking the man with him, he had effectively given him a holiday from the front. A lower-middle-class, New Army temporary in an ex-Regular Battalion, Owen seems to have been particularly keen that his batmen recognised the status conferred by a commission: part of his objection to the man was that he 'doesn't always "jump to" my orders!'[139] But there was an element of the familial, as well as of class tension, in this kind of grumbling; indeed, Owen, like many other officers, included his batmen within the wider networks of his family. When his batman went on home leave, Owen had no compunction in giving him an entrée to the family home, Mahim, even although the man had only just been assigned to Owen, and was 'a 'scratch' batman not my choice'.[140] Officers' complaints about their batmen were part of what made the relationship familiar, resembling as they did, pre-war complaints about the failings of domestic servants or – indeed – of their own mothers.

His menial role and inevitable failures made the batman a comic figure among the officers. Hale remembered the reaction when he and his fellow batmen, aggrieved because their right to be excused from parade had been over-ruled, staged a sit-down protest: 'They seemed to regard it as a sort of joke. After all, a batman himself is a subject for joking, when one comes to think of it, although he may not always see the point of the jest.'[141] Hale's observation was astute. In R. C. Sherriff's famous play of 1928, *Journey's End*, the comic action centres on the batman Mason's feeble attempts to make Army rations more appetising. When the ex-schoolteacher Osborne asks Mason, who is heating yet another meal of ration meat, 'What are you going to tempt us with tonight?', the joke is entirely lost on Mason.[142]

Despite all the difficulties and frustrations of class differences and inhospitable conditions, officers and batmen might come to feel a degree of mutual consideration, even affection. As their respective memoirs reveal, David Starrett and General Crozier were clearly fond of each other, though their relationship was both unusually long-lasting, and bolstered by the paternalistic traditions of the Regular Army. Starrett was at pains in his memoirs to counter the public image of Crozier as 'Mad Jack', stressing his kindness and forgiving attitude towards Starrett's own lapses of discipline and his bad temper. Crozier's feelings about Starrett were equally positive. He was 'the faithful one.'[143]

Closer relations between the batman and his officer were likely to develop in the trenches, where the weight of Army hierarchy was less visible and the batman's duties towards his officer were greater. In the trenches Coppard grew 'attached' to Captain Wilkie, who 'regarded me as a comrade.'[144] Hewins' affection for Captain Edwards had grown in the trenches, where 'we'd had many a chat'.[145] At the same time, when supplies were poor and loyalty to the officer might conflict with self-preservation, the *limits* of care were also exposed. After five months on the Western Front, the exposure to shelling, cold rations and the elements were taking their toll on both Captain Leland and his batman, Hilton. Leland writes to his wife on 13 July 1917:

> I am feeling a wee bit better but still very rotten. I have got what I hardly ever suffer from. A d---d bad headache and no appetite. Probably the sun has a bit to do with it, but I think that the stink, the flies, and the dust, are principally to blame. I feel very sick, and my temper is vile, and I pour with perspiration at the least annoyance.

Leland felt a little resentful of his batman, who, at the very moment when he was feeling poorly, was engrossed in his own problems:

> Hilton is damnably annoying, and never thinks of anything. He loses my handkerchiefs and collars, and I can get nothing clean to put on. You can imagine what that means when I come in tired and soaked to the skin with sweat. He sulks when I swear at him and says that he has a headache, or stomachache [*sic*] or some such nonsense, for he does nothing but overeat himself.[146]

Hilton's own maladies were actually rather similar to Leland's, but he could spare little sympathy for the batman. The two men seemed to be competing over who was the most deserving: what particularly riled Leland was that Hilton seemed to be taking the lion's share of their scarce rations.

Conditions continued to be difficult through the summer. Rations were short for much of the time and when Leland visited the dug-out of some officers in the Staffords, who laid on the 'finest dinner I have had for a long while', this only served to rouse resentment about his own domestic hardships, and Hilton's part in them. His own dug-out was a 'pig-stye'. Hilton 'is as big a fool as ever, and spends most of his time in the Estimanet, and making excuses to me for not being able to get this or that thing done. If he had not been so long with me I would have sacked him long ago, but I have no time or patience to train another man even if I could procure one.'[147]

Ten days later, taking pity on Hilton, Leland took him out 'for company' on another visit to the Staffords' dug-out. The spread they laid out made Leland feel 'I might have been a little God', but Hilton disgraced himself by getting lost on the way home and spending the night in a ditch. 'He is absolutely no use to me as he is very "windy". Shells are certainly raining very heavily upon us, but I do think ones [*sic*] servant should "stand by". He simply goes to ground, and nothing can unearth him.'[148]

When Hilton re-appeared in dug-outs, he was incapable of cooking. Leland asked him to make some soup, but it was 'awful stuff':

> He seemed to have mixed it with stable manure. He produced a bit of meat afterwards calling it steak. I asked what was wrong with it as it looked so enemic [*sic*]? He said that is what I made the soup out of, and there is nothing more. I am afraid I lost my temper with him. He has now got the hump.[149]

Though Leland was exasperated with Hilton, he thought he knew why the batman was behaving in this way, and was not censorious when Hilton asked to be let off sick: 'I am very sorry for him. He can't help it, but he does annoy me. He is not a coward, but his nerve has quite gone, and so, I'm afraid is mine!'[150] Eventually, after Hilton went missing, Leland decided that his groom, who is 'very kind and attentive to me', should become his batman. Rather than dismiss Hilton, Leland appointed him temporary groom.[151] Hilton was angry at his demotion, and naturally envied the new batman, but in fact Leland had treated Hilton relatively lightly by not reporting his absence, and not sending him back to the ranks. Leland was genuinely concerned for his batman. Their 'rough times together' had brought the relationship to the point of breakdown, but had also left a reservoir of loyalty on both sides.[152]

The officer and his batman faced the same dangers in the front line, and this, as much as traditions of service and deference, shaped the relationship. The batman was usually close to his officer's side during battle, and might be the first person to come to his assistance if the officer was wounded. Marshall, a Regular soldier in the Coldstream Guards, tended his officer when he was hit in the stomach by sniper fire. He helped carry Leveson-Gower back to the Casualty Clearing station, and was at his side in hospital when he succumbed to 'a sleep from which he never awoke'. He would 'see him laid to rest to-morrow.' The loss affected Marshall deeply. As he explained: 'I am an old soldier, having served in Africa under several Officers, and your son is the third

Officer I have been batman to in this Campaign, and I cannot find words to express my sorrow this night.'[153]

When Second Lieutenant H. A. Munro was killed trying to pull a booby-trapped German flag down from No Man's Land, his batman collected Munro's watch and diary to pass on to his family. He took up the diary where Munro had left off, explaining how Munro had died and how they had marked his death:

> Friday 11am. Under Lieutenant Disselduff we laid him to Rest in a little Churchyard side by side with some of his departed comrades of the 8th Argylls. A kind and thoughtful Master to B. Graham.[154]

Graham used the diary as a means of keeping Munro's family in touch, supplying information about their son's death that he knew they would be anxious to hear. The diary also became, in Graham's hands, a personal tribute to his officer.

Accounts of wounded batmen being tended to or visited by their officers are not unknown, but this type of loyalty was expected principally from the batman, not his officer.[155] After all, the officer had his platoon or company to look after, not just his batman. Acting on such assumptions, the families of officers often initiated correspondence with the batman after a son's death, assuming that he would have the fullest knowledge of his last moments, and trusting that his feelings of loyalty would extend to them.[156] Captain Edwards' father, stricken by grief, was willing to pay for contact with anyone who had been close to his son during the war. George Hewins, even although he usually exploited every possible chance of financial gain when dealing with middle-class people, decided on this occasion not to continue the correspondence. Perhaps he was unwilling take advantage of the bereaved father, in deference to Captain Edwards, who he regarded as a 'nice chap', although he never tipped. Or perhaps Hewins did not wish to be reminded of his own war, and the shell blast that had blown away his privates and made him infertile.[157]

Reggie Trench's batman, Albert Lane, a miner in civilian life, was in effect treated as a member of Trench's household. When it looked as if Trench might get home on a staff course in Aldershot, his wife Clare rented a house close by and suggested that Lane should live in.[158] On 21 March 1918, with the German advance in full swing, and just before both men were due to return to England, Lane was delivering a message behind the lines when he heard that Trench had been hit. Lane ran back up the line as fast as he could, to find Trench already dead, lying face down in the trench. He had been shot through the head. The Colonel had told Lane to take any personal effects from Trench's body so they could be given to his wife. Lane took the watch from Trench's wrist, and was getting the signet ring from his little finger when the stretcher bearers arrived and told him to leave the body alone. Lane watched as they buried Trench on the side of a sunken lane. He wrote to Mrs Trench: 'I never felt so awful in my life and have felt it very much indeed.'[159] Later that day Lane was taken prisoner. He kept Trench's watch concealed in his sock or in the sole of his shoe for the next six months while quarrying stone in a POW camp.

Lane visited Clare Trench after the war to tell her about Reggie's last moments and return the watch, its glass broken but otherwise in 'perfect working order'. Clare's daughter, Delle, recalls that her mother wore the watch until the very end of her life, when her wrist became too thin. Delle herself had no direct memory of what had happened to her father as she was only three at the time. It was Lane who, while staying nearby with relatives one year, visited mother and daughter in Eastbourne, and told Delle how her father had died. Shortly afterwards Delle wrote the account down, and it was this that, at the age of ninety-two, she now repeated for me.[160] Her gratitude to Lane, for passing on his recollections of a father she barely knew, animates her letter.

The urge to stay in touch did not necessarily diminish over time, as men settled back into civilian life. In the papers of Captain Carpenter is a photograph of two old men, probably taken in the 1970s, standing side by side in a small backyard, surrounded by roses, and dwarfed by a factory in the background. The man on the right is Carpenter, bent over a walking frame. He is of a more stocky build than his comrade, and wears a cardigan and open-necked shirt. His ex-batman is dressed more formally with a tie under his cardigan, pinned neatly to his shirt. He stands erect, a model of military bearing.[161] Much in the image cannot be explained: whose house is it, who contacted whom? However, the fact that officer and batman were in touch sixty years after the war, that they had turned themselves out for the occasion; and were at ease together in this domestic setting, suggests something about the continuing significance of their wartime contact.

How do we explain the sentiments that prompted the batman to keep in touch with his officer, or the officer's 'affectionate interest', as Leland called it, in his batman? What were the social and emotional sources of this care? Chapter 4 investigates the origins of these powerful systems of domestic labour and attachment in the family lives of civilian soldiers.

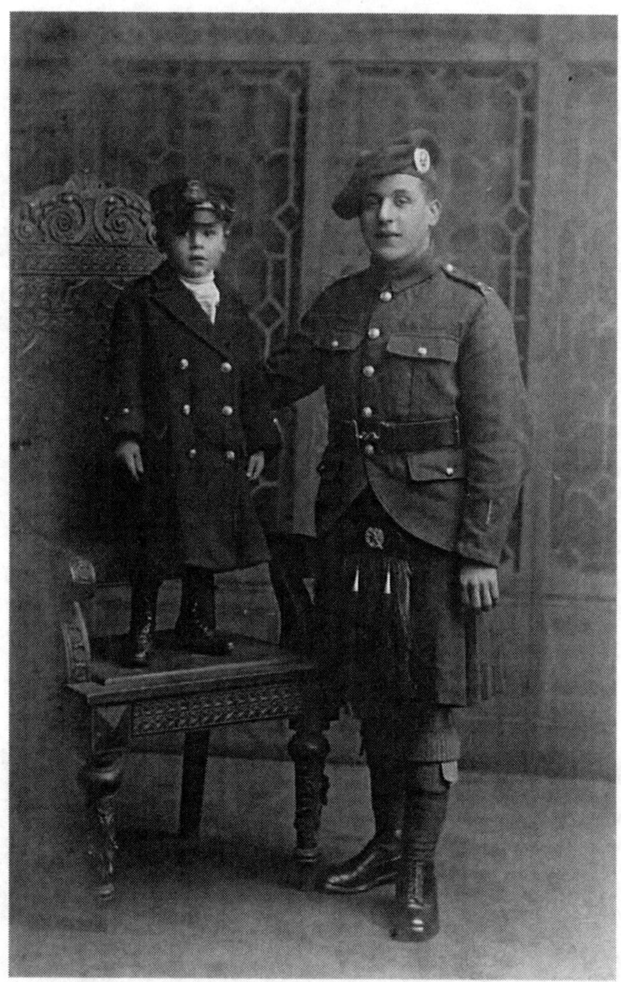

9 Arthur Hubbard in the uniform of the 1st London Scottish. The difference between the real soldier Arthur, and the boy playing at soldiers – possibly Hubbard's brother – is accentuated by the seat on which the latter stands, but they are separated in age by little more than a decade

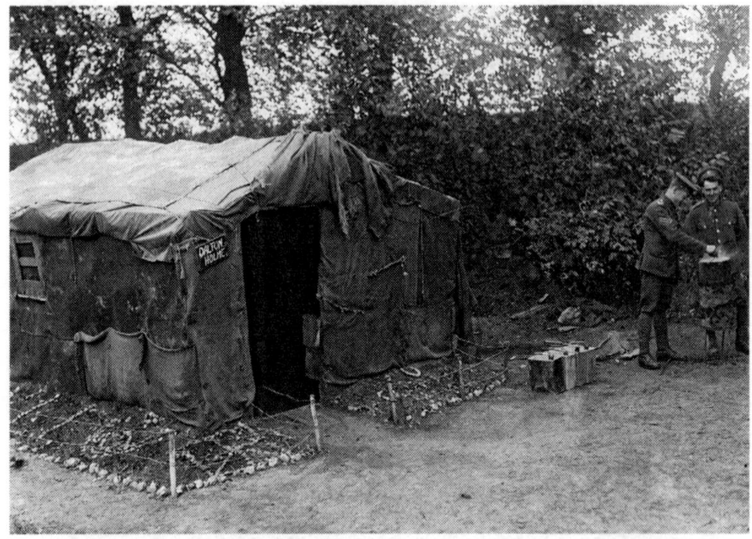


*10* A corporal of the King's Own Yorkshire Light Infantry prepares dinner outside his hut, 1917. Note the rockery and fence around 'Dalton Holme'

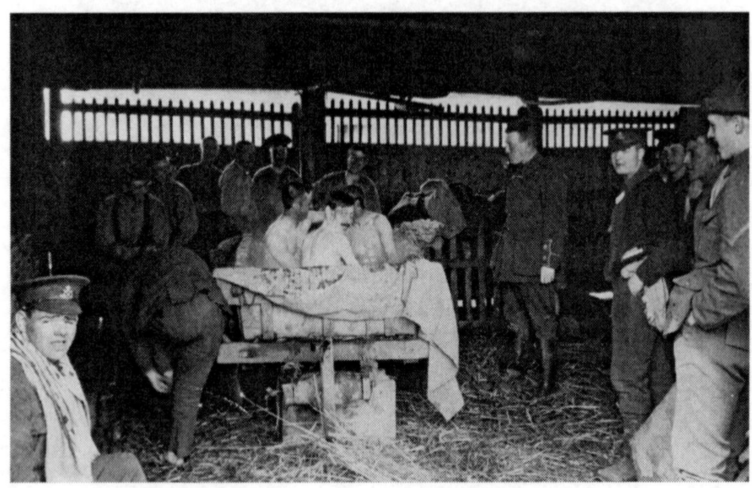

*11* Men of the 1/6$^{th}$ Battalion, South Staffordshire Regiment having a bath in an old cart, the water having been heated in biscuit tins, 1915

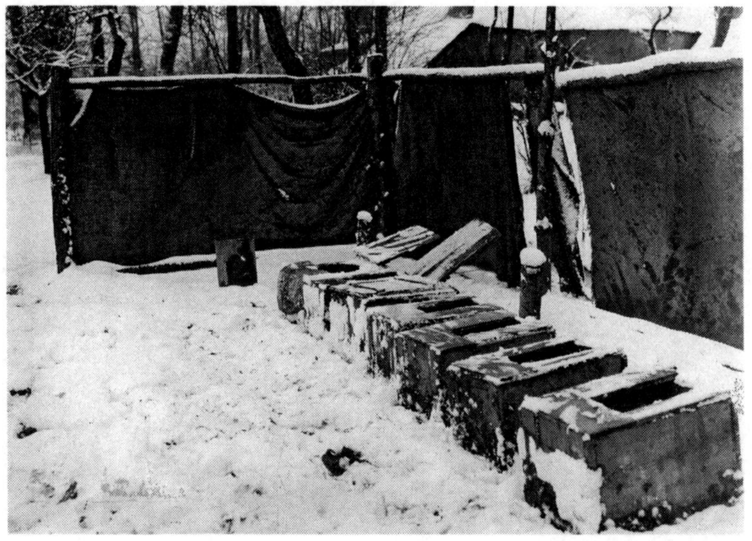

*12* Latrines at Lealvillers, 17 January 1917

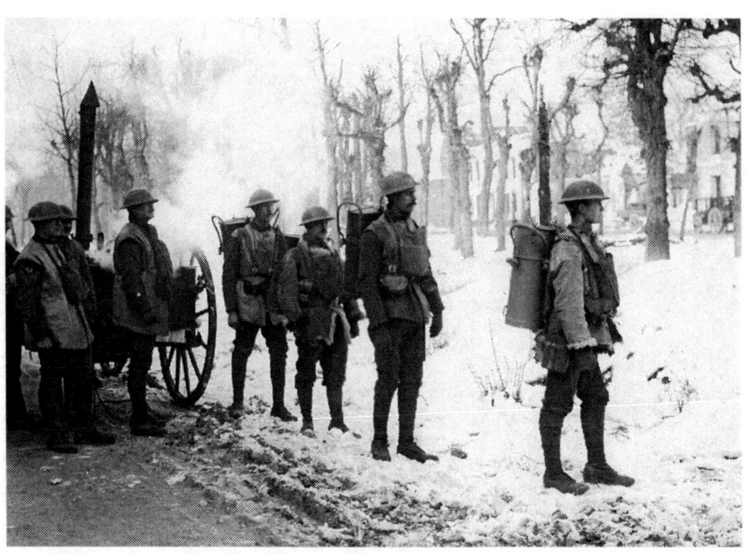

*13* A ration party carries soup containers from the field cooker, Arras, March 1917

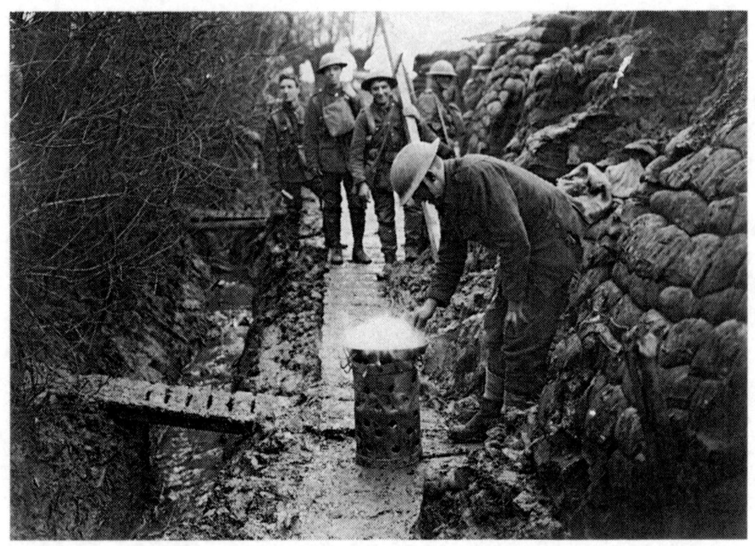

*14* Lancashire Fusiliers fry bacon on a brazier in a reserve trench, March 1917

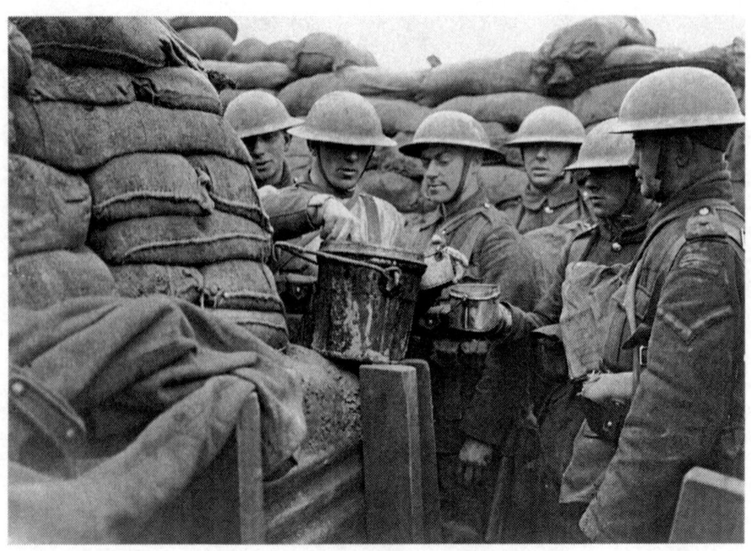

*15* Serving stew to men of the Lancashire Fusiliers in a front-line trench near Ploegsteert Wood, March 1917

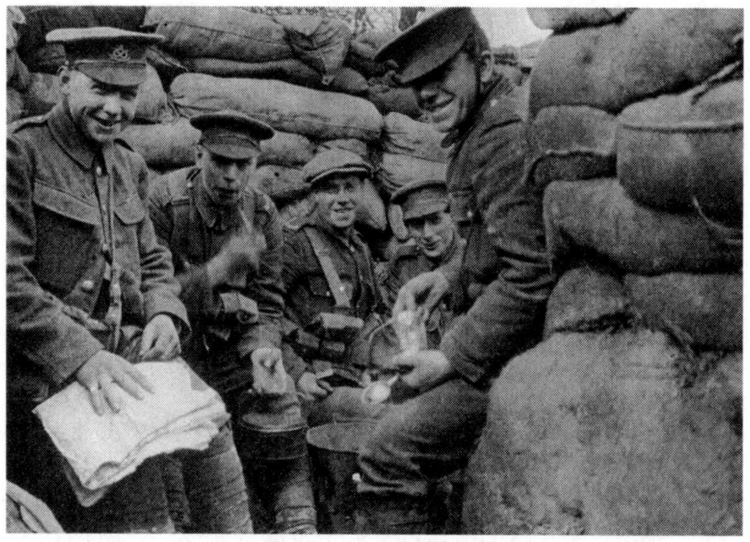

*16* Men of 'C' Company, 1/6th Batallion, South Staffordshire Regiment in No. 8 Trench, Messines Road, 1915

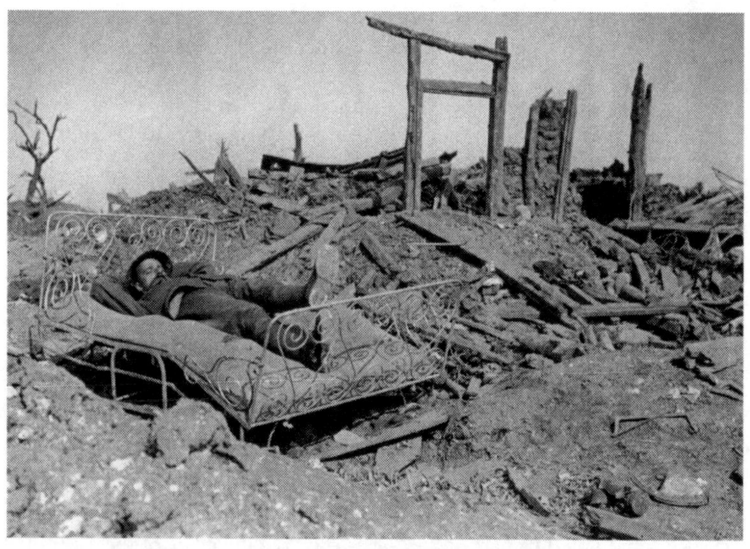

*17* Man sleeping on bed among ruins at Morval, September 1916

## Notes

1 R. Trench to mother, 15 February 1917, private collection.
2 Trench to mother, date illegible, March 1917.
3 Trench to mother, 30 April 1917.
4 Trench to mother, 10 May 1917. The domestic concerns of Reggie Trench are vividly described by his grandson, Anthony Fletcher, 'An Officer on the Western Front', *History Today*, Vol. 54, No. 8 (August 2004), pp. 31–7.
5 E. Leed, *No Man's Land. Combat and Identity in World War I* (Cambridge: Cambridge University Press, 1979), p. 195.
6 R. D. Mountfort to mother, 26 May 1916, IWM Con Shelf.
7 See R. Holmes on food, *Tommy. The British Soldier on the Western Front 1914–1918* (London: Harper Perennial, 2005), pp. 314–15.
8 T. Ashworth, *Trench Warfare 1914–1918. The Live and Let Live System* (London: Macmillan, 1980), pp. 24–5. '[T]he war lapsed' during breakfast, wrote Guy Chapman. *A Passionate Prodigality. Fragments of Autobiography* (New York: Holt, Rinehart & Winston, 1966), p. 29.
9 Trench to mother, 13 April 1917.
10 J. G. Fuller, *Troop Morale and Popular Culture in the British and Dominion Armies* (Oxford: Clarendon Press, 1991), pp. 48–9.
11 I. Bet-El, *Conscripts. Forgotten Men of the Great War* (Stroud: Sutton Publishing, 2003), p. 14.
12 D. Winter, *Death's Men. Soldiers of the Great War* (London: Penguin, 1979), p. 99; J. Ellis, *Eye Deep in Hell. Trench Warfare in World War I* (Baltimore: Johns Hopkins University Press, 1976), p. 51.
13 C. Carrington, *Soldier From the Wars Returning* (London: Arrow Books, 1965), p. 141.
14 On collapsing dug-outs see G. Greenwell, *An Infant in Arms. War Letters of a Company Commander 1914–1918* (London: Allen Lane, The Penguin Press, 1972), p. 71.
15 J. C. Dunn (ed.), *The War the Infantry Knew. A Chronicle of Service in France and Belgium* (London: Abacus, 1994). Introduction by Keith Simpson, p. xxv.
16 Dunn (ed.), *The War the Infantry Knew*, p. 314.
17 Dunn (ed.), *The War the Infantry Knew*, p. 318.
18 Trench to mother, 2 June 1917.
19 Winter, *Death's Men*, p. 59.
20 G. Talbot, *Gilbert Walter Lyttleton Talbot. Born September 1 1891. Killed in Action at Hooge, July 30 1915* (London: Chiswick Press, 1916), p. 51. Criticism of the soldiering skills of the Territorials, originally peacetime volunteers, was common among Regulars, although in fact Talbot's Rifle Brigade battalion, the Seventh, was actually formed as a Service Battalion in 1914 and was thus part of the New Army. On the ethos of the Territorial Forces see Gary Sheffield, *Leadership in the Trenches. Officer–Man Relations,*

*Morale and Discipline in the British Army in the Era of the First World War* (Basingstoke: Palgrave, 2000), pp. 156–9.

21 Winter, *Death's Men*, p. 100.

22 G. Coppard, *With A Machine Gun to Cambrai. A Story of the First World War* (London: Cassell, 1980), p. 68.

23 Bet-El, *Conscripts*, p. 113.

24 On the importance that food assumed see N. Gladden, *Ypres 1917* (London: William Kimber, 1967), p. 96. For discussion of the problems of provision and the reactions of rank-and-file soldiers to army rations see Rachel Duffett, '"I believe 'e'd sell 'imself for a tin o' toffee": The Significance of Food in the Memoirs of the Rank and File Soldiers of the First World War', MA dissertation, Department of History, University of Essex, 2005; and 'A War Unimagined: Food and the Rank and File Soldier of the First World War', in J. Meyer (ed.), *Popular Culture and the First World War* (Leiden: Brill, 2007), pp. 49–60.

25 See, for example, A. Hewins (ed.), *The Dillen. Memories of a Man of Stratford upon Avon* (Oxford: Oxford University Press, 1983), p. 142.

26 E. K. Smith, who served in the ranks of the Artists' Rifles prior to his officer training, described army food as 'no doubt absolutely wholesome, but one gets very tired of it especially when there is no variety to speak of.' E. K. Smith to mother, 9 February 1915, *Letters Sent From France. Service with the Artists' Rifles and the Buffs, December 1914–December 1915* (London: J. Cobb, 1994), p. 20. George Coppard recalled the unpopularity of plum and apple jam:

> Tickler's Jam, Tickler's jam,
> How I love old Tickler's jam,
> Plum and apple in a one pound pot,
> Sent from Blighty in a ten ton lot.
> Every night when I'm asleep,
> I'm dreaming that I am,
> Forcing my way through the Dardanelles,
> With a ton of Tickler's jam. (*With A Machine Gun*, p. 43)

27 P. Smith to Mother and dad, 18 September 1917, IWM 02/21/1. The standard of Army food may have been uneven, but it was generally only during particular military crises, such as the Spring retreat and Summer advance of 1918, when supply lines were not properly established, that men went hungry. See Bet-El, *Conscripts*, pp. 115–16.

28 Gladden, *Ypres*, p. 16.

29 Coppard, *With A Machine Gun*, p. 43.

30 D. H. Fenton to Willie, 8 August 1915, IWM 87/13/1.

31 Coppard, *With A Machine Gun*, p. 96.

32 E. M. Remarque, *All Quiet on the Western Front* (London: Vintage, 1996), p. 69.

33 F. Manning, *Her Privates We* (London: Serpent's Tail, 1999), p. 65, p. 172.
34 After a day or two in Barracks, jostling for food and drinking tea from a soup plate, Coppard, 'realised that I had left the simple decencies of the table at home.' *With A Machine Gun*, p. 2.
35 H. McCartney, *Citizen Soldiers. The Liverpool Territorials in the First World War* (Cambridge: Cambridge University Press, 2005), p. 181.
36 H. J. C. Leland to wife, 16 September 1917, IWM 96/51/1.
37 Gladden, *Ypres*, pp. 16–17.
38 F. Richards, *Old Soldiers Never Die* (Uckfield: Naval and Military Press, 1994), p. 198.
39 Coppard, *With A Machine Gun*, p. 55.
40 Dunn (ed.), *The War the Infantry Knew*, p. 253.
41 R. Christoper to mother, 9 September 1916, IWM 88/11/1.
42 C. Ramsdale to mother, 11 October 1918, IWM Con Shelf.
43 C. Christoper to mother, 16 December 1915, IWM 88/11/1.
44 Fenton to Willie, 20 August 1915. See also Coppard on the consumption of absent pals' parcels, *With A Machine Gun*, p. 45.
45 Richards, F., *Old Soldiers*, pp. 213–14.
46 A. P. Herbert, *The Secret Battle* (Thirsk: House of Stratus, 2001), p. 53.
47 Herbert, *The Secret Battle*, p. 54.
48 In *Her Privates We*, Bourne's comrades jeer as one parcel and letter after another is passed to him. '"Dyou want the whole bloody lot?", someone cried.' (Manning, p. 199.)
49 Willis Brown to mother, 15 June 1915, IWM 01/52/1.
50 Dunn (ed.), *The War the Infantry Knew*, p. 168.
51 Dunn (ed.), *The War the Infantry Knew*, pp. 203–4.
52 A. H. Trapmann, *Straight Tips for 'Subs'* (London: Forester Groom, 1916), p. 25.
53 A. Gibbs to mother, 2 January 1916, IWM P317.
54 Greenwell to mother, 24 May 1915, *An Infant in Arms*, p. 15. After buying supplies for the Mess, allotting huts to the NCOs, putting out all the valises of C. Company's officers – replete with hot water bottles – and generally making 'things look as cosy as possible', the Mess President Geoffrey Thurlow commented to Vera Brittain, 'Really I'm getting quite domesticated!' G. Thurlow to V. Brittain, 30 December 1916, in A. Bishop and M. Bostridge (eds.), *Letters From a Lost Generation. First World War Letters of Vera Brittain and Four Friends* (London: Abacus, 1999), p. 309.
55 R. Foulkes to Ma, 1 October 1915, IWM 82/4/1.
56 L. Hall to mother and father, 9 March 1917, IWM 96/57/1.
57 Gibbs to mother, Christmas Day 1915.
58 E. F. Chapman to mother, 25 February 1917, IWM Con Shelf.
59 L. Urwick to mother, 9 November 1917, private collection.
60 Winter, *Death's Men*, p. 99.

61 Carrington, *Soldier From the* Wars, p. 132, p. 170.
62 Trench to mother, 26 April, 30 April 1917.
63 Chapman, *A Passionate Prodigality*, p. 217.
64 E.g. Dunn (ed.), *The War the Infantry Knew*, p. 285.
65 E. K. Smith to mother, 6 October, 12 November, 22 November 1915, *Letters Sent From France*, pp. 105–6, p. 121, p. 125.
66 W. B. P. Spencer to mother, 26 December 1914, IWM 87/56/1.
67 Cited in A. Simpson, *Hot Blood and Cold Steel. Life and Death in the Trenches of the First World War* (London: Tom Donovan, 1993), pp. 141–2.
68 W. R. Bion, *War Memoirs 1917–19* (London: H. Karnac, 1997), p. 60.
69 Bet-El, *Conscripts*, p. 129; Fuller, *Troop Morale*, p. 61.
70 F. Merivale to mother, 21 December 1917, in J. H. Merivale papers, IWM P471.
71 J. H. Merivale diary, 30 December 1915, IWM P471.
72 Trench to mother, 10 May, 22 May 1917.
73 Trench to mother, 19 August 1917.
74 *Statistics of the Military Effort of the British Empire during the Great War, 1914-1920* (London: War Office, HMSO, 1922), p. 873; p. 580.
75 Trench to mother, 5 September, 9 September 1917.
76 Trench to mother, 14 February 1918.
77 A. Fletcher, 'Patriotism, Identity and Commemoration: New Light on the Great War from the Papers of Major Reggie Chenevix Trench', *History*, Vol. 90, No. 300 (October 2005), p. 542.
78 Trench to mother, 18 August 1917.
79 *Statistics of the Military Effort*, p. 581.
80 Trench to mother, 19 August 1917.
81 Trench to mother, 5 September, 9 September 1917.
82 Sheffield. *Leadership in the Trenches*, p. 100.
83 E. R. Hutt to mother, 24 July 1915, IWM 90/7/1.
84 Urwick to mother, 7 September, 18 September 1915.
85 E. F. Chapman to mother, 29 January 1917.
86 Sheffield, *Leadership in the Trenches*, p. 82.
87 Dunn (ed.), *The War the Infantry Knew*, p. 312.
88 Vernon Merivale to mother, 20 July, 29 July 1916.
89 Vernon Merivale to mother, 14 September 1916.
90 Fuller, *Troop Morale*, p. 82. The Second Royal Welch Fusiliers were very proud of their Battalion Canteen. See Dunn (ed.), *The War the Infantry Knew*, p. 184, p. 203.
91 Fuller, *Troop Morale*, p. 53.
92 F. Wollocombe diary, 4 March, 5 March 1916, IWM 95/33/1.
93 Dunn (ed.), *The War the Infantry Knew*, p. 287.
94 Coppard, *With A Machine Gun*, p. 60.
95 Gladden, *Ypres*, p. 17.

96 Gladden, *Ypres*, p. 53.
97 D. Starrett memoir, 79/35/1, p. 49.
98 Quoted in Fletcher, 'Patriotism, Identity and Commemoration', p. 546.
99 Quoted in P. Liddle, *The Soldier's War 1914–1918* (London: Blandford Press, 1988), p. 81. The officers in the Royal Welch Fusiliers carried their own packs when the Battalion was in full marching order, but all was not as it appeared, wrote Dunn, for 'it was not unknown for a subaltern's pack to contain nothing heavier than an inflated air-cushion.' Dunn (ed.), *The War the Infantry Knew*, p. 47.
100 D. Hankey, *A Student in Arms* (London: Andrew Melrose, 1917), p. 170. The division between self-serving and altruistic officers is also a theme in Sherriff's hugely popular play of 1928, *Journey's End* (London: Heinemann, 1981), the distinction being portrayed through attitudes to food. The counterpoint to Captain Stanhope, the conscientious public school officer, is Trotter, who has been promoted from the ranks. Trotter is constantly hungry and spends his time thinking about how he might obtain the best and largest portions of any food on offer, whereas Stanhope's mind is on his men.
101 Spencer to father, 15 January 1915.
102 Bion *WarMemoirs*, p. 109, p. 123. The psychoanalyst Paulo Sandler comments that characters like 'Aitches' carry characteristics that Bion disliked in himself, especially cowardice. P. Sandler, 'Bion's War Memoirs: A Psychoanalytical Commentary', http://psychematters.com/papers/psandler2.htm. Accessed 21 January 2005, p. 2.
103 Talbot, *Gilbert Walter Lyttleton Talbot*, testimony from Rifleman Dent, p. 46.
104 Owen to mother, 16 January 1917, in J. Bell (ed.), *Wilfred Owen. Selected Letters* (Oxford: Oxford University Press, 1985), pp. 213–14. Owen's poem 'The Sentry', begun at Craiglockhart and completed in September 1918, but based on the events at Beaumont Hamel, rues his failure to look after the blinded sentry. Owen 'forgot him there/In posting Next for duty, and sending a scout/To beg a stretcher somewhere, and flound'ring about/To other posts under the shrieking air'. J. Stallworthy, (ed.), *The Poems of Wilfred Owen* (London: Chatto & Windus, 1990), pp. 165–6.
105 McCartney, *Citizen Soldiers*, p. 164, table 7.2, p. 177.
106 J. Puttowski and J. Sykes, *Shot at Dawn. Executions in World War One by Authority of the British Army Act* (London: Leo Cooper, 1999), p. 78.
107 Sheffield, *Leadership in the Trenches*, p. 83.
108 Trench to mother 22 May 1917.
109 G. Fortune memoir, p. 7, IWM 04/5/1.
110 C. W. Taylor memoir, np, IWM 01/8/1.
111 Starrett memoir, pp. 10–11.
112 Hewins, *The Dillen*, p. 132.

113 Starrett memoir, p. 43; Coppard, *With A Machine Gun*, p. 71.
114 Owen to mother, 4 January 1917, in Bell (ed.), *Wilfred Owen. Selected Letters*, p. 208.
115 E. Marchant to mother, 30 May 1915, IWM DS/MISC/26.
116 Hewins, *The Dillen*, p. 134.
117 Coppard, *With A Machine Gun*, p. 69, p. 71.
118 A. H. Hubbard to mother and all, 9 June 1916, IWM Con Shelf.
119 P. Fussell (ed.), *The The Ordeal of Alfred M. Hale. The Memoirs of a Soldier Servant* (London: Leo Cooper, 1975), p. 149.
120 Fussell (ed.), *The Ordeal of Alfred M. Hale*, pp. 70–5.
121 Fussell (ed.), *The Ordeal of Alfred M. Hale*, p. 92.
122 Fussell (ed.), *The Ordeal of Alfred M. Hale*, pp. 77–82.
123 Fussell (ed.), *The Ordeal of Alfred M. Hale*, p. 161, p. 68.
124 Fussell (ed.), *The Ordeal of Alfred M. Hale*, p. 58.
125 Fussell (ed.), *The Ordeal of Alfred M. Hale*, p. 76, p. 86, p. 80.
126 Fussell (ed.), *The Ordeal of Alfred M. Hale*, p. 155.
127 Fussell (ed.), *The Ordeal of Alfred M. Hale*, p. 85, p. 64.
128 Fussell (ed.), *The Ordeal of Alfred M. Hale*, p. 86.
129 Coppard, *With A Machine Gun*, pp. 68–9.
130 Coppard, *With A Machine Gun*, p. 81.
131 A. Bishop, with T. Smart (eds.), *Vera Brittain. War Diary 1913-1917, Chronicle of Youth* (London: Victor Gollancz, 1981), p. 216; W. T. Hate, 'Diary of War', 10 March 1915, IWM 86/51/1.
132 Trapmann, *Straight Tips for 'Subs'* (London: Forester Groom, 1916), p. 24.
133 K. Simpson, 'The Officers', in I. Beckett and K. Simpson, *A Nation in Arms. A Social Study of the British Army in the First World War* (Manchester: Manchester University Press, 1985), p. 78.
134 Dunn (ed.), *The War the Infantry Knew*, p. 167.
135 H. A. Munro diary, 10 June 1915, IWM P374.
136 Owen to mother, 9 January, 10 January, 12 February 1917, in Bell (ed.), *Wilfred Owen. Selected Letters*, p. 210. p. 212. p. 220.
137 Fussell (ed.), *The Ordeal of Alfred M. Hale*, p. 84. R. C. Sherriff noted the importance of personal preferences in *Journey's End*. In one scene, Mason frets when he is unable to obtain pineapple chunks from the canteen and has to serve up apricots when 'I know the captain can't stand the sight of apricots' (p. 16).
138 Greenwell to mother, 23 September 1915, *An Infant in Arms*, p. 54.
139 Owen to mother, 4 January, 12 February 1917, in Bell (ed.), *Wilfred Owen. Selected Letters*, p. 208, p. 220.
140 Owen to mother, 8 October 1918, in Bell (ed.), *Wilfred Owen. Selected Letters*, p. 352.
141 Fussell (ed.), *The Ordeal of Alfred M. Hale*, p. 99.
142 Sherriff, *Journey's End*, p. 9.

143 Brig.-Gen. F. P. Crozier, *A Brass Hat in No Man's Land* (London: Jonathan Cape, 1930), pp. 202–3.
144 Coppard, *With A Machine Gun*, p. 68.
145 Hewins, *The Dillen*, p. 151.
146 Leland to wife, 13 July 1917.
147 Leland to wife, 24 September 1917.
148 Leland to wife, 5 October 1917.
149 Leland to wife, 21 October 1917.
150 Leland to wife, 22 October 1917.
151 Leland to wife, 2 November 1917.
152 Leland to wife, 14 November 1917.
153 Letter from Private G. Marshall to Lieutenant R.C.G.G. Leverson-Gower, 1 August 1917, in papers of R. M. Synge, IWM 99/15/1.
154 H. A. Munro diary, 22 September 1915; Letter from Neil Munro to Sheriff John Macmaster Campbell, 21 October 1915, IWM P374.
155 Hewins, however, was visited in hospital by Captain Edwards, *The Dillen*, p. 151.
156 See, for example, V. Brittain to E. Brittain, 27 January 1915, in Bishop and Bostridge (eds.), *Letters From A Lost Generation*, p. 226.
157 Hewins, *The Dillen*, p. 159.
158 A. Fletcher, 'TheWestern Front 1918: March 21st', unpublished draft, p. 4.
159 Fletcher, 'TheWestern Front 1918', np draft, p. 3.
160 Delle Fletcher to Michael Roper, 30 May 2007.
161 Papers of A. G. Carpenter, IWM 76/184/1.

# 4

# Learning to care

After five days of constant rain in trenches with 'dead things unburied', into which the Germans were pumping water from their own flooded trenches, Second Lieutenant Ernest Smith wrote to his mother: 'I have been having horrible dreams about my entire platoon convicted of something dreadful and being left out in the filthy rain all night with practically nothing on!!' He mentioned them again at the end of his next letter: 'More tomorrow. I must lie down now and hope not to dream of finding all my men lying out in the pouring rain with only underclothing on – as I did the other night!'[1]

Rather than having a hidden meaning, as Freud's theory of dreams would suggest, Smith's dream was a pretty direct expression of his worries. According to the Battalion Diary, the trenches near Hooge that his platoon occupied were in a 'very bad condition owing to the recent heavy rains, and still much damaged by the frequent bombardments + fighting this area has seen.'[2] Hoping to give his men more protection, Smith put them to work repairing the walls and building dug-outs, but Smith's own dug-out was the only one they had managed to keep dry, and he did not like to take shelter in it 'when the men have practically none'. He spent much of his time with his men, concerned that they could not 'stand it much longer without cracking up'.[3]

On the night before his dream, Smith had been sorely tested. He had discovered two of his men asleep on watch. Smith should have had them Court Martialled, but as the offence technically carried a death penalty if they were found guilty, he turned a blind eye:

> weakly I suppose – [I] brought them up for 'inattention only; as I knew they had hardly had any sleep at all for a long time and could not bring myself to take the worst view of the case – the punishment for which of course you know.
>
> Of course, if this were known, I should be hauled over the coals pretty severely, and I shall feel bound to go the whole hog next time as I told them, they being responsible for the safety of others beside themselves. This is a thing I have always dreaded – (not being a real soldier I suppose).[4]

It was not uncommon for junior officers to face the kinds of difficulties that Smith experienced in October 1915. The Second Lieutenant occupied the lowliest position in the commissioned ranks, and was just as often taking orders as giving them. Yet the 'boy officer', as the subaltern Donald Hankey called him, 'in addition to facing death on his own account, has to bear the responsibility of the lives of a hundred other men.'[5] Often he was younger than the men he was commanding and less experienced. Smith, aged twenty-two and serving in The Buffs, a Regular Battalion with a distinguished history, was an amateur among professionals.

He had been a reluctant recruit to the commissioned ranks. When, halfway through his training in the Artists' Rifles, it was turned into a reserve unit from which other regiments could recruit officers, Smith initially decided not to apply for a commission as 'It is not a thing I feel personally fitted for'. The strict Army rituals did not appeal to him; he was amazed when a sentry was punished for having his boot laces done up the wrong way.[6] At Cadet School, however, he came to appreciate the 'housewifery and general thoughtfulness and management' shown by the NCOs, and to feel that commanding a platoon would be a more 'human' job than High Command, as he would be responsible for the 'comforts and good spirits of the men.'[7] All the same, Smith and his fellow temporary officers were uneasy among the Regulars in the Battalion, who 'are all too military for us and will talk of nothing else and we like to break loose occasionally.' He also felt the artificiality of his authority over the men, many of whom were '"old originals"'.[8] On joining his platoon he had found them 'slack', having been without an officer for a couple of weeks. Smith thought it 'necessary' – as much so as to establish his own credentials as to improve the men's habits – 'to face the situation and show them from the outset that it would not do. Accordingly, I delivered a speech in a severe tone which was very largely assumed, had they known it.'[9] They probably did know it.

Smith reproached himself for not being tougher on the sentries who had been asleep at post, but many a temporary officer, faced with the military consequences of court martial, made the same judgement.[10] Temporary officers tended to be more sympathetic than Regulars to the tribulations of the men, and more forgiving of their lapses of military code.[11] In part, this less authoritarian style reflected their limited capacity to exert discipline over other recruits who had, as Gary Sheffield puts it, 'counted for something' in civilian life.[12] In Smith's dream, however, the consequences of lenience are disastrous for the very men whose safety and good opinion he hopes to maintain.

In the dream, moreover, it is not the Germans who punish the men but Smith's own Commanding Officers, and this reveals another of the young temporary officer's difficulties, caught between loyalty to his class and to his men. When he first joined up Smith was typical in being unused to the close proximity of working men. During his training in the Artists' Rifles he kept a keen eye on their habits. He wondered what it would be like to sleep in a tent packed with 'dirty regulars'. During a dinner held for an Irish regiment he watched in horrified fascination as the men, lacking spoons, consumed their soup by lapping it up or 'reducing it to a pudding consistency with bread'.[13] Three months into his service in France, Higher Command seemed infinitely more remote than his men, but identify as he might with them, in his dream Smith could do nothing to shield them from shells and the 'filthy rain'. It is the men's nakedness amidst the mud that makes the scene one of acute 'psychic anxiety', to use Santanu Das' phrase.[14]

Smith's dream reveals how deeply felt the subaltern's responsibilities could be, and it prompts us to ask: how did these young officers, soldiers of a largely civilian Army, often with little experience of life apart from their homes and schooling, learn to look after their men? What models of care did they fall back on? And what enabled rank-and-file soldiers to keep going even when, as Smith put it, they had 'lost all the go?' What previous experiences did each draw on to get through?

Recent histories of the British Army in the Great War, reflecting the growing dialogue between social history and military history, have begun to ask this question. John Bourne has shown how working-class culture provided the Army with a 'bedrock of social cohesion.'[15] The working-class recruit was used to drudgery and to helping his comrades out, and he knew how to take orders and cut some slack for himself.

When investigating the civilian resources that helped soldiers to survive, historians have tended to underplay the significance of the private sphere. Thus while John Bourne suggests that the home was one source for the solidarity shown by civilian rankers, it merits less attention in his discussion than the neighbourhood, workplace and mutual associations.[16] Studies of where officers got their ideas of leadership from also tend to concentrate on the public sphere. John Keegan argues that volunteer officers 'saw to the men's food, health, cleanliness' because they had been taught to do this as boarders at public school.[17] Gary Sheffield highlights the importance for military leadership of public school values such as chivalry, athleticism and self-sacrifice, but downplays the prewar contact between social classes within the household, claiming for example that relationships with servants were 'not generally conducive to intimacy'.[18] The public schools undoubtedly provided the subaltern with models of how to relate to the rank-and-file soldier, but so too did relationships with servants, the latter being all the more powerful because they often went right back to infancy, and involved intimate emotional and physical needs.

The neglect of household and family relationships is surprising given the relative youth of recruits in the British Army. For young officers and rankers alike, the closest emotional bonds were with sisters and brothers, mothers and fathers, aunts, uncles and grand-parents. The Army, of course, was also, like the family, a domestic institution. It fed, clothed and sheltered them. When the soldier took out his sewing kit or 'housewife' to mend his tunic, heated up his rations on a Tommy cooker, or tried to rid himself of the ubiquitous louse, he performed a domestic task, sometimes with help or advice from his mother. How things had been done at home influenced how, in this largely non-professional Army, things would be done at war.

Smith's dream indicates how the military and domestic situations could be linked. It is after all *his mother* to whom he relates his dream, and he writes to her knowing she will appreciate how hard it is to ensure that those in one's charge are kept warm, dry and safe. But he is communicating his own feelings to her, as well as reporting on the state of his men. In the letter describing his dream Smith reflects on why 'I always write more when we are having the most uncomfortable time – I suppose it is because I naturally think more of you all then, and writing is the next best thing to actually talking to you.'[19] The subaltern had to try and subordinate his own needs to his men's, but this could also increase his *own* need for comfort. Smith's dream bears out the insight of the military psychiatrist W. H. R. Rivers, who observed that it was the officer's 'knowledge . . . that the honour of their military unit and the safety of their comrades depend on their efficiency which forms by far the most potent factor in the production or maintenance of anxiety states.'[20]

The upbringing of temporary officers like Smith had a profound impact on the way they commanded their men, though the effects did not always benefit military efficiency. Anxious as many officers were about their responsibilities, the rank-and-file soldier actually depended little on his officer for day-to-day survival. Smith was typical of the temporary officer in needing the good opinion of his men and in sometimes over-estimating the degree to which his efforts counted.[21] A study of the homes these men came from suggests why it mattered so much to them that they should be liked, and be seen as indispensable by their men, and how it was that rankers got by even when their officers were incompetent or felt over-burdened.

## Looking after the men

The officers in Kitchener's Army brought a range of life experiences to the job of military command, drawn as they were from across the British middle class. Early in the war, only a man who had been to one of the best public schools would be likely to get a commission: nearly all the boys who joined up after leaving Manchester Grammar School at the start of the war went into the ranks.[22] Though most of the men who were made junior officers during the rush to volunteer did not actually have a country estate and independent means, their commissions confirmed their civilian status as 'gentlemen.' In 1915 the War Office set up new criteria for selection, so that normally a man would serve in the ranks before being selected for an Officer Cadet Battalion.[23] Ability came to count for more and, increasingly, men from minor public schools and grammar schools became junior officers. By the end of the war even some skilled workers were getting commissions and the majority, in Martin Petter's careful assessment, 'came from outside the traditional "officer class"', the largest group being 'what Masterman called "the suburbans."'[24]

R. C. Sherriff was typical of the kind of 'temporary gentleman' who would be recruited after 1915. His father had scraped and saved to afford the ten pounds a term fee for Kingston Grammar School, and Sherriff had worked as an insurance clerk in 1914 before enlisting in November 1915 with the Artists' Rifles.[25] Ernest Smith also joined the Artists' Rifles, but his family, living in Onslow Gardens in London, right next to Highgate Wood, his father an ex-mining engineer and self-employed businessman, was probably a cut above Sherriff's. Both, however, were the kinds of men about whom the term 'temporary gentleman' might be used by others, not just to signify that they were serving for the duration, but as a pejorative label which identified their origins on the fringes of the middle class. Wilfred Owen, his father a stationmaster who became assistant to the Superintendent of the Joint Railways, also fits the picture of the post-1915 officer intake; though the lumping together of men who had been in pre-war times deeply sensitive to small class differences produced a characteristic disdain on Owen's part towards the 'quite temporary gentlemen', 'glorified NCOs' and 'privates and sergeants in masquerade' who were getting commissions late in the war.[26]

These shifts in the social composition of the commissioned ranks mattered because the family culture of the better-off, public school officer was likely to be quite different from that of the clerk. While the one had grown up in a household which did not just consist of the immediate family and contained its own internal social distinctions, the atmosphere of the other was emotionally intense and exclusive, not just because there were fewer servants, but because the families of the lower middle class tended to be particularly small. Richard Church, brought up in a semi-detached house in Battersea, his father a post-office clerk, marvelled at 'how different are the family relationships, how much closer and fiercer the intimacies, in the lower-middle-class homes, from those in the classes above, where servants, boarding schools, wider intellectual interests, came between parents and children, to make their affections more formal and restrained.' Church singled out mothers as crucial to the different emotional dispositions of the lower-middle- and middle-class man: his own mother had been 'almost sensual' towards him; and this kind of environment tended to produce men who were 'over-emotional, unadventurous, matriarch-ridden.'[27]

One might think that a cosseted, mother-centred upbringing such as this would make unpromising material for a commissioned man, yet, as Smith's habit of taking his mother into his confidence shows, the roles of subaltern and mother were not entirely unalike. Indeed, contemporaries sometimes remarked on the maternal aspects of caring for the men. Checking on his men during heavy shelling, one subaltern saw himself as 'like a mother going round her children's bedrooms in a great thunderstorm . . . Metaphorically I tucked each detachment up in bed, told them they would be all right'. Quoting this passage, Richard Holmes puzzlingly describes it as an instance of 'paternal' feeling, and his assumption about the paternal nature of care of the men is widely shared.[28] As military historians now do, military training handbooks during the war struggled to accommodate the more feminine aspects of the officer's role with traditional conceptions of the soldier. *Straight Tips for 'Subs'* warned that although the subaltern should get to know his men, he should keep a certain emotional distance. He must not 'do it on the lines of a mothers' meeting'.[29] 'Basilisk', the author of another military training guide, explained that the subaltern must not 'dry-nurse' his men, but should 'be a father to them all the same.'[30] The very proximity of maternal functions to the subaltern's role led these commentators to compare them, but the association then had to be discounted so as to preserve the manliness of the officer's station. The elements of practical domestic management that officers were required to perform did not fit neatly into a paternal model.

The habit of describing the subaltern's work as 'housewifery' or 'mothering' was more than a linguistic quirk, for there were structural similarities between these roles. Both were domestic managers of a kind. Where a middle-class mother might oversee the weekly domestic routine, supervise washing, plan menus, order supplies and manage budgets, the subaltern's tasks ranged from overseeing trench repairs or sentry duty to ensuring that the rations arrived and that the men were kept as clean and warm as possible. The junior officer instructed his NCOs and the men how to carry out these tasks, as the mother instructed her servants, and both could find it taxing to organise large numbers of frequently changing personnel.[31]

There were some affinities, too, between the emotional qualities required of a subaltern and of a mother. Both were responsible for the minor punishments, the Company Commander having the power to levy fines, confine to barracks, order extra fatigues, or refer on to the Commanding Officer all those below the rank of corporal.[32] Each kept order within the household, platoon or company, but was also expected to be sympathetic. Mothers, commented the Victorian advice writer Sarah Ellis, tended to exhibit more 'nicety and tact' in the 'minute affairs of domestic life' than fathers, and were more sensitive to 'individual feeling'.[33] Tact and attention to feeling were also capacities that the subaltern was encouraged to develop. He needed to be able to imagine how he would feel in the men's situation, as Smith did when observing that his men were cold, tired and demoralised. 'Basilisk' thought sympathy should be the 'keynote' of the officer's dealings with his men.

He defined sympathy not as pity, but as a capacity to '"to feel with", to place yourself in the position of another, to see things through his eyes, to grasp his point of view, his thoughts, his feelings and difficulties.'[34]

The attitudes that officers were expected to show in their care of the men were actually rather similar to those that they expected mothers to show *them*. They not only wanted their practical needs to be met, but to be anticipated: for socks and underwear to be sent when the supply was exhausted, for remedies and for their treasured 'comforts' to arrive at the very moment of need. Meeting wants on time – sometimes without even having to be asked – showed that their mothers were thinking of them. Roland Mountfort was delighted when, shortly after requesting 'a few little luxuries', he received a parcel from home. 'I think the more of the parcel inasmuch as it was despatched before you received my last letter', he explained.[35] 'I need not tell you what I want', wrote Graham Greenwell to his mother, 'because you always know best and anticipate me.'[36]

Junior officers and mothers both occupied an intermediate – and ambiguous – position within the hierarchies of family and Army. Though she 'ruled the roost', the wife was formally subject to her husband, while the subaltern was answerable to higher command. Both were responsible for the physical reproduction of life, but had little formal authority. 'The trench officer', remarked Second Lieutenant Lyndall Urwick to his mother in 1915, 'combines a heavy responsibility with extraordinarily small powers of control'.[37] At the same time, his role in looking after the men gave the subaltern a certain moral authority, as it did the mother. Though men like Smith feared being called to account by their senior officers, their duties were self-evidently crucial to the war effort. However, the position of senior officers, or 'Red Tabs' as they were called – like the position of the middle-class father in the Edwardian home, when mothers carried so much weight in domestic matters – was harder to justify. Both possessed ultimate authority but were an 'absent presence', the father's role being defined as much by provision outside the home as by his place within it; the senior officer's by the fact that he directed battle from behind the lines.[38]

When paternal authority was remote, it could carry the blame for difficulties. It was the distance of high command from the front line that made it a target of scorn among young subalterns. As Lyndall Urwick remarked in a letter home:

> I am constantly at a loss out here because in the case of the old colonels & people of that sort, their minds don't seem to work rationally at all. They never seem to hold the same view on any given subject for two minutes at an end. It all seems a kind of jerky illogical process compound [*sic*] three parts of prejudice & one part of liver.[39]

Reggie Trench was equally suspicious of the movements of the Brass Hats as he was of the Germans. When one of his sentries spotted a General moving about close by, Trench got a man to train his field-glasses on the Brass Hat 'as one never knows what these fellows will do if not carefully watched!'[40] Graham Greenwell was furious when reprimanded by the Commanding Officer for allowing his men to sleep in the forward trenches with their boots off (this violated the principle of readiness), the more so because the General's 'stinker' had been written when he was 'safely entrenched in his office.'[41]

The senior officers were fair game because – as their subordinates saw it – they knew little of the front-line soldier's lot. Their incompetence sometimes put men at risk, yet protection was supposed to be the keystone of paternal authority. While fathers were meant to be, in John Tosh's apt military metaphor, 'the first line of defence against intrusion or danger', in the First World War they put sons in their place.[42]

## Selflessness and service

Given that care of the men required a certain maternal sensibility, what lessons could the young junior officer take from his own mother? The upper-middle-class son might have had a more distant relationship to home than the clerk or skilled labourer, but he was also prone, perhaps *because* of this remoteness, to rather elevated and moralised conceptions of both motherhood and military service.

Reflecting the broadening of Christian principles from the church to secular society at the end of the nineteenth century, and from altar to hearth, it was principally from their mothers that young boys received their moral education.[43] They learnt to be sensitive to others' needs and feelings, and to regard introspection as a malaise.[44] While Robert Graves' nurse undertook the 'practical' aspects of looking after him, his mother, who was descended from a prominent Bavarian family that included the historian Heinrich von Ranke, took charge of his spiritual training. She instructed her five children (there were another five from Graves' father's first marriage) in the scriptures, censored their reading and instilled in them a sense of public spiritedness. She told them stories about 'inventors and doctors who gave their lives for the suffering . . . and saintly men who made examples of themselves.' The Graves children were brought up to 'benefit humanity in some practical way.'[45] Susan Owen, though from a less rarefied background (her father had been a successful ironmonger), acted in a similar way towards her children. Her family were evangelicals and from a young age Wilfred prayed and studied the scriptures with her. The notes in the margins of Susan's bible suggest the significance which she placed on the mother as the source of Christian compassion: 'As one whom his mother comforteth, so I will comfort you; Wilfred Feb 16th 03.'[46]

Maternal love in middle-class families was deeply spiritual. Marie Leighton used to go up and see Roland after the nurse had put him to bed, a habit that began when he was two and continued even when he was on home leave from the war. She would watch him say his prayers, they would sing songs and talk, and 'Sometimes we stayed quiet all the time that I was there, having only our hands clasped.' She felt that they 'were never quite so completely in touch with each other when we did not get these talks.'[47] Through this contact Roland had acquired a 'touch of the feminine', and 'reverence for womanhood.'[48] Marie Leighton was firm with Roland, so that he would learn to consider others: 'I never yielded to him, not even in those babyhood days, for I wanted him to grow up to be a fine specimen of manhood, and I knew that if he was to do that he must know that his mother was not weak.' If he misbehaved she would refuse to visit him at bed-time.[49] As boys became men, their love for their mothers demonstrated the civilising virtues of selflessness. When Vera Brittain met Marie Leighton for the first time, she commented that 'a man who cares deeply for his mother can be trusted very far.'[50] A close bond with a mother was evidence in itself of concern for others, a quality which influenced notions of manliness as much as motherhood.

Such an elevated and moralised code of personal conduct was not easily squared with what subalterns had to do in the war. Violence could not be openly countenanced. Men wrote to their mothers not of killing but of sacrifice; aggression was sublimated into the rhetoric of suffering. It was also difficult to voice personal distress, as emotional energy always had to be directed to the care of others. Ernest Smith was at a loss to describe to his mother his first experience of battle, at Hooge in August 1915. He had undergone 'a truly terrific bombardment', and was then moved up into a trench which had recently seen violent fighting. Rather than describe the scene, Smith praised his comrades. The Medical officers had been exceptionally brave, and so had his friend Ferguson: 'leading his own men under the most excessively trying conditions, he did more than his duty, hurling bombs and holding the men together in the most wonderful way, the Captain cannot say too much for him'. Smith, in concentrating on the altruism of his comrades, strove to ward off depressing thoughts:

> Personally I soon got used to seeing nasty things, and one seemed to forget everything else, but a desire to help as much as possible. I wish I had been able to do more real good, but anyone else's efforts seemed to pale before the absolutely marvellous energy of these men, surely there is some good even in war if it provides scope for things of this sort!! anyhow [*sic*], that is the way I prefer to look at it.[51]

The ethos of selflessness raised the stakes: it injected a religious note into the care of the men and could turn the subaltern himself into a Christ-like figure. Inspections of the men's feet commonly gave rise to biblical references, illustrating the subaltern's devotion. Donald Hankey described an officer lancing a boil on a ranker's foot: 'It seemed to have a touch of the Christ about it, and we loved and honoured him the more.'[52] Just prior to going up the line for the first time Owen wrote to his mother of 'praising the clean feet, but not reviling the unclean', here perhaps evoking Christ's washing of his disciples' feet after the last supper.[53]

When a parcel from his mother had arrived mid-way through the attack at Hooge, Smith shared it with his men as they 'were very short' of food. Its contents could not have gone far among a platoon of fifty to sixty men, but the significance of his help for the needy, and its resemblance to the biblical story of feeding the five thousand, would probably have crossed his mother's mind.[54] There was an equally grandiose quality in the stories of officers who carried their men's packs when they were tired or ill. When his 'friend and best officer', Second Lieutenant Alliban, was listed as missing, Reggie Trench's glowing tribute evoked the Road to Calvary:

> I have heard his voice at the rear of the Company encouraging men + helping them along – have seen him carrying one or two rifles in addition to his own equipment and later have seen him when out of sight of the men lying exhausted with lack of sleep + general fatigue. His spirit was indomitable.[55]

Suffering and sacrifice were everywhere, and covered over the violations of Christian morality which, at times, the subaltern must commit.

Maternal selflessness set a standard of service which few subalterns could live up to. While it produced plenty of men who, like Smith, Trench and Owen, were conscientious about their duties, it did not equip them with the practical skills of care. Its impact was paradoxical, for a selfless mother was likely to produce children who were unaware of the labour that ensured their own comfort, and who had little sensitivity towards others' needs. This was astutely observed by Beatrice Webb, whose sister had remarked to her:

> 'I can't see where exactly I have gone very wrong, for I have always loved them and worked day and night for their comfort.' This was a mild statement of her deserts from the standpoint of a self-devoted mother and wife. Alas! Poor sister: where you erred was in doing too much for them . . . you made your children regard life as one constant ministration to their physical comfort and self-complacency . . .[56]

Webb, though a pacifist, might have found unlikely allies among the Regular officers of the Welch Fusiliers, who believed that the well-heeled soldiers who volunteered early in the war had been too cosseted at home to look after their men properly. At the same time these temporary officers were deeply imbued by their mothers with ideas of Christian selflessness. They had high ideals of service, and high expectations of themselves. John Tosh's observation about the late-Victorian middle class, that once they left home sons 'did not on the whole live by the morality they had learned at their mother's knee', did not hold true in the war, but at the same time, military service constantly exposed gaps between the elevated ideals these sons had grown up with, and the reality of keeping men fit for killing.[57]

## Domestic service

Most of the men who became junior officers in the war would have come from homes with servants. Because servants usually lived in and had been around them as long as they could remember, these relationships shaped their feelings about people beyond their own class. In middle- and lower-middle-class homes it was common to employ at least one servant and the families of many skilled workers also had a servant to help with the cooking, washing and cleaning. Servants often left a powerful and lasting impression on the children in these kinds of households; not least because one of their main jobs was to help with the childcare. Wilfred Owen, for example, had a nurse-maid, and in one of the family photographs she and his mother sit with his younger siblings Harold and Mary on their laps, while the five-year-old Wilfred stands between the two women.[58] The importance attached to childcare in households where there were only one or two servants is reflected in the names they were known by, such as 'nurse-maid' or 'mother's help'.[59]

It was among the better off that the servant's emotional impact on children was probably greatest. In these kinds of houses, servants not only assisted parents in childrearing, but to some extent took over their functions. A nanny or nurse would carry out the practical care of children, supported by an array of other staff that might include a cook, maids and perhaps a governess. One of five surviving children, Reggie Trench had two nurses and three servants in his family home.[60] Nannies occupied a unique place between the other servants and the family. Young children sometimes shared a bedroom with their nanny or nursemaid, or their bedrooms might be closely connected so that the nurse could keep watch over them. Nannies taught them to read and write, and took them for walks, giving them contact with street life and working people beyond the genteel environs of the home.[61]

Winston Churchill's affection for Nanny Everest is well known. She, Churchill's son wrote, was the 'principal confidante of his joys, his troubles, and his hopes'. She fed, washed and dressed him, nursed him through his childhood illnesses, and slept in his room until Churchill was eight.[62] Ronald B, born in 1902 and brought up in a household with three servants, did not see much of his mother. She was 'out a lot' on Church activities and social visits, or preoccupied with her 'at home' days. Though 'sure she was a jolly good mother to us', he felt closer to his nanny, whom he nicknamed 'Tommy'. She 'had a great deal of affection for me and if the truth be told I had perhaps more affection for my nanny than I had for my mother because I saw and lived with and had a lot more to do with my nanny. We were very close together, she treated me almost as her own child.' Like Churchill, as a child Ronald B slept in the same bedroom as Tommy and she stayed with the family until her retirement, when they set her up in her own house.[63] It was not unusual for children to refer – as Ronald B did – to their nanny as a 'second mother'.[64]

Many of the better-off men who served as junior officers in the war had enjoyed close relationships with their nannies. Roland Leighton's nurse stayed with the Leighton family until her death during the First World War. When Roland left for boarding school she worried that he would have a bilious attack, since 'E' always feels it in the inside when his nerves is upset.'[65] As a baby Gilbert Talbot was 'devoted' to his nanny 'Uty', reported Lavinia Talbot, and even when he was at Winchester School and Oxford she would come and visit him.[66] Ralph Bickersteth, an officer in a Leeds Pals' Battalion, wrote to his nanny as he drew close to the front. His letter reveals the associations that a subaltern might feel between his own early care, and his present situation: 'All the officers mess together now and sleep at houses round, but quite close. I sleep with two other officers on the floor, but on a mattress, and very comfortable it is too.'[67] Writing to his nanny about how he slept at the front probably felt natural to Bickersteth, as she may well have put him to bed as a child, and have slept – as his fellow officers now did – 'quite close' by.

The experience of being looked after by nannies and other servants created complicated attitudes towards working people. It could give rise to strong feelings of loyalty and gratitude, though children had little ability to reciprocate the care they had been given. Churchill was deeply upset when he learned, aged eighteen, that his parents were considering dismissing Nanny Everest, and wrote to them 'She is an old woman – who has been your devoted servant for nearly twenty years – she is more fond of Jack and I than of any other people in the world, so to be packed off in the way the Duchess suggests would possibly, if not probably, break her down altogether'. He was with Nanny Everest when she died, and later paid for the upkeep of her grave.[68]

The intimacy that existed between children and their nannies could extend beyond the nursery to other domestic staff. At the memorial service for George Vernon, who had lived with the Charteris family at Stanway prior to his enlistment, the 'immaculately professional butler' broke down in tears. The butler, Cynthia Asquith explained, 'couldn't bear not to have been there to look after him at the end after having "mothered" him through so many illnesses'.[69] The emotional distance and social segregation between parents and children in wealthier households could mean that a child felt more comfortable with the servants than their parents: Ronald B thought he and his brothers and sisters had 'perhaps more fun in the kitchen than we had elsewhere.'[70] Children and servants might conspire together to keep a servant's indiscretions from parents, or to protect children from getting into trouble.[71]

The subjectivity of middle-class sons was frequently split between the attitudes of their own social class and attachment to the world of their carers. The emotional effect of this split was profound, as the attachment to a servant did not cancel out, but was itself formed by, relations of superiority and subservience. Children – especially in larger households where nannies and servants did much of the mothering – needed to win over their affections against the smouldering resentment that servile relationships produced.

## Military service

Many aspects of military service mimicked the emotional economy of domestic service. The association is apparent in the way that batmen and officers regarded each other. The batman B. Graham clearly considered himself as much a personal servant as a soldier, describing his officer, Lieutenant Munro, as 'A kind and thoughtful Master to B. Graham.'[72] Similar to a nurse-maid or mother's help, the batman was often regarded as a 'second mother'. In a letter to a Scottish friend, Lieutenant Munro's brother wrote of how Graham had attended his officer 'like a mother.'[73] Paying tribute to a fellow batman's care of his officer, David Starrett explained how the man had 'nursed him like a child'.[74] When Guy Chapman got drunk on 'so-called milk punch' at a Battalion dinner, the 'wholly reliable George Knappett' led him to bed.[75] At times like these it was the officer who was the dependent party and the batman who had to act *in loco parentis.*

Relationships across the ranks repeated the split feelings and loyalties of the subaltern's early life. On the one hand, in relying on working people to dress, eat and even put him to sleep, the middle-class son was not just practically but emotionally dependent. On the other hand, personal service made him feel superior. Many subalterns found their men's personal habits repugnant and commented freely on them. The new recruit Graham Greenwell disliked physical drill because his men, 'though all good fellows and very keen, perspire freely!'[76] Even the most conscientious officer was apt to find material for comedy in the ways of his men. Munro's diary included a selection of typical opening lines from the men's letters home, presumably gleaned from censoring them. His first example found humour in the stock phrase 'Hoping this finds you as it leaves me in the pink'; a second, in a directness of expression that an officer would never dare adopt: 'Dear Mother. I am getting on alright, but life out here is a pure bugger!'[77]

That the men were frequently the butt of officers' humour was widely observed within the Army. The popular subaltern '*never rags his men*' (italics in original), wrote Captain Trapmann in his military manual, re-released as a second edition during the war with a new chapter on

'How to treat your men'.[78] A lecture produced by the Censorship and Publicity Section of the War Office contained a stern warning against discussing the contents of the men's letters:

> There are some who even go so far as to joke over the private affairs of their men. Such proceedings cannot be too strongly condemned and most certainly tend to destroy the confidence of the men in their officers. You should never forget that the private affairs of the men must be regarded as absolutely confidential, and every officer should reflect upon what his own feelings would be if his private letters were made the subject of ribald conversation in the mess or orderly room.[79]

Some temporary officers, it seems, could not be relied on to respect their men's privacy, despite the gross intrusiveness of censorship, but that might not be surprising when, within their own households, servants had had little privacy and their personal foibles would be discussed openly among the family.

Officers could be disdainful of their men but they could also like and even envy them. When censoring letters they were sometimes struck by the men's strong feelings towards their loved ones, and their directness in expressing them. The letters of Lionel Hall's men 'are always full of kisses XXX – and odd expressions of endearment', while among Owen's men, 'the number of XXX to sisters and mothers weigh more in heaven than Victoria Crosses'.[80] When Anthony Eden's trusted sergeant died, he was astonished to learn from reading his men's letters home how fond they were of their NCO. It was their capacity for affection that he noted: 'That week every letter contained a reference to Park's death, which was natural enough. More extraordinary was the warmth and, more particularly, the understanding of the extent to which their sergeant had spent himself on their behalf.' [81]

Middle-class reactions to displays of emotion such as this were ambiguous. The ranker's demonstrative nature could be admired but it also defined him as not genteel. An officer from the Royal Welch Fusiliers reported a conversation between two rankers. One had recently seen his friend die violently and was describing the circumstances to a comrade. The story of the man's bereavement, commented the officer, would no doubt be told again and again and 'always with the same senseless obscene garnishing.'[82] Marie Leighton, looking over a letter sent to her son Roland by a 'vulgar' ex-lover, remarked that there 'were actually crosses for kisses, as if the letter were from a tweenymaid!' (the tweenymaid was a lowly servant). [83] Vera Brittain was clearly a more suitable partner, for she shared her future mother-in-law's distaste for showy expressions of emotion. Brittain was deeply disapproving when she saw the 'sloppy kisses' given by a Captain to his sister and mother as they parted on the station platform; this officer's lack of 'calm, controlled behaviour' marked him out as a temporary gentleman.[84] Precisely because the officer himself was supposed to show restraint in matters of feeling, he was prone to disparage, but was also drawn to, the ranker's supposed emotionality.[85]

Censoring letters, officers learnt how deeply the men's affections lay in their own families, but nevertheless they could not help but look for signs that they too were liked, and they anxiously scanned letters home for clues. Wilbert Spencer, just about to go into his second tour of the trenches, felt he was 'getting to know my men and I think they like me. Anyhow it appeared so in one of their letters which I had to censor.'[86] Graham Greenwell's desire to win over the affections of his men was revealed in a letter he wrote to his mother shortly after joining his platoon. He had been censoring their letters and noted the many 'very touching' remarks about his predecessor, who had been killed a week earlier.[87] Spontaneous acts of kindness assumed great significance. While his men were shoring up his billet, Reggie Trench overhead one of them say 'come on lad – we must make the bloody skipper more comfortable – he deserves it.'[88]

Reggie Trench was probably more realistic than many about the limits of his mens' regard for him. In a letter to his mother he made a telling distinction between love and trust, a distinction that a younger subaltern may not have appreciated: 'No, you are quite wrong, the men do <u>not love</u> or even like me but I think they will follow me. Very few men and I'm not one of them – can keep good discipline and popularity. I think I have the first but know I have not got the second.'[89] Reggie Trench was an unusually good officer because he understood that his men's trust rather than their love was what mattered. But Trench, in his late twenties, was an older and more experienced soldier than many, having joined the Inns of Court Officers' Training Corps in 1909 after graduating from Oxford, and becoming a Second Lieutenant in 1912.[90]

The summer camps that Trench went on each year after 1909, and his role early in the war, training prospective officers in the Inns of Court Corps, would have given him a close knowledge of how to manage the domestic routines of soldiering, but his background and personal situation may also have helped. Reggie's family circumstances set him apart from some other subalterns. He was married, and had a daughter, Delle, on whom he doted. He would write little letters addressed to 'Miss Chenevix Trench' though she was only eighteen months old when he arrived on the Western Front in February 1917.[91] At the same time that Reggie Trench was receiving long letters from his wife Clare about the trials and tribulations of caring for Delle, he was writing back to her and his mother about the feeding, health and hygiene of his men. Younger officers, having so recently been the focus of their parents and their servant's concerns and still needing their love, their heads full of abstract ideals of service and selflessness, did not find it easy to adjust to the mundane realities of looking after the men's practical wants.

Most, though anxious to fulfil the mission, simply lacked the life experience of a man like Reggie Trench. The letters of condolence written by Yvo Charteris' comrades could not help but betray his immaturity. Yvo was nineteen and had been in France for barely a month when he died. His Commanding Officer Gerald Trotter perhaps gave away more than he intended when he wrote that Yvo 'was shaping up so well as an officer', while Yvo's sergeant clearly saw himself as the better soldier despite his subordinate rank: 'During the period he was with me, I took great interest in giving him the benefit of my experience, which dates back from when the war commenced.'[92] Most telling was the behaviour of Yvo's men, who had '"chipped" him by singing "and a little child shall lead them"'.[93]

Yvo Charteris was not unusual in carrying heavy responsibilities so young. Because of the casualty rates among officers, by 1917 many companies were being commanded by men aged twenty or under.[94] Among the Second Lieutenant's fifty or so men, or the 200-odd commanded by a Captain, some would have been older than he.[95] Their NCOs were often older and more experienced soldiers. Captain Trapmann advised new subalterns to defer to the Sergeant-Major's greater knowledge of military matters, and warned, 'Do not attempt to "put him in his place."'[96] Recalling his Sergeant-Major, Lyndall Urwick commented in 1970 that 'I still blush with shame when I think what an unlicked cub he must sometimes have found me.'[97] The gap between formal and actual authority might chafe among NCOs, as it did when Lance-Corporal George Coppard was forced to take care of a new Second Lieutenant. Although 'Mr X' was actually two or three years older than Coppard, 'I felt responsible for teaching him the ways of trench life.' The man quickly proved 'physically and mentally incapable of making good.' Under heavy shell-fire he retreated to a dug-out, blocking access for the stretcher-bearers and wounded men. He burst into tears, refused the food that

Coppard had prepared, and would not leave the dug-out for a call of nature, so 'I was obliged to empty his slops.'[98] The subaltern's terror forced Coppard into the roles of nurse and chamber-maid.

In Ernest Smith's case, too, the formal relations of rank and the emotional relations of service were sometimes at loggerheads. Smith treated Sergeant Mould, who was older than he and had children of his own, rather like a parent. Mould, Smith told his mother, 'is a splendid fellow and takes great care of me, the difficulty is to persuade him to sleep at all!' He was the 'most wonderful person for rapid waking that I have ever struck and quite makes me ashamed of my own drowsiness whenever he has to wake me suddenly.'[99] Smith's parents acknowledged how Mould had helped their son by keeping him in cigarettes, and when it seemed that Mould might go for a commission and leave the Battalion, Smith was 'very distressed.'[100] Smith had 'confided in me in everything', Mould later wrote to Smith's mother.[101] Men like Smith had trouble enough looking after themselves, let alone looking after the men.

Officer training which, by the end of the war, was extended from a month to a year, helped the prospective subaltern learn how to care for his men. In the Artists' Rifles, Smith would have been given a lecture instructing him that 'your first job is to get to know your men, look after them'.[102] Military guides and handbooks emphasised the same thing. *Duties for all Ranks* explained that he must learn to 'care for their [the men's] comfort and well-being.'[103] A Sandhurst examination paper from December 1916 included a question that asked candidates to imagine their platoon arriving at their billets from the trenches, wet and cold. 'Before going to your own quarters', it asked, 'what will be your duties as platoon commander, with regard to your own platoon?'[104] Like many subalterns, Ernest Smith followed closely the advice he had been given during his officer training. After reaching France he asked his parents to send over his Field Service pocket books and his manual, 'Infantry Training 1914'. On joining his platoon he requested a roll book with which to record the names and addresses of his men's next of kin, knowing that he might soon have to write to a bereaved wife or mother.[105]

Though many a temporary officer was conscientious about putting his military training into action, little in his upbringing prepared him for the reality of being responsible for the lives and deaths of men. Brought up from birth with servants, these young men were emotionally as well as practically dependent on working people, and they found it difficult to shake off these habits. The NCO and the batman took the place of their servants. The words 'loyal' or faithful' that officers used to describe men of the 'Other Ranks' were the very same ones they applied to servants. And whereas at home they had deflected the servant's potential resentment towards them by making themselves lovable, they now sought to win over their men's affections. Turning a blind eye to lapses of military discipline, or getting their parents to send out cigarettes for the men, were ways of compensating for the fact that they did not feel themselves to be 'real' soldiers, as Smith put it. They hoped instead to make the men like them. For good or ill, domestic service, with its emotional reference points facing back towards childhood, rather than the – as yet untried – adult identities of employer or public official, provided the emotional template of the officer's relations with his men.

* * *

Just after stand-to on 20 December 1915, Ernest Smith was working his way back along the line after visiting his men when a shell burst right in front of him. There had been heavy shelling and rain and many of the trenches, according to the Battalion Diary, were 'unoccupiable [*sic*] and the line held chiefly by isolated posts.'[106] These posts gave Smith little protection from the shell blast, and fragments entered his abdomen and head. Sergeant Mould, Smith's batman, and the stretcher-bearer stayed with him in the trench all day, as it was too exposed, and the route back too muddy, for him to be moved in daylight. The surgeon at the Casualty Clearing Station operated on Smith to try to repair the hole in his intestine, but he suffered a fatal brain haemorrhage just as the operation was nearing completion.

To Smith, being in the advanced trench must have felt as if his disturbing dreams of last October had come true. It was only 2 ft deep, so he and his men were fully exposed to the German shells. They were also, in Sergeant Mould's words, 'up to one's neck in mud caused by constant rain', just as they had been in the 'filthy rain' of the dream. In these trenches, however, it seems that Smith was determined not to look passively onto the scene. He had continued visiting the detached posts through the night although the Battalion was being 'crumped with heavy howitzers', killing three private soldiers and wounding nineteen.[107]

Smith had remained attentive towards his men, but he was puzzlingly careless of himself. In Mould's letter to Smith's parents, he included some details about the circumstances of Smith's death that they must have found deeply discomfiting:

> Smith as brave as ever, visited the Posts, and on returning I saw he was smoking a cigarette, I said to him 'Mind the cigarette sir', knowing that the glow could be seen. Immediately I had said that Mr Smith got down putting the cigarette out . . . No sooner had he got in the trench than I heard the whistle of shells. Mr Smith, Cpl. Collins and I stood together, I shouted 'get down' and the next moment a shell burst 2 yds. behind and Mr. Smith said 'I am hit'.[108]

What was Smith doing smoking a cigarette in the dark, making himself clearly visible in an unprotected area that had been shelled through the night? His actions look like those of the rank amateur he had been in August, yet Smith, having served six months in trenches, was now a seasoned soldier. Was this a show of bravado or something else? The ever-watchful Sergeant Mould saw the danger immediately, why did Smith not? The stress of his tours of the trenches may have produced a kind of exhaustion which made him careless. Other temporary officers reported a similar attitude during prolonged spells in dangerous trenches; it was something different from bravery, or setting an example to the men. Siegfried Sassoon was wounded in a bombing raid near the Hindenberg Line when, against the advice of his corporal, he advanced into a sap-head (a small trench dug forward of the front trench-line) and, finding it quiet, 'decided to take a peep at the surrounding country.' His 'foolhardy attitude' grew more intense after he was wounded: his 'over-strained nerves had wrought me up to such a pitch of excitement that I was ready for any suicidal exploit.'[109] Wilfred Bion recalled a similar feeling after getting separated from his men during an attack. Fearing that they would lose their nerve, he got out of his trench and walked over the top to reach them, and was knocked over more than once on the way. It was an act of 'sheer unadulterated lunacy . . . the maddest and most dangerous thing I ever did', but by this point in the war 'I cared too little about the whole business to mind the idea of getting killed.'[110]

The ideal of service to others, which had been instilled by mothers from an early age, added to the pressure of command.[111] It could encourage reckless behaviour among exhausted young subalterns. Paradoxically, it was only in death that the devotion Smith so hoped to inspire among his men, was fully expressed. Sergeant Mould wrote to Smith's parents that his passing had 'cast a gloom on us all. The men loved him and I have never felt the same since. I have tried but could not take any interest in my work since. No-one knows only myself how the men worshipped him. His last thoughts on leaving the trench was for them.'[112] The personal inscription on Ernest Smith's headstone reveals how much this tribute would have meant to his parents, but it reminds us too that the high-minded ideal of service could be lethal: 'The Lord Said Well Done/Thy Good and Faithful Servant.'[113]

## Looking after themselves

It was not only the 'Old Originals' in Smith's platoon who were better prepared for Army life than he; the same applied to many civilian rank-and-file soldiers. In some ways the usual relationships between resources and social class were turned on their head in the trenches, since the poorest recruits to the ranks possessed some survival skills that their social betters did not. For the unskilled labourer the privations of the trenches were probably less of a shock than they were to the clerk or skilled manual worker.

The ranks of the wartime British Army were far from homogeneous, and recruits who in civilian life had jealously guarded their class distinctions were forced to live cheek-by-jowl. There were some 'gentleman rankers' who joined up early in the war when commissions were hard to come by; clerks and shop-keepers; engineers and craftsmen, miners and farmers; agricultural labourers and the casually employed poor. But it was the urban working classes who formed the mainstay. Over half the men who served in the British Army between August 1914 and February 1916 (out of a total of 1,743,000) were in the industrial sector. Although these figures include supervisors and managers, the vast majority would have been skilled, semi-skilled and unskilled manual workers.[114] More than three times as many men in the British Army were drawn from the industrial sector as from finance, commerce and the professions combined, the latter sectors containing a high proportion of white-collar workers. It was not just their civilian occupations that distinguished the clerk from the engineer or the farm labourer; their home lives were equally diverse.

For one thing, family size varied widely according to social class and region. In general the poorest tended to come from the largest families, reflecting the inverse relationship between prosperity and fertility.[115] In 1900, birth rates in the largely middle-class area of Hampstead were around 183 per 1,000, compared with 273 per 1,000 in Bethnal Green.[116] It was not unusual for a working-class child to have four or more siblings, whose ages might be spread out over as much as twenty years.[117] The 'hugger-mugger' atmosphere of the lower-middle-class home, by contrast, was due in no small measure to the fact that children in these families often had only one or two siblings.

The poorest families and those in cities were the most over-crowded. In London, one in six lived in housing where there were more than two people to each room.[118] Agricultural labourers in England were also over-crowded, and it was rare for a cottage to have more than two bedrooms.[119] When Charles Taylor, a tunnel construction worker, signed up in April 1915, fourteen people were living in his mother's six-roomed house in South London, and he slept on the couch in the front room. Officers sometimes wondered how the men managed to get to sleep in primitive billets or funk holes, but many had never enjoyed the privacy of a separate bedroom. While the clerk might have found it bewildering at first to have to sleep twelve to a bell tent in the Army, the semi-skilled working man Charles Taylor probably did not; and he was used to putting away his bedding by day.[120] 'It is a hard life we live', reflected the ex-private Thomas Hope as he described pushing his way into a crowded dug-out to get some rest, but 'the ability to look after oneself and rough it are assets. Softness is played upon.'[121]

Ill-fitting Army clothes might not have disconcerted the poor in the way that they did the better off. Jack Cornes, for instance, growing up in the village of Shobdon in rural Hertforshire, wore his older brothers' cast-offs and grown-ups' clothes cut down to size, while his Army boots were probably no less comfortable than the 'heavy hobnailed boots of strong leather' he had been used to wearing on his father's rented small-holding.[122] Though few would have come across anything like the mud of trenches, it was the poorest that lived the closest to dirt. It was not unknown for rural cottages to have earthen floors, and urban children from rough and respectable homes alike would have helped scrub floors and doorsteps in the battle against dirt. Many working-class houses would have had plumbed toilets by 1914, but cesspools at the back of the garden were still in common use: of the 10,000 or so houses in the working-class town of Rochdale in 1906, only 750 had WCs.[123] The private soldier from Rochdale was probably less embarrassed than the London clerk by having to use latrine saps dug hastily off the side of the trench, or a pail or helmet, and would not have blanched afterwards at having to wipe himself with the *Daily Mail* or his shirt tail.[124] He might have endured the grime of the trenches on his body better too, since in houses that lacked plumbed water beyond the kitchen, it was difficult to bathe regularly, while the more prosperous, by the war, would have had cold and in some cases hot water, piped through the house to a bathroom.[125]

Unlike the clerk or craftsman, the unskilled labourer was also used to working in all weathers, as he would again in the trenches. The fastidious personal habits which counted for so much as a mark of respectability in peace time could be a disadvantage in the war.

Working-class housing was generally not just more cramped and harder to keep clean, but less separate from its neighbours than in the middle class. A tenant in a Birmingham back-to-back complained that every 'sound can be heard in the next house. We ourselves can hear those next door sweeten their tea.'[126] More space allowed families who were better off to enjoy leisure and privacy indoors. Harriet Vincent's situation (her family owned two boarding houses close to the docks near Cardiff), with a mother who 'never was outside the home' and a father who would spend his leisure sitting indoors, would have been unthinkable in the cramped homes of the poorest.[127] In crowded houses, mothers wanted children out from under their feet, so they played in the street among larger groups. A Bolton girl whose mother was a weaver remembered the boys playing football in the street, and huddling into a circle on a Saturday to play pitch and toss while she looked out for police.[128] Children did odd-jobs in the neighbourhood, child-minding, getting fuel, shopping and doing delivery jobs. Support could go beyond the immediate family to others, and it was not unusual to have non-kin members living in a house.

The rich associational culture encouraged by these relatively loose household forms provided the working-class ranker with useful survival skills in the war. Anna Davin comments on the 'fear of being alone and a pleasure in company which, whether adaption or cause, must have made the crowded homes more tolerable.'[129] The men's sociability that so impressed officers, and their capacity to get along in large groups, had its roots in the family and household.[130] This can be seen in the pleasure they took during the war in special meals, and in the food that they shared among themselves, as they had with friends and neighbours before the war.[131]

One way in which the more financially secure benefited was that they were likely to be better travelled than the poorest; and hence to find the dislocation of service abroad less disorientating. For all that the agricultural labourer was inured to draughty and damp housing, he was likely steeped in a traditional and very local culture, his travel limited to where he could go on foot, unused to mass entertainments like cinema or music hall and finding even the visit to the nearest market town 'something of a momentous event.'[132] For the son of a skilled urban worker or clerk, travel might be part of his leisure, going to the theatre, cinema, or boy scout troop meeting, boating, fishing, or bicycling, as Richard Church and the iron moulder's son Frank Benson did.[133]

Most rankers, though their mothers did much to look after them as adults, were more practised in housework than their officers. They knew how to clean, launder, sew and cook. Children would help out even in better-off families within the working class. Boys would be set tasks by their parents: cleaning boots on a Saturday, turning the handle of the mangle on washing day, chopping wood or lugging coal and, (in homes that lacked plumbing), fetching water.[134] From about the age of fifteen the First World War veteran Henry Valentine used to 'do all the mangling the iron [*sic*], the washing up and all that. Used to do the lot.'[135] Children did many of the tasks that a servant would do in the middle-class home; and they frequently looked after each other, the difference in age between the oldest and youngest being up to half a generation.[136] They may have nursed younger siblings through illness. The 'calloused surface' of wartime comradeship that gave way to 'rough, protective care' when danger was around, had its antecedents in pre-war friendships and relationships with brothers and sisters.[137]

The majority of rank-and-file soldiers would also have earned money from a young age. For the more prosperous and respectable this was a way of teaching industriousness, but for the poorest it was a necessity.[138] Among sons in particular, their earnings were a matter of pride. The son of a South London coal heaver with ten brothers and sisters truanted from school to sell firewood door-to-door, and stationery in a pub off Farringdon street. He 'never used to get anything out of our parents . . . They never had enough for their beer.'[139]

If a harsh physical environment provided useful survival skills for the poorest Army recruit, the same cannot be said about nourishment. The healthiest recruits were likely to be clerks and skilled workers, while there were high rates of rejection among the urban working class.[140] After the introduction of conscription it was found that the teeth of four out of five adult men were so bad that they could not eat properly.[141] Agricultural labourers were among the least well nourished despite working on the land. Though by 1902 their expenditure on meat was as great as on bread, their diets were deficient in protein.[142] It was harder for men who had been under-nourished to withstand the physical stresses of Army life, but at the same time, the lack of variety in the Army diet would not have been novel for them, and as calorific tables and subjective impressions confirm, they might have fed better than at home. The casual labourer George Hewins, for one, thought the food was 'fairly good when you could get it', and 'more'n we was used to'.[143] Men like Hewins were probably not the ones to complain about Tickler's jam or bully beef.

The ability to scrounge, and the sharing of the spoils among friends and family, also helped soldiers from poorer backgrounds. When Percy Smith took some potatoes and beans from a ruined village in order to make some 'some good hot suppers for the boys', he might have been doing the kind of thing he had as a boy in the farms around Linbury and Leagrave, then largely rural settlements on the edge of Luton.[144] It would be easy to idealise these solidarities but they were fragile and hardship could just as easily cause a man to look after himself first as encourage generosity. Children of the poor might not only thieve from people outside their neighbourhood but from their own.[145] On the Western Front there was an equally blurred line between what was fair game and what was not. Articles of George Coppard's kit kept getting stolen during his time at training camp, and after having a couple of deductions from his pay for the losses, he decided 'the only thing I could do was a bit of counter-swiping'.[146] Some of the men in the Royal Welch Fusiliers threatened to spoil Christmas Day 1916 for their comrades in 'A' Company when they 'made off with the dixies when the cooks' backs were turned.'[147]

Hardship could stunt empathy towards others. Constant shortages could make mothers short-tempered and hard to live with, prone to nagging and outbursts of violence.[148] A Liverpool mother who had given birth to nineteen children (seven of whom survived), and whose husband was a drunkard, coped through the kind of stern discipline the future ranker would encounter among his NCOs:

> She was very strict . . . She'd have a little stick, a little thing what they called the cat o' nine tails on the table, and if we was all sitting down to our meals then we mustn't speak, you had to get on with your meals, and no putting off your plate on the other one's plate what you didn't like . . . You had to eat it.[149]

Rose Albert remembered how little sympathy her mother, who was on her own, had for her children: 'I don't want to hear your troubles, you know', she had said.[150] George Coppard spoke of how the hardships of the trenches made them fractious: 'We would often quarrel violently over nothing. We would rage over little things. Our life was dominated by small, immediate events . . . A slight deficiency in the rations would arouse mutinous mutterings. An extra pot of jam in the ration bag would fill us with a spirit of loyalty and patriotism.'[151]

Poverty could make relationships brittle, but the children of the poor, no less than the children of the better off, lived in their mother's world. Richard Church described how, as a boy, his

> universe was still centred in my mother's fragrant person: her lap, caress, her hair and eyes so curiously the same nut-brown colour, warm and glowing. The garments she took off – the apron, the dropped handkerchief – shone for a while with her light, and I would touch them with rapture, beside myself with love. She and these detachable attributes were like the sun and his flakes of fire. The further I got from her, the colder and darker fell my living days and nights.[152]

A boy from one of the gangs that roamed the back streets of Battersea, inspiring terror in respectable children like Richard Church and his brother, may not have expressed his affections in such a rapturous style, but he was probably just as attuned to his mother's moods and feelings; and with a strong sense too of what it cost her to bring him up.[153] Children in working-class households tended to marry late, the average for men being around twenty-seven and twenty-five for women, which meant that after starting work they could be living in the parental home for up to a decade before setting up their own household. [154] They relied on their mothers to cook meals, purchase clothing and so on, though they contributed to the household financially. When Charles Taylor returned home on leave, his mother slotted straight back into the familiar routines, boiling his clothes and delousing him.[155] Whereas the sons of prosperous middle-class families were sent to boarding school from around age eight, London's working-class mothers 'kept each of their sons close to them for almost two decades.'[156]

Within the working class the well-springs of stoicism were as much maternal as paternal, in contrast to the lower middle and middle classes, who praised stoicism as an aspect of manliness, and who established institutions such as the public schools, boys' brigades and boy scouts, devoted to its inculcation. Children with hard-pressed mothers learned to be uncomplaining. If food was short they tried not to protest, and they tended not to burden mothers with their own troubles. 'None of us wears his heart on our sleeves. We was brought up to keep us moans and us groans to ourselves', recalled one man of his working-class childhood.[157] Hardship and consideration towards the mother tended to produce a capacity for what one working-class writer called 'mute endurance'.[158]

This attitude impressed many a platoon officer during the war. They noted the men's capacities to stay 'cheerful' in the most miserable situations. E. K. Smith, writing home after battle at Hooge described how the bombardment 'resulted in a great strain on the nerves which the men stood wonderfully well, and did not need much steadying from me.'[159] At home, humour was a way of defusing hardship and buoying up loved ones; and it played a similar role in boosting morale during the war.[160] Edward Chapman wrote to his mother in typically patronising class idiom of the 'little fellow in the Company, who is always making jokes and keeping everybody laughing. I should like to appoint him my Jester, and keep him at Company headquarters to keep my spirits up!'[161]

Growing up amidst dearth, children often possessed a strong desire to make their mothers' lives easier. Ellen Ross has noted how the memoirs of working-class Edwardian children are 'at least partly structured by gratitude'.[162] 'I believe my mother was one of the most absolutely unselfish women who even breathed', wrote a working-class man in his memoirs.[163] For a young man, the pride in earning his own wage was not just related to the status it gave him among his peers, but because it allowed him to make his mother more comfortable.[164] The take-up of Separation Allowances during the war, which were often organised with help from sons, showed how many men had been contributing to their mothers' support before the war.[165]

How did this kind of background affect the men's relationships with their officers? The social and emotional worlds of officers and men faced inwards, towards their own. The officer might feel some affection for the rankers in his platoon, seeing them as 'MY MEN' and talking freely about how 'intimately' he knew them, but to the ranker even the most approachable officer was a pretty distant figure.[166] Out of the line a man could not even approach his platoon or company officer directly, but must relay his request for an interview through the NCO.[167] These differences never disappeared even in the front line where discipline was more relaxed.

At the same time, the shared experience of hardship and danger in the trenches could result in feelings that, whilst not based on knowledge of each other's personality and situation, were nonetheless affectionate. 'Some of my best men are very awkward on parade', wrote Chapman from the front line, but 'I cannot get angry with them for it. When you have ducked to the same shell with a man over and over again, you develop a sense of comradeship, which you couldn't get in any other way.'[168]

Most rankers would not have talked of their officers as comrades, but as long as an officer was doing his best to look after them, they would accept his leadership. The veteran ranker Norman Gladden, who was not afraid to criticise the officers, wrote admiringly of Captain West. West, a professional man in civilian life, did not exhibit the traditional qualities of an officer. Although brave, he was of a gentle temperament, 'never, in fact, raising his voice in anger'. He 'always treated us with consideration.'[169] Gladden and his comrades 'loved' Captain West, but the ranker's feelings towards a bad officer could be equally extreme. A Major on home leave spoke of 'officers, and these not a few, who are conceited cads, and behave so badly to the men that the men detest them. It is no uncommon thing to hear a growl in billets – "So and so is a brute. Wait till I get him in front of me in action, and I will put a bullet into him."'[170] When rankers were critical of their officers, it was usually because they were inconsiderate towards them. Alfred Hale laid the blame for his misery in a Royal Flying Corps training camp at the feet of the Commanding Officer. If Captain Ross 'had been a little less of an almighty tin god, thought a little less of his own comfort and a little more of other people's, things might have been very different.'[171]

Officers in the line were frequently bad-tempered, taking out their stress on the men, as hard-pressed mothers had done. 'The nervousness, strain and irritability of his officers could be responsible for a lot of what Tommy had to put up with. In the final analysis he was always the butt', wrote the ranker George Coppard.[172] Wilfred Owen, on joining his Battalion in France, noted that 'On all the officers' faces there is a harassed look that I have never seen before'.[173] A private might chafe under the hot temper of his officer, but, as with the exasperated outbursts of a mother, he could see the strain he was under. He shared the subaltern's distrust of senior officers: when Gladden's 'quiet and gentlemanly' Captain was bawled out by the adjutant for allowing his men to be dismissed early from parade, the men 'were genuinely sorry for our immediate leaders and did our best to share the humiliation being suffered on our behalf.'[174] The ranker's sympathy towards his officer was strengthened by their shared resentment of High Command. George Coppard reckoned that General Haig did not have the confidence of his men because he was 'so completely remote from the actual fighting'. The men were 'wholly loyal to their own officers, and that was as far as their confidence went. It was trust and comradeship founded on the actual sharing of dangers together.'[175]

The structures of feeling that allowed rankers to survive the Western Front were as much the product of their experience within the home, as of authority relations within the workplace or the Army. The men from less well-off backgrounds who made up the mainstay of the 'other ranks' entered the trenches with a long history of being uncomplaining, and of cooperating with those in authority. This is not to say – much as the subaltern might have wished it – that the ranker who felt deep affection for his officer was typical. Rather, it is to suggest that his consent to the authority wielded by his officers was conditioned by his experience of growing up, including his feelings towards his mother.

*  *  *

Shortly after arriving in France, Lionel Hall wrote home to his parents 'we are a very cheerful crowd – officers and men. We play all sorts of children's games with the men. There is something wonderfully pathetic about the private soldier in France. He is just a child, sometimes querulous, but always trustful.'[176] Officers frequently thought of their men as child-like; and indeed, the emphasis the British Army put on ensuring the men's comforts reflected its distrust in their ability to look after themselves. The British rank-and-file soldier, Bourne notes, was 'mollycoddled'.[177]

But this stereotype of the dependent ranker frequently bore an inverse relationship to reality. It was young men such as Hall, fresh from the playing field of the public school, financially independent for the first time, showered with parcels from home and unpractised in the care of others, who were the more like children. When the Welsh miner Rowland Luther joined the Army at nineteen – around Hall's age – he had been working for five years, was earning £2 a week, and was about to train as a Colliery manager.[178] It is one of the ironies of leadership during the war that the private soldier was often better at looking after himself than the officer who was supposed to look after him.

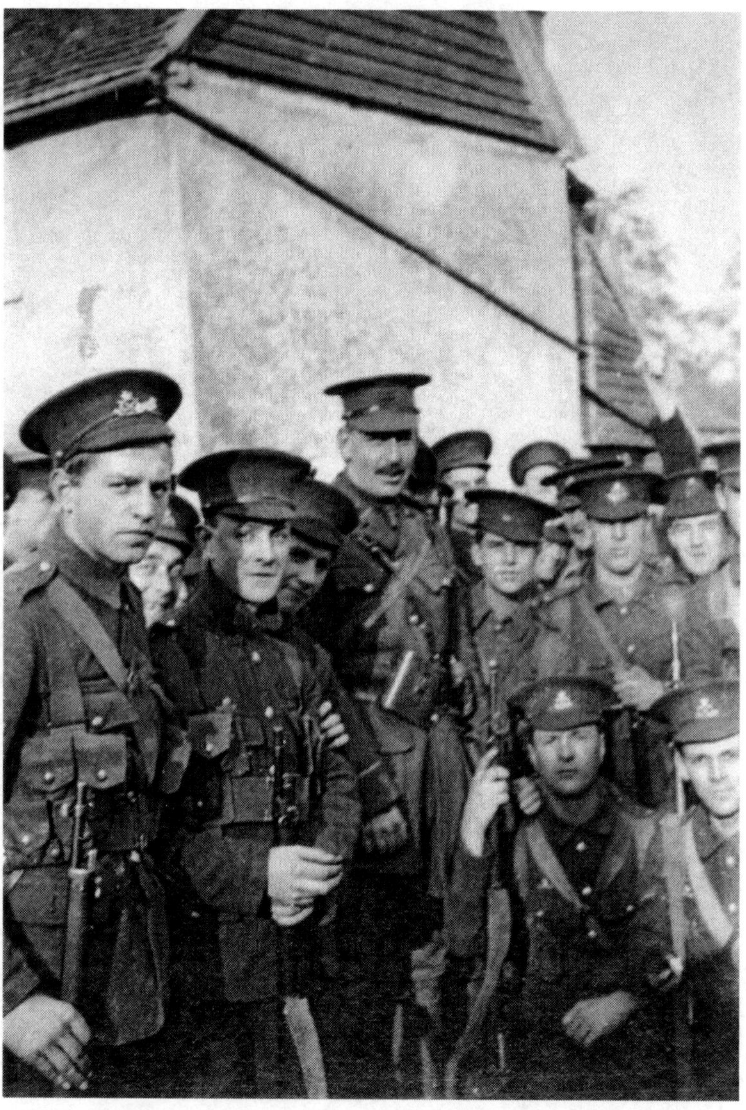

*18* Lieutenant Finnis and men of the 1/6th Battalion, South Staffordshire Regiment, 1915

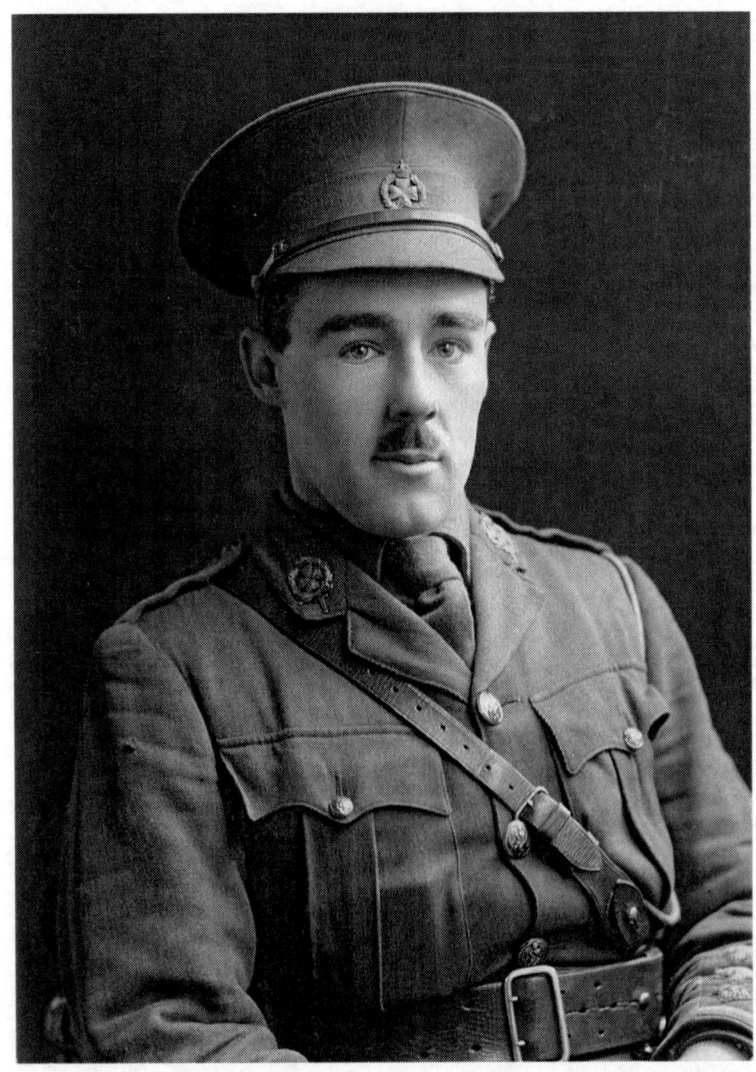

*19* The two identities of Reggie Chenevix Trench: soldier, 1914–15 . . .

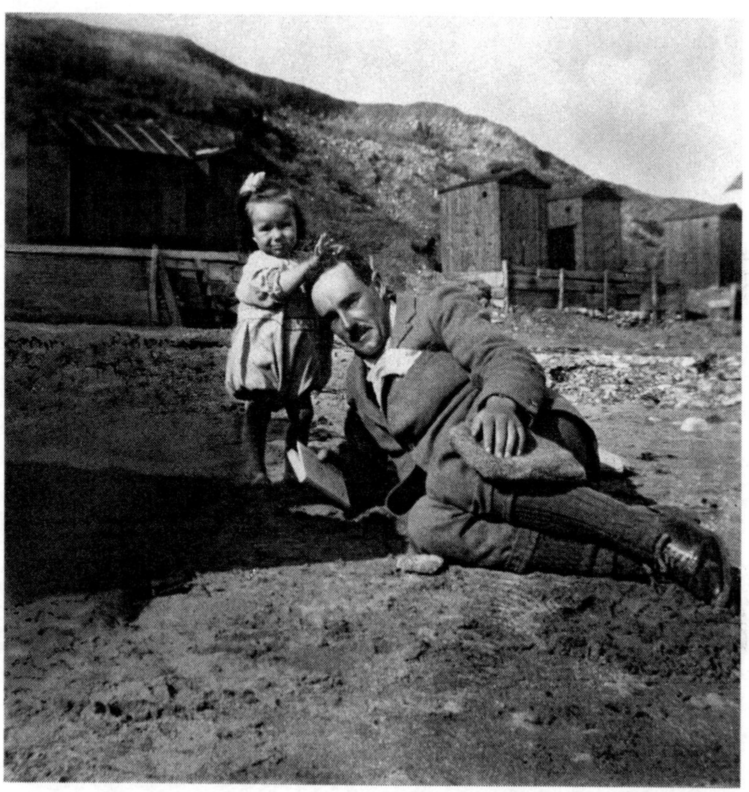

*20* . . . and father, at Charmouth beach, July 1917, with daughter Delle

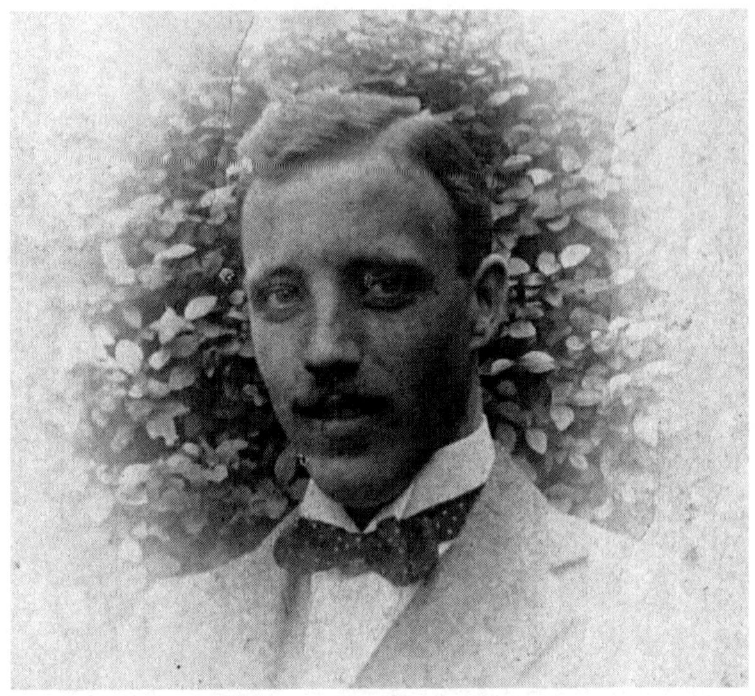

*21* Portrait of Ernest Smith

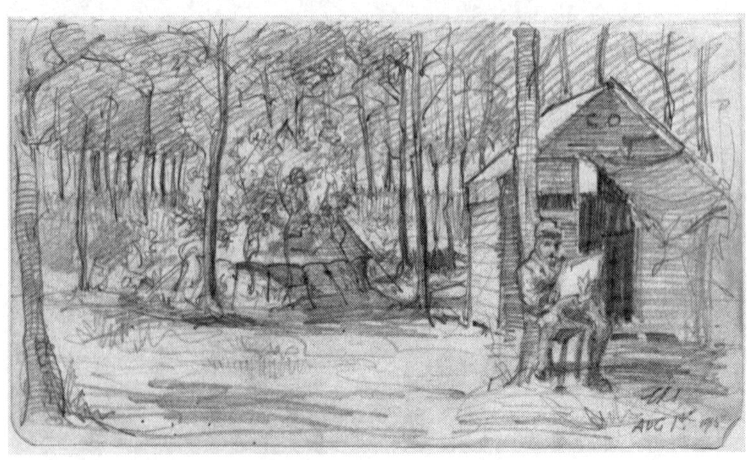

*22* 'August 1st 1915', sketched by Ernest Smith as he made his way up to the front line for the first time

## Notes

1 E. K. Smith to mother, 29 October, 1 November 1915, *Letters Sent From France. Service with the Artists' Rifles and the Buffs, December 1914–December 1915* (London: J. Cobb, 1994), p. 115, p. 118.
2 1st Battalion, The Buffs Diary, 22 October 1915, National Archives WO95/1608.
3 E. K. Smith to mother, 1 November, 27 October 1915, *Letters Sent From France*, p. 116, p. 113.
4 E. K. Smith to mother, 28 October 1915, *Letters Sent From France*, p. 114.
5 D. Hankey, *A Student in Arms* (London: Andrew Melrose, 1917), p. 112.
6 E. K. Smith to mother 20 January, 4 February; 3 April 1915, *Letters Sent From France*, p. 14, p. 18, p. 42.
7 E. K. Smith to mother, 21 April; Smith to father 22 June 1915, *Letters Sent From France*, p. 46, p. 66.
8 E. K. Smith to mother, 16 September, 3 August 1915, *Letters Sent From France*, p. 93; p. 75. See Janet Watson on the volunteer soldiers' unease among Regulars. *Fighting Different Wars. Experience, Memory and the First World War in Britain* (Cambridge: Cambridge University Press, 2004), p. 51.
9 E. K. Smith to mother, 9 August 1915, *Letters Sent From France*, p. 77.
10 Gary Sheffield, *Leadership in the Trenches. Officer–Man relations, Morale and Discipline in the British Army in the Era of the First World War* (Basingstoke: Palgrave, 2000), p. 88.
11 The word 'tact' is used in more than one military history to describe the volunteer officer's leadership. D. Winter, *Death's Men. Soldiers of the Great War* (London: Penguin, 1979), p. 64; Sheffield, *Leadership in the Trenches*, p. 74. Second Lieutenant Graham Greenwell felt uncomfortable sitting on the Court Martial of a 'poor devil' who had drunk his comrade's rum ration, for he 'sympathised with him sincerely.' Greenwell to mother, 8 February 1917, *An Infant in Arms. War Letters of a Company Commander 1914–1918* (London: Allen Lane, The Penguin Press, 1972), p. 152. By contrast, General Crozier, a veteran of the South African campaign, disapproved greatly of the 'humane principles' shown by one of his New Army Majors, who refused to enforce a death sentence on a man found asleep on sentry duty. Brig.-Gen. F. P. Crozier, *A Brass Hat in No Man's Land (London: Jonathan Cape, 1930)*, p. 148.
12 Sheffield, *Leadership in the Trenches*, p. 75.
13 E. K. Smith to mother, 5 January; 21 March 1915, *Letters Sent From France*, p. 7, p. 36.
14 S. Das, *Touch and Intimacy in First World War Literature* (Cambridge: Cambridge University Press, 2005), p. 35.
15 J. Bourne, 'The British Working Man in Arms', in H. Cecil and P. Liddle, *Facing Armageddon. The First World War Experienced* (London: Pen & Sword, 1996), pp. 341–2.

16 Bourne, 'The British Working Man', pp. 346–7.
17 J. Keegan, *The Face of Battle* (London: Jonathan Cape, 1976), p. 274.
18 Sheffield, *Leadership in the Trenches*, pp. 43–50, p. 70.
19 E. K. Smith to mother, 29 October 1915, *Letters Sent From France*, p. 115.
20 W. H. R. Rivers, *Instinct and the Unconscious. A Contribution to a Biological Theory of the Psycho-Neuroses* (Cambridge: Cambridge University Press, 1920), p. 221.
21 J. G. Fuller is surely right that officers were liable to 'misjudge' the esteem in which they were held. *Troop Morale and Popular Culture in the British and Dominion Armies* (Oxford: Clarendon Press, 1991), p. 53.
22 M. Petter, '"Temporary Gentlemen" in the Aftermath of the Great War: Rank, Status and the Ex-Officer Problem', *The Historical Journal*, Vol. 37, No. 1 (March, 1994), p. 136.
23 Petter, 'Temporary Gentlemen', p. 131, p. 137.
24 Petter, 'Temporary Gentlemen', p. 139.
25 R. M. Bracco, *Merchants of Hope. British Middlebrow Writers and the First World War* (Oxford: Berg, 1993), p. 155, p. 165.
26 W. Owen quoted in Petter, 'Temporary Gentlemen', p. 140.
27 R. Church, *Over the Bridge. An Essay in Autobiography* (London: William Heinemann, 1955), p. 22.
28 R. Holmes, *Tommy. The British Soldier on the Western Front 1914–1918* (London: Harper Perennial, 2005), pp. 577–8. Gary Sheffield remarks on how, in their officer-training courses, temporary officers were taught, and internalised, 'the paternalism and *noblesse oblige* which was the hallmark of the Regular officer.' *Leadership in the Trenches*, p. 59. See also D. Winter, *Death's Men*, p. 61.
29 A. H. Trapmann, *Straight Tips for 'Subs'* (London: Forester Groom, 1916), p. 49.
30 'Basilisk', *Talks on Leadership Addressed to Young Artillery Officers* (London: Hugh Rees, 1921), p. 25.
31 On the work involved in running a household see Carol Dyehouse, 'Mothers and Daughters in the Middle-Class Home c. 1870–1914', in J. Lewis (ed.), *Labour and Love. Women's Experience of Home and Family 1850–1940* (Oxford: Blackwell, 1986), p. 32.
32 Holmes, *Tommy*, pp. 556–7. On mothers and discipline see J. Tosh, *A Man's Place. Masculinity and the Middle-Class Home in Victorian England* (New Haven: Yale University Press, 1999), p. 92.
33 S. Ellis quoted in Tosh, *A Man's Place*, p. 91.
34 'Basilisk', *Talks on Leadership*, p. 13. 'Perhaps the golden rule which covers all tips on the treatment of men', stated another guide, is 'to place yourself in the man's position, and then do as you would be done by.' Trapmann, *Straight Tips for 'Subs'*, pp. 49–50.
35 R. D. Mountfort to mother, 26 September 1915, IWM Con Shelf.

36 Greenwell to mother, May 24 1915, *An Infant in Arms*, p. 15.
37 L. Urwick to mother, 17 October 1915, private collection.
38 J. R. Gillis, *A World of Their Own Making. Myth, Ritual and the Quest for Family Values* (New York: Basic Books, 1996), p. 73; Tosh, *A Man's Place*, p. 86.
39 Urwick to father, 21 April 1915.
40 R. Trench to mother, 2 June 1917, private collection.
41 Greenwell to mother, 25 May 1917, *An Infant in Arms*, p. 182.
42 Tosh, *A Man's Place*, p. 85.
43 The ideal of selflessness, and its teaching by mothers, was especially important in evangelical families. See Tosh, *A Man's Place*, pp. 112–14.
44 As Stefan Collini remarks, 'emotional entropy [was] assumed to be the consequence of absorption in purely selfish aims.' *Public Moralists. Political Thought and Intellectual Life in Modern Britain* (Oxford: Clarendon Press, 1993), p. 65.
45 R. Graves, R., *Goodbye to All That* (Harmondsworth, Middx.: Penguin, 1960), p. 18, pp. 31–3.
46 Susan Owen quoted in D. Hibberd, *Wilfred Owen. A New Biography* (London: Weidenfeld & Nicolson, 2002), p. 19. Gilbert Talbot's mother recalled that 'As a child and boy he was delightful to teach from the Bible.' G. Talbot, *Gilbert Walter Lyttleton Talbot. Born September 1 1891. Killed in Action at Hooge, July 30 1915* (London: Chiswick Press, 1916), pp. 37–8.
47 Anon., *Boy of My Heart* (London: Hodder & Stoughton, 1916), p. 145, p. 141.
48 Anon., *Boy of My Heart*, p. 32.
49 Anon., *Boy of My Heart*, pp. 30–1, p. 91.
50 V. Brittain, in A. Bishop, with T. Smart (eds.), *Vera Brittain. War Diary 1913–1917, Chronicle of Youth* (London: Victor Gollancz, 1981), p. 138.
51 E. K. Smith to mother, 13 August 1915, *Letters Sent From France*, pp. 80–1.
52 Quoted in S. Das, *Touch and Intimacy*, p. 7.
53 W. Owen to mother, 10 January 1917, in J. Bell (ed.), *Wilfred Owen. Selected Letters* (Oxford: Oxford University Press, 1985), p. 212.
54 E. K. Smith to mother, 13 August 1915, *Letters Sent From France*, p. 81.
55 Trench to mother, 10 May 1917.
56 Quoted in B. Caine, *Destined to be Wives. The Sisters of Beatrice Webb* (Oxford: Oxford University Press, 1988), p. 157.
57 Tosh, *A Man's Place*, p. 114.
58 Wilfred's father is absent from the scene. Hibberd, *Wilfred Owen*, p. 33, pp. 76–7.
59 The variety of terms is revealed in the oral history project by P. Thompson and T. Lummis, 'Family Life and Work Experience Before 1918, 1870–1973' [computer file], 5th edition (Colchester: UK Data Archive [distributor], April 2005. SN: 2000).

60 A. Fletcher, 'Richard Chevenix Trench and his Legacy: An Appreciation by Anthony Fletcher', unpublished paper, p. 25.
61 L. Davidoff, *Worlds Between. Historical Perspectives on Gender and Class* (Cambridge: Polity Press, 1995), p. 112.
62 J. Gathorne-Hardy, *The Rise and Fall of the British Nanny* (London: Arrow, 1972), p. 26.
63 Thompson and Lummis, 'Family Life and Work', interview 142, pp. 4–5, p. 8, p. 11.
64 Davidoff, *Worlds Between*, p. 110. It was not necessarily the case, however, that children who were close to their nanny were less close to their parents. Affections for servants, as Elizabeth Buettner notes, 'complemented or competed with parent–child intimacy.' *Empire Families. Britons and Late Imperial India* (Oxford: Oxford University Press, 2004), p. 113.
65 Anon., *Boy of My Heart*, p. 34, p. 132.
66 Talbot, *Gilbert Walter Lyttleton Talbot*, p. 10.
67 R. Bickersteth to nurse, 8 May 1915, The Bickersteth War Diaries and the Papers of John Burgon Bickersteth, Vol. 2, p. 555, Churchill Archives Centre, GBR/0014/BICK.
68 Gathorne-Hardy, *The Rise and Fall*, pp. 27–8. As Davidoff notes, it was children who were most likely to maintain contact with servants in later life. *Worlds Between*, p. 33.
69 C. Asquith, *Diaries 1915–18* (London: Hutchinson, 1968), pp. 98–9.
70 Thompson and Lummis, 'Family Life and Work', interview 142, p. 3.
71 See for example Thompson and Lummis, 'Family Life and Work', interview 178, p. 8; interview 247, p. 22–3.
72 H. A. Munro diary, 22 September 1915, IWM P374.
73 Letter from Neil Munro to Sheriff John Macmaster, 21 October 1915, IWM P374.
74 D. Starrett memoir, p. 14, IWM 79/35/1.
75 G. Chapman, *A Passionate Prodigality. Fragments of Autobiography* (New York: Holt, Rinehart & Winston, 1966), p. 209. Warwick Deeping, in his autobiographical novel, describes another domestic scene after battle: Finch 'makes me lie down. He unlaces and pulls off my muddy field-boots, and covers me with the blanket. I have a strange feeling of being a child in the hands of a strong, and capable nurse.' *No Hero – This* (London: Cassell, 1936), p. 271.
76 Greenwell to mother, 1 October 1914, *An Infant in Arms*, p. 2.
77 Munro diary, 10 June 1915.
78 Trapmann, *Straight Tips for 'Subs'*, pp. 49–50.
79 War Office, General Staff Censorship and Publicity Section, 'Lecture on the Postal Censorship Orders' (London: Censorship and Publicity Section, General Staff, 1918), p. 19.

80 L. Hall to parents, 9 March 1917, IWM 96/57/1; W. Owen to mother, 4 January, 10 January 1917, in Bell (ed.), *Wilfred Owen. Selected Letters*, p. 208, p. 212.
81 A. Eden, *Another World 1897–1917* (London: Allen Lane, 1976), p. 85.
82 J. C. Dunn (ed.), *The War the Infantry Knew. A Chronicle of Service in France and Belgium* (London: Abacus, 1994), p. 176.
83 Anon., *Boy of My Heart*, pp. 62–3.
84 Brittain, *Vera Brittain*, pp. 230–1.
85 Well-to-do social commentators before the war were sometimes prone to idealise the affections of working people in the same way. Charles Booth, for example, thought the children of the wealthy were emotionally impoverished by comparison with the working class who, though less likely to survive to adulthood, were 'free from the paraphernalia of servants, nurses and governesses.' Quoted in A. Davin, *Growing Up Poor. Home, School and Street in London, 1870–1914* (London: Rivers Oram Press), p. 20.
86 W. B. P. Spencer to father, 24 December 1914, IWM 87/56/1.
87 Greenwell to mother, 27 May 1915, *An Infant in Arms*, p. 16.
88 Quoted in A. Fletcher, 'An Officer on the Western Front', *History Today*, Vol. 54, No. 8 (August 2004), p. 33. See also Edmund Blunden's poem 'The Watchers', which recalls a 'gruff sentry's kindness'. *Undertones of War* (London: Penguin, 2000), pp. 233–4.
89 Trench to mother, 13 May 1917.
90 Biographical details are given in A. Fletcher, 'Patriotism, Identity and Commemoration: New Light on the Great War from the Papers of Major Reggie Chenevix Trench', *History*, Volume 90, No. 300 (October 2005), p. 532.
91 Delle Fletcher to Michael Roper, personal communication, 30 May 2007.
92 M.C.W. Charteris, *A Family Record* (London: Curwen Press, 1932), pp. 333–4.
93 Charteris, *A Family Record*, p. 313.
94 Sheffield, *Leadership in the Trenches*, p. 91. Fuller notes that the youth of public school officers was a cause of discontent among some rankers. *Troop Morale*, p. 54.
95 A platoon might even be constituted in the majority by men who were older than their officer. Of the twenty-one men listed in the Platoon Roll Book for 'D' Company 8th Northamptonshire Regiment for 1916, almost half were older than thirty, whilst only three were under twenty. IWM Misc. 60/911.
96 Trapmann, *Straight Tips for 'Subs'*, p. 23.
97 L. Urwick, 'Apprenticeship to Management. An Autobiography of Lt. Col. L. F. Urwick', 1970, in private possession, p. 85.
98 G. Coppard, *With A Machine Gun to Cambrai. A Story of the First World War* (London: Cassell, 1980), p. 118.

99 E. K. Smith to mother, 16 October, 18 September 1915, *Letters Sent From France*, p. 118, p. 109.
100 E. K. Smith to mother, 29 October, 19 December 1915, *Letters Sent From France*, p. 115, p. 138.
101 Sergeant Mould to Mrs Smith, date unknown, *Letters Sent From France*, p. 142.
102 Quoted in Sheffield, *Leadership in the Trenches*, p. 90.
103 B. Hood, *Duties For All Ranks. Specially Compiled For the New Armies and Volunteer Training Corps from the C.O. to the Private* (London: Harrison & Sons, 1915), p. 14.
104 Quoted in Sheffield, *Leadership in the Trenches*, p. 59.
105 E. K. Smith to mother, 21 April, 3 August 1915, *Letters Sent From France*, p. 47, p. 76.
106 1st Battalion, The Buffs Diary, 20 December 1915.
107 1st Battalion, The Buffs Diary, 20 December 1915.
108 Sergeant Mould to Mrs Smith, 24 January 1916, *Letters Sent From France*, pp. 141–2.
109 S. Sassoon, *The Complete Memoirs of George Sherston* (London: Faber & Faber, 1972), pp. 444–5.
110 W. R. Bion, *War Memoirs 1917–19* (London: H. Karnac, 1997), p. 106.
111 Janet Watson points out how the service ethos could compound the stress of combat among soldiers; this was particularly true of subalterns, who were supposed to set an example to their men. *Fighting Different Wars*, pp. 47–8.
112 Sergeant Mould to Mrs Smith, 24 January 1916, *Letters Sent From France*, pp. 141–3.
113 E. K. Smith's headstone is at Ljissenthoek Cemetery, row II A. 19.
114 J. M. Winter, *The Great War and the British People* (Basingstoke: Macmillan, 1985), Table 2.3, p. 34.
115 Davin, *Growing Up Poor*, p. 16.
116 E. Ross, 'Labour and Love: Re-Discovering London's Working-Class Mothers, 1870–1918', in J. Lewis (ed.), *Labour and Love. Women's Experience of Home and Family 1850–1940* (Oxford: Blackwell, 1986), Table 3:1, p. 76.
117 Davin, *Growing Up Poor*, p. 16.
118 P. Thompson, *The Edwardians. The Remaking of British Societyy* (London: Routledge, 1992), p. 34.
119 Thompson, *The Edwardians*, pp. 35–6.
120 C. W. Taylor memoir, np, IWM 01/8/1.
121 Quoted in D. Winter, *Death's Men*, p. 57.
122 J. Cornes, 'The Village and Other Recollections', p. 3. In private possession.
123 J. Burnett, *A Social History of Housing, 1815–1985* (London: Methuen, 1986), p. 214.
124 On latrines in the trenches see D. Winter, *Death's Men*, p. 104.

125 Burnett, *A Social History of Housing*, pp. 214–15.

126 Thompson, *The Edwardians*, p. 34.

127 Thompson, *The Edwardians*, p. 119. The relative spaciousness of lower-middle- class homes, comments Geoffrey Crossick, helped promote 'a family centredness, a degree of privacy and isolation that was impossible for most working class families.' 'The Emergence of the Lower Middle Class in Britain': A Discussion', in G. Crossick (ed.), *The Lower Middle Class in Britain, 1870–1914* (London: Croom Helm, 1977), p. 27.

128 Thompson, *The Edwardians*, p. 68.

129 Davin, *Growing Up Poor*, p. 56.

130 As Bourne observes, the Army was like the working-class neighbourhood in that it 'provided an overlapping network of communities beyond the primary group' (i.e, the platoon section or household). J. Bourne, 'The British Working Man', p. 349.

131 E. Ross, *Love and Toil. Motherhood in Outcast London 1870-1918* (Oxford: Oxford University Press, 1993), pp. 30–1. On the emotional significance of food shared between men, see R. Duffett, 'A War Unimagined: Food and the Rank and File Soldier of the First World War', in J. Meyer (ed.), *Popular Culture and the First World War* (Leiden: Brill, 2007), pp. 53–5.

132 Thompson, *The Edwardians*, p. 40.

133 Thompson, *The Edwardians*, p. 131, p. 140.

134 Davin, *Growing Up Poor*, p. 164, pp. 176–7, p. 186.

135 Thompson and Lummis, 'Family Life and Work', interview 419, p. 13.

136 Davin, *Growing Up Poor*, p. 175. The testimonies of this generation, Ellen Ross comments, are full of domestic tips: 'the intricacies of diapering a baby, getting a wash white, or making a tasty stew for under sixpence.' Ross, *Love and Toil*, p. 153.

137 Winter, *Death's Men*, p. 57.

138 Davin, *Growing Up Poor*, pp. 164–5.

139 Thompson, *The Edwardians*, p. 62.

140 Jonathan Wild goes so far as to call clerks the 'ideal physical specimens for soldiering.' 'A Merciful, Heaven-Sent Release?: The Clerk and the First World War in British Literary Culture', *Cultural and Social History* Vol. 4, No. 1 (March 2007), p. 76.

141 Thompson, *The Edwardians*, p. 18.

142 J, Burnett, *Plenty and Want. A Social History of Diet in England from 1815 to the Present Day* (London: Scolar Press, 1979), p. 152, p. 154.

143 A. Hewins (ed.), *The Dillen. Memories of a Man of Stratford upon Avon* (Oxford: Oxford University Press, 1983), p. 142.

144 Percy Smith to Mother and Dad, 18 September 1917, IWM 01/21/1.

145 See Davin, *Growing Up Poor*, pp. 185–6.

146 Coppard, *With A Machine Gun*, p. 7.

147 Dunn (ed.), *War the Infantry Knew*, p. 174, p. 221.

148 Ross, *Love and Toil*, p. 150; J. Burnett, *Destiny Obscure. Autobiographies of Childhood, Education and Family from the 1820s to the 1920s* (London: Allen Lane, 1982), p. 235.
149 Thompson, *The Edwardians*, p. 60.
150 Ross, *Love and Toil*, p. 151. See Melanie Tebbutt on the way that poverty could erode sympathy. *Women's Talk? A Social History of 'Gossip' in Working Class Neighborhoods 1880–1960* (Aldershot: Scolar Press, 1995), p. 112.
151 Quoted in Winter, *Death's Men*, p. 56.
152 Church, *Over the Bridge*, p. 3.
153 Church, *Over the Bridge*, pp. 13–17.
154 Ross, *Love and Toil*, p. 63; Thompson, *The Edwardians*, p. 65.
155 Taylor memoir, np.
156 Ross, *Love and Toil*, p. 153.
157 Thompson and Lummis, 'Family Life and Work', interview 181, p. 31.
158 Quoted in Ross, *Love and Toil*, p. 152.
159 E. K. Smith to mother, 13 August 1916, *Letters Sent From France*, p. 79. For other examples see Fletcher, 'Patriotism, Identity and Commemoration', p. 546.
160 See Ross on the role of humour in working-class families, *Love and Toil*, p. 129.
161 E. F. Chapman to mother, 18 May 1917, IWM Con Shelf, p. 74.
162 Ross, *Love and Toil*, p. 24.
163 Quoted in D. Vincent, *Literacy and Popular Culture. England 1750–1914* (Cambridge: Cambridge University Press, 1989), p. 63.
164 For examples of this pride see Ross, *Love and Toil*, p. 160; L Jamieson, 'Limited Resources and Limiting Conventions: Working-Class Mothers and Daughters in Urban Scotland c. 1890–1918', in J. Lewis (ed.), *Labour and Love. Women's Experience of Home and Family 1850–1940* (Oxford: Blackwell, 1986), pp. 52–5, p. 58.
165 S. Pederson, 'Gender, Welfare, and Citizenship in Britain during the Great War', *American Historical Review*, Vol. 95, No. 4 (1990), p. 985; Jamieson, 'Limited Resources', p. 88. See also Chapter 2 above on Separation Allowances, pp. 105–6.
166 Quote from E. K. Smith to mother, 18 May 1917, *Letters Sent From France*, p. 74.
167 K. Simpson, 'The Officers', in I. Beckett and K. Simpson, *A Nation in Arms. A Social Study of the British Army in the First World War* (Manchester: Manchester University Press, 1985), p. 68.
168 E. F. Chapman to mother, 17 May 1917.
169 See N. Gladden, *Ypres 1917* (London: William Kimber, 1967), p. 83, p. 110.
170 Rev. A. Clark, *Echoes of the Great War* (Oxford: Oxford University Press, 1985), p. 203.

171 P. Fussell (ed.), *The Ordeal of Alfred M. Hale. The Memoirs of a Soldier Servant* (London: Leo Cooper, 1975), p. 100, pp. 112–13.
172 Coppard, *With A Machine Gun*, p. 69.
173 W. Owen to mother, 4 January 1917, in Bell (ed.), *Wilfred Owen. Selected Letters*, p. 208. Frederic Manning described how, in the build-up to battle, the officers grew more agitated: 'now there was continual wind-up. A hot and exasperated officer would suddenly appear outside the huts, and the men were fallen in to receive his orders.' F. Manning, *Her Privates We* (London: Serpent's Tail, 1999), p. 199.
174 Gladden, *Ypres*, p. 83.
175 Coppard, *With A Machine Gun*, p. 76.
176 Hall to parents, 9 March 1917.
177 J. Bourne, *Britain and the Great War* (London: Edward Arnold, 1989), p. 221.
178 R. M. Luther memoir, IWM 87/8/1, p. 2.

PART III

# Falling apart

# 5

# Love and loss

On 22 April 1915, as David Fenton was following Jim Noone up a communication trench after twenty-four hours in the line, Jim suddenly reeled to the left and, with a 'choking sob', slumped to the ground unconscious. He had been hit in the back of his shoulder and the bullet had probably punctured his lung. Fenton bent down beside his friend on the trench floor and 'held him in my arms to the end, and when his soul had departed I kissed him twice where I knew you would have kissed him – on the brow – once for his mother and once for myself.'

After Jim's death Fenton gathered together his personal possessions for Mrs Noone. He had hoped to get her a lock of Jim's hair but it was too dangerous to carry his body back to billets. They 'buried him where he fell, so I must disappoint you in this respect.' Fenton promised that if he did not 'join him in the meantime', after the war 'I will show you and yours his grave.' He ended his letter with a tribute and a request. Jim had been 'the life of the section, a universal favourite and a true, pure and faithful friend. So, Mrs Noone, I join my tenderest sympathy with you in your great loss.' He would also be 'greatly favoured' if Mrs Noone had 'anything of his which you could spare for me to wear.'[1]

Fenton here constructs a triangular scene, in which mother and friend are brought together by their love of the same man. The scene is deeply touching, but Fenton is careful to insulate Mrs Noone from its horror. He describes Jim's death in a precise and spare manner, explaining how the bullet 'came out about four inches below his throat, and must have pieced his lung.' There is no mention of blood, though the bullet had passed through one of the most blood-intensive organs in the body and may well also have hit major blood vessels. The sound of a man dying for breath – it was not for nothing that lung wounds were called 'sucking wounds' – is elevated into a poetic 'choking sob'.[2] Noone is saved from pain by becoming unconscious almost immediately, and, though this is not unlikely given the place of entry of the bullet, deaths from lung wounds were often drawn out as the level of oxygen in the blood fell to a lethal point.[3] Fenton controls Mrs Noone's emotional proximity to the scene, screening her from horror. He creates what Carol Acton, in her study of mourning in modern warfare, calls an 'abstraction of the body', which guards against the excessive pain of mothers, and thus makes it possible to continue fighting.[4]

The self-possession and composure in Fenton's prose is remarkable considering that his Battalion, the 1/4 Duke of Wellington's (West Riding Regiment) had landed at Boulogne only a week earlier and this was most likely Fenton's first experience of the front-line.[5] Fenton was also the youngest of the three in the triangle, being just twenty, a full five years younger than his friend. Before the war it would have been highly unusual for such a young man to break the news of a death as Fenton did here. His calm, controlled tone, which imparts the facts and carefully moves Mrs Noone to grief, approximates that of a husband and father perhaps. Yet at no point does Fenton address Jim's father, though he is presumably among the 'you and yours' who would be taken to visit Jim's grave after the war. Fathers are kept outside the triangle. If in some ways Fenton seems to shoulder a burden beyond his years, in others he seems to want mothering, as he intimates in his request for some of Jim's clothes to wear. Fenton's own mother had died when he was young and his step-mother was also dead. No mother would grieve for him if he should die, and his tender letter was perhaps animated as much by this thought as by the soldierly duty of one comrade towards the family of another.

If his tone is manly, at the same time the tenderness that David Fenton admits towards Jim is far removed from the stoic image of the soldier. He holds and kisses his friend, but this intimacy is made permissible partly because he acts on *behalf* of Noone's mother. Admitting Mrs Noone into the scene gives David Fenton someone he can confess his love to – mother and friend can mourn together or 'join' in their loss, as he puts it – but it also removes any thought that this friendship was anything other than 'pure'. The statement that Jim was a 'universal favourite' does the same thing, picturing Fenton's affection, not as singular, but as something felt by the whole section; as comradeship. The 'intensification and quickening of male bonds' that Santanu Das notes during the war, is thus placed back within familiar understandings of friendship and gender.[6] Indeed, not only is any taint of 'homoerotic frisson' safely removed, but the tale becomes an exemplary one of comradeship and empathy towards the grieving mother, for Fenton's letter was published in the local paper, where it appeared under the heading 'Sympathetic Letter from Lance Corporal D. H. Fenton'.

Although fathers were given no place in the scene, John Fenton was proud enough of his son's thoughtfulness to make his own copy of the letter to Mrs Noone, which he kept with his son's private letters. The impersonal inventory which John Fenton received when David himself was killed four months later, listing the photographs and 'letters etc' found on his body, show us why David's letter might have mattered so much to a parent.[7] There is no record in the IWM files of John Fenton receiving letters of condolence anything like as intimate as his son's letter to Mrs Noone.

In their reactions, soldiers and their families inevitably drew on the pre-war conventions surrounding death. For example, it is Fenton's evocation of the Pietà holding the dying Christ in her arms that makes his account so moving.[8] He asks Mrs Noone for clothing that belonged to his friend, a request that was not unusual among working-class families, as a way of incorporating within oneself the identity of the dead.[9] He extends his sympathy to the mother, and assumes that her loss stands for everyone's, as people usually did when a child died in Edwardian Britain.

At the same time, conditions on the Western Front made it impossible to carry out many of the normal rituals of burial and mourning, and it thrust new and frightful responsibilities on men like Fenton. If a man died in action his comrades sometimes had to bury him where he fell. A party would be detailed to leave the cover of the trenches at night and dig a hurried grave, afraid all the while of being spotted in the Very lights (flares used for communication and illuminating targets). Graves were sometimes only a couple of feet deep; an existing shell-hole might be used, and they often held more than one body.[10]

Crosses for dead comrades would be fashioned from scraps of wood or metal, and a brief service would be held over the grave. When his friend was killed on the Somme, Private Roy Ashford stuck the man's bayonet into the ground at the head of the grave, and placed his steel helmet over it.[11] By the end of the war the Western Front was dotted with small and improvised graves such as this, but the rituals of disposal and the recording of death became more institutionalised when, in March 1915, the Graves Registration Commission was established. After 1915, a chaplain or officer was supposed to report the position of the grave and an officer from the Graves Registration Unit would then place a wooden cross at the site, to which a mass-produced metal strip with the man's name, regiment and rank would be affixed.[12] More and more bodies were buried behind the lines as the war went on, and already by 1916 there were 300 cemeteries on the Western Front.[13] The bureaucratic organisation of death had reached such a scale by the final years of the war that large burial plots were dug in advance of major operations.[14]

When a body could be brought back behind the lines, the rituals of burial were more elaborate. Padres would hold a service, and the grave might be marked out with stones and covered with flowers. Even in the back areas, however, the dead were not safe, as many cemeteries were within range of German artillery. At a cemetery near an Aid Post at Hillside, the body of a Royal Welch Fusilier was reputed to have been re-buried twice in one day.[15]

Soldiers sometimes went to great lengths to recover their dead, risking their own lives in the effort.[16] When Lieutenant Gilbert Talbot was killed, his brother Neville, an Army Chaplain, interviewed those who had been close to Gilbert in the moments before his death. Gilbert, he was told, had been hit in the neck as he struggled to cut the barbed wire. His batman attempted to get the officer off the wire and lay him on his back but a bullet had passed through the batman's finger (which later had to be amputated); and then through Gilbert's cigarette case and heart. At least two men were injured trying the retrieve the body. Having established how and where he died, Neville set out to see for himself. Once the battle subsided he went over the top in the cover of night, where he was able to feel for Gilbert's pocket-book and prayer book, badge and wristwatch, and 'stroke with his hand the fair young head that he knew so well'.[17]

Occasionally the retrieval of bodies took place on a larger scale. Christmas Day 1914 began for the seventeen-year-old officer Wilbert Spencer with the sound of German soldiers calling out 'Happy Xmas', after which his men stuck up a board wishing them 'Gluchliches Wermachten' [*sic*]. Two German soldiers then came half way out into No Man's Land, calling for an officer. Wilbert clambered out of the trenches to speak with them, and found they were willing to have an armistice for four hours. His men followed him out of the trenches and went over to shake hands with the German soldiers, each wishing the other the 'compliments of the season'. But the cessation of hostilities had another, far from festive purpose:

> Then they carried over the dead. I won't describe the sights which I saw and which I shall never forget. We buried the dead as they were. Then back to the trenches with the feeling of hatred growing stronger after what we had seen. It was strange after just shaking hands and chatting with them. Well it was a very weird Xmas day.[18]

Often bodies could not be retrieved. J. M. Winter estimates that around half of those who died in action were 'unidentified or unidentifiable'.[19] For parents a missing body was particularly upsetting because it was impossible to grieve properly, but for the soldier it was often the 'unidentifiable' missing that caused most distress.[20] John Middleton saw a direct hit on a dug-out which left two men 'unrecognisable and only to be identified by their discs'; the previous day a 'heavy' had hit a trench mortar howitzer party and 'Two again were killed outright – one could not be found.'[21] The remains of eleven men killed in a dug-out did not even fill a sandbag, but were nonetheless given a burial service by the Padre.[22] 'Unidentifiable' deaths like these might mean that a man had to scrabble around in trenches shovelling up dismembered limbs and other body parts. Though untold in letters home, these incidents might be recalled later, as in Edmund Blunden's 1928 prose memory of a Lance-Corporal hit by a shell without warning as he was warming up his tea, which leads Blunden to ask, 'For him, how could the gobbets of blackening flesh, the earth-wall sotted with blood, with flesh, the eye under the duckboard, the pulpy bone be the only answer?'[23]

Bodies might remain 'unidentified' for a number of reasons. When a man had been killed after going over the top, sometimes the most that his comrades could do before passing on was to close his eyes or cover his face.[24] Men who had initially been buried with their identification might become 'missing' if the site was not properly registered and shelling later disturbed the grave. Naked bodies were sometimes recovered from No Man's Land, the uniforms and identification having been stripped by German raiding parties. The Royal Welch Fusiliers were warned to watch out for impostors in Middlesex Regiment uniforms after one such incident.[25]

Once a man had been buried his comrades usually gathered together his personal effects and sent them back to his loved ones. Not all possessions found their way home. Charles Carrington was appalled to hear from the salvage party which returned from No Man's Land with the body of his friend, the commander of 'C' Company, that 'some keen pilferer had taken his signet ring and had cut the finger off to get it.'[26] When Norman Gladden's friend Harold Eldred was fatally wounded at

Ypres, his parents could not understand why Eldred's gold wedding ring was not returned with his other effects. Gladden could, 'for robbery of the dead was but an incident of war not considered a crime – as, of course, it was.'[27] Theft from the corpse of an ally mattered not only because it dishonoured the ideal of comradeship, but because it threatened to expose to parents the dirty secret of what it meant to live among the dead.

## Passing on the news

The initial responsibility for passing on information to the next-of-kin lay with the dead man's Commanding Officer. Subalterns dreaded this job. Often exhausted and perhaps mourning their own loss, they could find it difficult to muster sympathy for the family. Ralph Bickersteth, who was serving in a Leeds Pals' Battalion, lost two 'excellent' men in the space of twenty-four hours. His Lance-Corporal, who had recently become a father, was 'killed within two yards of me' by a sniper and Bickersteth was left feeling 'fed up to the world absolutely.' Rather than write to the man's widow himself, he asked his father, the Canon of Leeds, to visit her: 'I simply am at a loss to know what to say and I fear the effect on her would be so bad. Tell her he was splendid, fearless, and set on doing his duty.'[28]

Bickersteth was only twenty-one at the time and unmarried, so the task must have felt daunting. But his failure to write was not born of indifference; and the rather formulaic tribute he asked his father to convey was not a lie. Bickersteth had seen his men killed close-up and keenly felt what the loss would mean to the Lance-Corporal's wife, for 'As I say, she is only just a mother.'[29] He felt too upset to write himself, and judged, probably correctly, that his father was more experienced, and in a better state than he, to break the news.

Condolence letters took time to compose because the writer had to convey a sense of personal connection to the dead person.[30] When writing to the families of other commissioned men, officers normally drew on their personal knowledge of the man, having quartered with him in billets and dug-outs. Captain H. Campbell Ashenden was familiar with the personal circumstances of Mrs Hague, her son Harold having 'often chatted to me over his personal matters + I remember him coming home from his leave in March + speaking of his father's illness + his ultimate grief at his death.'[31] Here, the officer was acknowledging the double grief of the mother. Others, although showing the emotional reserve expected of an officer, indirectly conveyed the depth of their own distress by reporting on the reactions of the men. 'So fond were the men of him that some of them actually wept when they heard of his death – + these were strong brave fellows', a subaltern wrote to Wilbert Spencer's father after Wilbert was killed at Neuve Chapelle.[32] Personal knowledge of the dead officer's family made sympathy feel the more genuine.

Officers generally lacked this kind of knowledge about the family lives of the men in their platoon or company, and this showed itself in their condolence letters. Despite the number of letters they might have to write after battle, many did try to convey something of the dead man's character, and show sensitivity to what his family might be feeling. Higginson's Commanding Officer singled out his sporting prowess, which had made him 'very popular' among his officers and comrades.[33] He wrote a second letter to Mrs Higginson, explaining that her son had been 'laid to rest by the side of three of his comrades who were killed at the same time', and directing her to the Registration of Graves Committee so she could learn the exact location of the grave.[34] A subaltern might recount actions or events in which the dead man had taken part, knowing how important it was to parents that the son had counted for something among his comrades. Second Lieutenant Tabberer wrote to Mrs Tomlinson of her son:

> I feel I must write a line to say how upset I am about your great loss and how I feel for you in it. I am in charge of No. 7 platoon, and can honestly say there was not a cheerier fellow in the whole platoon. It was only the other night I asked two picked men to come out on patrol with me, and he was one of them.[35]

In one case, a Commanding Officer who had served with a ranker early in the war, wrote a letter of condolence to the dead man's mother three years later upon hearing of the man's death.[36]

Not all were as conscientious. Alf Swettenham's mother wrote to the Colonel asking for any information about his death, but the reply that Major Davis gave on the Colonel's behalf was brief and discouraging: 'I regret I am unable to furnish any information concerning the Death of your Son.' Davis bluntly referred her on to the Directorate of Graves Registration and Enquiry.[37] The condolence letter was least adequate when a man had died shortly after joining the platoon. When Private Harry Carter was killed less than two weeks after arriving in France, his officer, Captain Collart, must have been at a loss to know what to write. Carter had been brought down by two bullets through the brain, he explained, so he 'possibly . . . hardly felt the shots.' Collart stressed to Mr and Mrs Carter that their son had not died alone. He himself had been beside Harry 'within a few seconds & he was quite unconscious'. Collart was able to offer reassurance about the circumstances of Harry's death but he struggled to find expressions which could assuage the deep personal loss faced by these parents: 'I am very sorry to lose him as he was a very promising lad, and gave no trouble – he was one of our youngest.'[38] The information about Carter's age was probably gleaned from the next-of-kin records and Collart had clearly got to know more about Carter after his death than he had done in life. Even so, the Carter family valued this last testament from their son's Commanding Officer enough to have it typed out and copied.

The sheer scale of the casualties meant that it was sometimes impossible to avoid perfunctory condolence, but the fact that death had become so routine was itself upsetting. There had been fifty casualties in John Millar Scott's Company during the Battle of Loos, and he found it 'a distressing business opening private letters, and writing what little is known of the casualty on the back.'[39] 'I've been writing dozens of letters to people whose relatives have been killed or wounded – a painful job', wrote the Reverend Parry-Okeden during the Spring Offensive in 1918.[40] Mass death strained to breaking point the whole idea of the personal letter of condolence.

In addition to the Commanding Officer, the dead man's comrades would often write to express their sympathy. They knew that the officer, who might have many such letters to write, might take two or three days to get around to the task. Appreciating that their letters might be the first to arrive, comrades took the responsibility for breaking the news of a son's death. Prowse and Warner were gentle with Mrs Tomlinson: 'We have some very bad news to communicate to you, and must ask you to take courage and bear up as best you can.' They continued: 'Between 5.30 and 6 o'clock this morning, Jim was shot in the head. He was rendered unconscious at once, and after lingering . . . for a few minutes, passed peacefully away.'[41] There was no fancy prose in this letter, no attempt to elevate the death into sacrifice or create a screen between the mother and a violent death. Tomlinson's friends broke the news in the way they would had they visited her in person, and they anticipated what she would be feeling.

Others were unfamiliar with the conventions of the condolence letter and struggled with the correct tone. The opening lines of W. Gray's letter would scarcely have prepared Mrs Dunning for the news to follow:

'Just a few lines hoping to find you in the best of health as it leaves Cooper and myself at the time of writing. I regret to inform you that your son Arthur was killed by a shell.'[42] Discomfiting though it was to write to the family, it ultimately felt worse to avoid the duty. Gladden neglected to write to the next-of-kin after his mate Jimmy Downs died on the Somme, but his 'woeful failure' worried him for months afterwards. When his second close friend, Harold Eldred, died of his wounds at Ypres, Gladden had 'no intention of shirking', and sat down to write his 'unwelcome note in halting self-conscious English to the two dear middle-aged publicans in Peckham who were his parents'.[43]

For a parent, the thought that a man had suffered a lingering and painful death was a cause of particular anguish.[44] Ella Bickersteth described her reaction after learning that her son Morris had been killed at the Somme: 'All yesterday we were so wondering how our darling son was killed and hoping he had not suffered long hours before he died.'[45] After learning that her husband's body had been left in No Man's Land, Dorothy Etherston wrote to Colonel Stephens 'I only pray he was killed <u>instantly</u> + did not suffer – but that of course I cannot know.'[46] Soldiers who had to write to bereaved families were acutely conscious of these anxieties. Time after time when reading condolence letters, phrases appear such as 'It is comforting to think that his end was not a painful one.'[47]

There was an element of concealment in such phrases, for deaths from weapons such as shrapnel, which caused massive tissue damage, were often neither peaceful nor quick, and as John Keegan remarks, there were unprecedented numbers of critical wounds in the First World War.[48] Higginson's friends, in their efforts to comfort his mother, perhaps unwittingly underscored the violence of his death when they explained that he was 'killed by a shell it only bursting only a yards away from him [*sic*] he died almost immediately it happened at 1 oclock A. M. on 11/8/17'.[49] The emotional pain suffered by the bereaved was believed to bear a close relation to the physical pain suffered by their loved one. Thus W. H. R. Rivers believed that his treatment of a shell-shocked soldier reached a turning point when he reminded the man that although his friend's death had been extremely shocking, he was at least 'spared the prolonged suffering which is too often the fate of those who sustain mortal wounds. He brightened at once.' But Rivers' kindly reassurance could do nothing to change the event that had brought the man's neurosis about in the first place, seeing his friend 'blown into pieces with the head and limbs lying separated from the trunk'.[50]

When a comrade wrote that death had been instantaneous he hoped to avoid having to relate just these sorts of horrific details, but the effort at concealment did not necessarily convince. Geoffrey Wainwright's fortitude in death was commended by his Commanding Officer but it was clear to Geoffrey's mother that the death had been neither quick nor painless. She quoted from the Commanding Officer's letter: '"unfortunately he was not taken to the Hospital til the next morning; I don't think he suffered much pain, at any rate he did not say so, but never whispered a word, + bore it like a man"'. Mrs Wainwright saw straight through the Commanding Officer's praise of Geoffrey's manliness: 'Can you understand, what I feel about his having been out all night, in that bitter weather, + in such agony?', she wrote to the poet Katherine Tynan.[51]

It was consideration towards parents that encouraged censorship. John Millar Scott was deeply affected when his NCO was killed on a wiring party by a sniper. Robertson lay 'lifeless, cold, his face smeared with blood', but these details were expunged from his letter to Robertson's mother, to whom Scott wrote 'as delicately as I could. She is over sixty, I believe, and her husband is dead.'[52] When the suffering of the wounded man could not be concealed, emphasis shifted to the personal qualities he had shown in bearing up to pain. An officer who had travelled with Hedley Payne on a German hospital train explained that although Hedley was 'Terribly wounded, + paralyzed from the waist down, he was still as smiling and gay + cheerful as if nothing at all were the matter with no compassion for himself, and nothing but confidence + hopefulness as to the future . . . I couldn't help feeling what a fine fellow he was, and hoping + trusting that his courage and grit would pull him through.'[53] The Medical Head of the hospital where Frank Wollocombe was sent with a severe leg wound acknowledged that he had been in 'much pain', but emphasised how Frank was 'very patient in spite' of this.[54] Terms that had once described heroic action on the battlefield were now applied to the mortally wounded. Roland Leighton's 'Colonel says "the boy was wonderfully brave", and the Chaplain "He died at 11 p. m. after a very gallant fight"', reported Vera Brittain in her diary.[55]

The ambiguous tones of letters of sympathy were matched by equally ambivalent reactions among families. Because the son had died away from home and there was no body, there was a strong impulse to seek information about the circumstances of death and during the war a number of voluntary agencies were set up to facilitate this. The activities of the Red Cross Bureau in searching for missing men have been widely discussed, and were particularly important in countries like Australia where the time-gaps in communication made it impossible to track down information while it was fresh in comrades' minds.[56]

The parents of British soldiers were often able to rely on direct contact with the son's military unit. The middle class had particularly good access to information about the circumstances of death, the parents of officers normally receiving a telegram, a letter from the Commanding Officer and at least one other officer; and frequently letters from NCOs, batmen and soldiers serving in the platoon as well. When Roland Leighton was killed, his family was sent information by the Hospital Chaplain, his Colonel, two Captains and Roland's batman. The quest for information was not limited to letters. Relatives of the dead officer might also encourage visits from men in his platoon or company, hoping to gain further information or just to be in contact with someone who had been close to him in his last hours. The survivor seemed to carry some trace of the loved one's being; it was as if, by creating a relationship with them, the deceased might not be wholly lost.[57]

Sometimes the range of contacts that the better-off were able to cultivate only added to the confusion and frustration. On 14 September 1916 Frank Wollocombe's parents were told their son had been shot through the middle of the back and killed; but the next day the Medical Head of the hospital at Corbie explained that he had been hit in the leg and had died two days later of sepsis.[58] After Eric Makeham was reported missing, his father managed to establish from 'scanty and very conflicting, accounts' that he had been on a bombing attack on Messines Ridge when he was hit by machine-gun fire. Eric's comrades had moved him to a shell-hole for protection, but had been unable to carry him away when German soldiers suddenly appeared from the next shell-hole. For 'months' the Makehams 'cherished the conviction that, at the close of the war, our boy would return – perhaps not seriously disabled.' They eventually received an official communication from Berlin stating that Eric had died, but despite his father's '[u]nremitting efforts . . . through every known agency, to obtain further details', the date, cause of death and place of burial 'were, and still are, all unspecified.'[59]

Women not only tracked down information about their own loved ones, but helped set up channels of communication between soldiers and bereaved families. In the early months of the war, the wife of Colonel Stephens, who ran the Comforts Fund for the Second Battalion of the Rifle Brigade, organised charitable collections for dependent mothers and subsequently she chased up their claims for the Separation Allowance. As the war continued, however, Mrs Stephens spent more of her time supporting the wives and mothers of killed and missing men. The volume of correspondence ebbed and flowed with the actions of her husband's unit and her carefully kept records were tinged with black after March 1915, when the Second Battalion lost eight officers and 250 Other Ranks at Neuve Chapelle.[60]

Mrs Stephens needed bureaucratic mechanisms to deal with casualties on this scale. The Quarter-Master kept her up to date with the names and addresses of wives and mothers in the Battalion, and she wrote to many explaining that she would be happy to seek information on their behalf. Agnes Johnson wondered if Mrs Stephens could track down her husband's belongings, and Ruby Barker also wanted help to retrieve 'the few things he had out there at the time of his death, I should treasure them.'[61] Such pleas suggest that the Army may have been more assiduous in its protection of the officer's property than the ranker's. Mrs Willis wrote asking if it was possible to have her husband 'put in our churchyard close by.'[62] Rose Toomey wrote to Mrs Stephens hoping that 'Col Stephens will return back to you safe and well as it must be an anxious time for yourself also if it is not asking too much if you have anything Black to dispose of it would be very acceptable as I found it rather expensive lately + I never insured my dear husband.'[63] The Comforts Fund's files include many such piteous letters from bereaved wives and mothers, written in excessively polite and formal prose, thanking Mrs Stephens for her condolences, and unfailingly considerate of her worries, with a husband of her own at the front.

Their distance from the place of death and their inability to see the body created an intense need among these mothers to discover more about the circumstances of death. This is powerfully conveyed by Mrs Gilbey, whose son was killed at Neuve Chapelle when he stopped to tend to a wounded man. Her tone is by turns angry and pleading; she can only just keep control over her prose and the force of her grief comes through in passionate underlining. Above all she wants news, and she rails against the assumption that she is too fragile to learn the worst:

> When he could (and I know how terribly occupied he must be) if he would guard all my darling's letters, books or any little personal things + send them <u>direct</u> to me. I have had a letter from Captain Cocks, which he wrote the first moment he could to tell me . . . but I should be <u>deeply</u> grateful to you, if you could tell me, or find out for me <u>everything, little thing,</u> you possibly could – <u>where my darling's</u> buried – <u>who</u> saw him after <u>he was</u> wounded? When did he 'pass on' <u>was he in a Hospital</u>, or where? Tell me please, <u>please</u>, if you can <u>anything</u> – when he was wounded and if

> he was conscious – you may think me heartless + cruel, but I long to know everything – everything – Any information you can give me . . . + do not spare my feelings in the very least please. I can stand everything + anything. Thank you so much for helping me – I cannot write more just now.[64]

Evidence of the son's last moments, however, when it finally came, could be deeply distressing. Little could bring a mother, father or sibling as close to a son's death as the things he had on him, and the clothes he was wearing when killed. Personal articles such as these had always been symbolically significant in death, but they assumed even more importance in the war because, in the absence of mortal remains, they were – as David Fenton understood – the only physical evidence there was of what had happened.[65]

When his son's kit was sent back to him, R. Anderson wrote to Katherine Tynan the next day. 'I unpacked it and went over everything – every mud-stained, war-torn item. Can you understand what that meant? Of course you can. There was a letter to me – a letter he could not post because he was hit the evening he wrote it – but there it was + I send you a copy of it.'[66] When Roland Leighton's kit and personal effects were returned to his family, they were able to learn much from it about the circumstances of his death. His tunic showed the point of entry of the bullet that killed him, a tiny hole just below the right-hand bottom pocket, and an exit right on the back-bone. His vest, breeches and even his braces were soaked in blood – the bullet had blown out his back – and they could see from this that he had lain on his back for some considerable time after being hit.[67] His filthy clothing smelled not of 'ordinary mud; it had not the usual clean pure smell of earth, but it was as though it were saturated with dead bodies – dead that had been dead a long, long time.' Mrs Leighton had seen more than she cared to, and wanted this particular evidence banished from her sight and memory:

> Mrs Leighton said 'Robert, take those clothes away into the kitchen, and don't let me see them again; I must either burn or bury them. They smell of Death; they are not Roland, they even seem to detract from his memory & spoil his glamour. I won't have any more to do with them.'

Mr Leighton took Roland's tunic away to bury in the garden, and the family threw open the windows and soon 'felt better, but it was a long time before the smell and even the taste of them went away.'[68] Close inquiry could threaten to undo a mother's comforting vision. It was as if, by ordering the destruction of his clothes, Mrs Leighton could banish the reality of killing and dying, and Roland could live on, a perfect image of the soldier-hero.

Many bereaved mothers were thought to have been made ill by their grief. Mrs Starky wrote to Mrs Stephens that she was not capable of a proper letter as 'you see i am in bed very ill at present i will write again.'[69] The 'blow has been so severe' wrote Isa Quarry, that her daughter had 'taken me away for a change.'[70] Vera Brittain's father called her back from France to England in April 1918 after her mother suffered a '"complete general breakdown"'.[71] After her son died, a poor London mother who had already lost nine of her thirteen children, 'took to her bed for good'.[72] Try as they might, there was ultimately little that family members and comrades could do to protect mothers. They saw through the omissions in condolence letters, and some had a strong desire to find out more. Yet it was ultimately the death itself, not the circumstances of it or the blood-soaked personal effects, that threatened to drive them mad.

## The order of grief

Women in late Victorian and Edwardian society were seen as having a special role in relation to death. In middle-class households, nurses and servants laid out the body; this task, Pat Jalland tells us, 'almost always fell to women'.[73] In working-class neighbourhoods, women helped each other with the practical arrangements, raising burial funds, laying out the corpse and organising the wake. It was through these activities, Julie-Marie Strange explains, that women offered each other sympathy.[74]

Families of all class backgrounds kept the body in the home for up to ten days after death, so people could view it and say goodbye before the coffin was closed. This ritual placed the body within the wife or mother's sphere, and her grief was acknowledged as visitors paid their respects.

Women were assumed to be less able than men to contain their grief.[75] Until the last quarter of the nineteenth century they were discouraged from attending burial services for fear that they would break down, and even in the 1890s Lady Colin Campbell felt that they should attend only if they could 'keep their grief within due bounds.'[76] The identification of women with grief was reflected in the customs which surrounded mourning. Middle- and upper-middle-class women were expected to withdraw from public engagements, widows wearing drab silk and crape for up to two years, mothers for a year. The suits worn by men were barely altered by mourning. They wore only a black mourning coat, and bereavement did not affect their public activities.[77]

During the war, the bereaved mother's removal from the body of her son, and her inability to take a direct part in the rituals of death and burial, made *symbolic* markers of her loss the more important. In 1927, almost a decade on from the war's end, many women attending the service at the Cenotaph on Remembrance Day were still dressed in deep mourning.[78] In addition to the public markers of their loss, they constructed private memorials. Mr and Mrs Swettenham were not able to locate their son Alf's body after he died in action on 23 October 1918, and consequently there was no grave. Mrs Swettenham, lacking a site of memory, constructed a memorial in her front room, putting a photograph of Alf in uniform, his two war medals, bronze medallion and pressed poppies into a frame and mounting it on the mantle wall, where it remained until she died in 1929.[79]

Consolation letters might be addressed to the father as the head of household, but many were written to the mother because of the special bond which she was thought to have with her children. By comparison, the father's place in mourning was ill defined. Though he might grieve deeply, the ability to keep control over his emotions was valued, and thus Leslie Stephen could write: 'The man who is occupied with his own interests makes grief an excuse for effeminate indulgence in self-pity.'[80]

Fathers often saw their main role as being to support the bereaved mother.[81] After Lord Edward Cecil's son was reported missing, he wrote a deeply touching letter to his wife that, at the same time, assumed that there was a hierarchy of grief. A mother's attachment to her children was the most profound in her life, whereas men had other responsibilities besides those to their children:

> I cannot tell you how awfully I feel for you. There is nothing in the world so terrible as this must be for you. In comparison my own seems so much less. I have my work and though I love George as much as any father loves his son yet of course I know that a mother's love is like nothing else on earth.[82]

Despite Lord Cecil's soothing words, the grief of a father could be just as profound as a mother's, but was not socially sanctioned. There were fathers within Lord Cecil's own circle, not least Rudyard Kipling, for whom the death of a son caused almost unbearable grief.[83] Family members and friends often noted the distress of fathers, but seemed unsure how to react. A father who could not hold back his grief was unmanned and it was difficult to know whether to leave him to himself or how to offer comfort. After Yvo Charteris was killed in early 1915, just weeks after he had gone out to the front, his sister Cynthia Asquith noted the reactions of her parents. Her mother was initially 'quite calm', but her father (even though Yvo was possibly not his own son) was 'most piteous – heartbroken and just like a child – tears pouring down his cheeks and so naively astonished.'[84] After losing a second son during the war, a bereaved father told the Irish poet Katherine Tynan that he wanted to 'go away into a wilderness and howl my miserable soul out'.[85] Grieving could be a lonely experience for these fathers when the networks of mourning and support functioned through mothers.

It was not only fathers but sisters, brothers and aunts whose grief might fall into the shadow of the mother's. Ellen Dickson kept up a correspondence with Mrs Stephens after her nephew, Captain Burton, died of his injuries in a Base Camp hospital. Burton's mother had been allowed to visit him in France and sit at his bedside, and later so had his brothers and father. But Ellen, stuck back in Britain, had to rely on Burton's mother, who was 'very nice + like a good woman altho' full of her own deep grief', had taken the time to keep Ellen informed. Ellen had been reading a letter from her 'with fairly hopeful news' when a wire arrived announcing Burton's death. It 'was a great shock to me for I loved him dearly. He was wounded by a bullet [also] from a shrapnel [*sic*] on the brain so there could have been no hope.'[86] She wrote again to Mrs Stephens to try and explain why she was so upset: 'I cannot describe to you what a bitter grief + shock it is to me as both have been like my own son's [*sic*] + I have had them so much with me.' No account of a mother's grief needed to be given, but because this aunt – who called her nephew 'my dear boy' and who clearly *felt* like a mother towards him – was outside the immediate family, she thought she must explain the intensity of her distress.[87]

The idea that a mother's loss symbolised and subsumed everyone else's owed something to the Christian traditions associated with mourning. As Regina Schulte has shown in her work on Käthe Kollwitz, the Pietà image placed mother and son in an exclusive relationship. It elevated the mother's loss as the supreme sacrifice and pushed fathers and other relatives aside.[88] The Pietà ideal was not only upheld by mothers but by fathers, too, as we can see from the memorial book to Second Lieutenant Eric Noel Makeham which was compiled by his father and published in 1917. The book was dedicated to Eric's 'MOTHER Whose Faith and Fortitude, Sustaining My Own Through Many Darkened Days, Have Brought It Into Being'. The volume concludes with a further testament to primacy of a mother's grief:

> In my mind, throughout this prefatory task, has run, in an inevitable undertone, the sad, sweet music of the Gospel story. In that story, the figure of Mary the mother emerges ever more clearly, and holds a place at once proud, lonely, and pathetic, while that of Joseph fades into a shadowy memory. And so, in my last and very tender thought, the mother of my boy stands, solitary in the sacredness of her grief, in the wonder of her love.[89]

Makeham pays a lavish tribute to his wife as a mother here, but where does it leave him? The association with Joseph makes the father an even lonelier and more 'pathetic' figure than the mother, old and forgotten, his love not commemorated; and he is not even a blood relation but a stand-in.

In the Vladslo cemetery near Ypres, Käthe Kollwitz's famous sculptures of grieving parents, produced in the 1920s, look onto the grave of their son Peter. They show us how far Kollwitz had moved from the Pietà vision of mourning, and they make us think about the way that other, more obviously Christian memorials privilege the mother. Father and mother are beside each other but on different plinths. The father clasps his arms around himself; the mother is bent forward and pulls her shawl around her. He is not reaching out to comfort her, as Makeham and Lord Cecil advocate, but is absorbed in his own grief as he looks out onto the ninth stone cross, under which lies his own son Peter, killed in October 1914. The two figures are surprisingly small as you look at them from the cemetery entrance, as if shrunken by their loss. Despite their separateness they convey a more symmetrical relation to grief than the heightened maternal symbolism of the memorials which were, as we shall now see, produced by middle-class parents in Britain.

## Mothers' memorials

When the Unknown Warrior was buried at Westminster in 1920, special provision was made for bereaved women, effectively displacing the wives of dignitaries and Society women. Mothers were given priority over widows at the ceremony, and among the applicants for tickets were 7,605 women who had lost one or more sons. [90] The tomb was visited by between half a million and a million people in the first week. In its coverage of Armistice Day in 1927, the *Daily Mail* noted that there were 'many mothers in that long file; some gripped at the wooden rail a little as they half turned to look at the tomb. Some bent and laid wreaths or bunches of flowers.'[91] Separated from the body of their loved one, they could imagine that the Unknown Warrior was their own son.[92] Through rituals such as these, personal tragedy was aligned with the idea of national sacrifice. Maternal loss, as Susan Grayzel notes, took on 'a deeply political overtone', subsuming to an extent the mourning of others.[93]

Ex-servicemen also had to make room for women, who increasingly from the late 1920s were to be found in France and Belgium on pilgrimages to the graves of sons, lovers and husbands. They were given a privileged place at the Menin Gate memorial ceremony in Ypres in 1928, and the popularity of the pilgrimage among women, some 3,000 of whom made the journey from Britain that year, took the organisers by surprise. Free tickets were given by the British Legion to 'absolutely poverty stricken women who have lost many sons in the War and are anxious to see their graves.'[94] As well as going on the British Legion organised tours, mothers paid private visits to the graves of their sons. They were sometimes seen carrying bundles of letters or other mementoes. They might kiss the headstone, have their photograph taken by it, or take back home a sprinkling of soil from the burial plot.[95] These visits were expensive, costing in the mid-1920s at least £4, more than the average weekly wage for an industrial worker, many of whom in any case did not get paid holidays.[96] A woman interviewed for The Edwardians project in the 1970s, asked if her mother had ever had a holiday, replied only once, and that was to 'see the grave of my brother what was killed in 1916.' This mother had travelled without her husband and other children, probably to save expense.[97]

Women's place in the rituals of mourning was not achieved without challenge. Some veterans had mixed reactions to their visits to the battlefields, feeling a sense of ownership of the sites they had defended for four years, and believing that the experiences of the mourners were gaining more public attention than those of the survivors.[98] There were heated debates in the mid-1920s about the rights of women, particularly mothers, to wear their sons' medals on remembrance occasions. As one mother explained in an interview at the Cenotaph just before Armistice Day 1926, 'I lost two sons in the war. I will wear the DCM and the MC they won whether the Home Office forbids me or permits me.' Such discussions about the wearing of medals demonstrated, Adrian Gregory remarks, that 'the bereaved mother was the pre-eminent subject of Armistice Day.'[99]

Military headstones also record the mother's prominence among the mourners. In the early 1920s when the Commonwealth Graves Commission was consolidating the dead on the Western Front into military cemeteries, it departed from its principle of uniformity in response to the 'individualist lobby', which had been calling for the return of soldiers' bodies to Britain.[100] Families were permitted to add a personal inscription of up to 66 letters to the headstone, initially at a cost of 3½ d per letter, but after protests about the cost the Commission later made the charge voluntary.[101] Around half of all identified headstones have an inscription.[102] These vary widely, as Bruce Scates observes in his study of Australian examples, but many speak eloquently of a mother's loss. Some mourn her absence from the scene of his death. Private A. Virgo's of the Royal Sussex Regiment reads: 'Could We Have Raised/His Dying Head/ And Heard His Last Farewell.' Others record the desire that a mother might lay out the body: 'No Mother Near To Close/His Eyes/Far From His Native Land he Lies' is the inscription on the grave of Private E. J. Johnson of the Royal Welch Fusiliers. It is not unusual to find the man's home address on a stone. The inscription on Second Lieutenant W. E. Harris' grave reads 'Elder son of W. J. and E. Harris of 43 Monks Rd Exeter', this evocation of a very specific place standing out among the massed and uniform rows of headstones. While many inscriptions mention mothers and fathers, others evoke an exclusive bond between mother and son. The headstone of Gunner C. H. Parmenter, RFA, reads 'Ever In My Thoughts, Mother'; that of Pte H. Marshall, Duke of Wellington's Regiment, 'Beneath The Soil/In Sweet Repose/Is Laid/Mother's Dearest Pride.'[103] The private discussions about what should go on the stones are lost to us, but the inscriptions themselves hint at how, in many grieving families, mothers' grief ranked first.

Mothers also tended to dominate memorial books.[104] Occasionally produced before the war when an adolescent son died, such books appeared much more frequently during and after the war. Often they were privately printed, the cost of production restricting them to upper-middle- and upper-class families, who circulated them among family and friends. Some were produced while mothers were still in the midst of grief. Marie Leighton's *Boy of My Heart*, published anonymously in 1916, was begun almost immediately after Roland died at Christmas 1915, and the intensity of her work on the book probably contributed to her breakdown.[105] Others took longer. Mary Constance Charteris was seventy when she published *A Family Record* in 1932. The 400 pages of her memorial book, which includes diary extracts, letters from her two sons and their comrades at the front, reminiscences from her daughter Mary and testimonials from friends, present a contrast to the slim volumes produced during the war.

What can these memorial books tell us about the culture of bereavement among the middle class, and the place of the mother within it? Pat Jalland argues that parents felt a particular need to produce additional memorials because the headstones, memorial tablets and remembrance rituals 'had been so woefully inadequate.'[106] Yet it was less the failure of ritual than the manner of death – its violence, the reversal of normal generational patterns, and the distance of the bereaved from the son's body – that impelled families to do something to commemorate the loss. No single memorial could exhaust grief.[107]

The typical raw material for these books was the son's correspondence from school and the war, which mothers or fathers, and sometimes sisters, had already copied into a clearer hand or got typed up.[108] It was common for families to do this, but where memorial books differed from transcriptions or other private notes on letters was that the son's own words were usually supplemented by commentaries from ministers, teachers and peers. In this way the son's biography was turned into an exemplary life. Gilbert Talbot was 'rather *special* amongst all the others' wrote Mrs Kay-Shuttleworth, the wife of Talbot's Commanding Officer.[109] Mrs Leighton recorded a friend's comment about Roland as a small child: 'He's got a sort of kinghood about him'.[110] 'Our Arthur was . . . a radiant being', wrote Isabel Small of her nephew.[111] The tendency to elevate these young men's personal and moral qualities was the greater because they had no legacy of their own in the form of children or a contribution to public life.

The image of the son that mothers created was not aggressively patriotic; there was little in these books about the winning of glory in battle. They extolled a more localised and gentler idea of service than is sometimes assumed in studies of the First World War, which tend to see service as synonymous with patriotism.[112] Maternal service is defined, in the work of Susan Grayzel, Nicoletta Gullace and others, in terms of the relinquishing of sons to the nation, something that gave mothers themselves – vicariously – a new place in civic life and a new claim on citizenship.[113]

But service to the nation is not the guiding ideal in memorial books. Rather, they extol service to company or platoon. The son, in the most elevated examples, is transformed into a Christ-like figure, the rank-and-file soldiers into his flock. Memorials look back on the son's pre-war life and his war experience for instances of selflessness. 'He was so absolutely unmercenary and self-sacrificing', wrote Herbert-Theodore Mayo in the family tribute to his brother.[114] A subaltern's moral character was revealed most clearly in his conduct towards his men. When it came to making sense of a life cut short, the ranker's feelings towards his officer mattered as much as those of other commissioned men, and consequently families often solicited testimonials from batmen, NCOs and others in the platoon or company. Eric Makeham's 'wonderful boys', wrote his father, 'gave him their unstinted devotion.'[115] The tribute that A. P. Pargiter wrote for his friend's father appears again and again in memorials and condolence letters: 'His men loved him and would follow him anywhere.'[116]

Mothers looked for examples of 'moral courage' that would help them come to terms with their loss.[117] '[H]ow I loved the "we" and the "our"!', wrote Roland Leighton's mother, looking back on his letters to her. 'He always has identified himself with his men, so that they know that he cares for them, and they would follow him, as his colonel put it, "anywhere and into anything"'.[118] After having interviewed Gilbert's batman, Lavinia Talbot was able to state that 'He dwelt on his great care for his men – as to health, comfort, etc – he always saw to all being as well arranged as was possible for them before he turned in himself, not leaving it to the sergeants till he felt satisfied all was right.'[119] These were details she needed to know. By endorsing the ideal of service to the men in this way, such mothers perhaps unintentionally encouraged the carelessness of self which cost many a subaltern his life. Lavinia Talbot proudly recited the advice given by Gilbert's Colonel: 'Remember you are responsible for 54 lives; not 55 – your own doesn't count.'[120]

Courage of this kind was thought to have its roots in the family. Home was the moral touchstone. 'His home-people, of course, came first', commented 'G.P.D', a master from Harold Parry's old school. [121] Looking back on his early letters from the front, Mary Charteris thought that 'the strange scenes in which he found himself, seemed only to intensify his love for his family and home'; he continued to write long letters to his family and his nanny.[122] Loyalty to mothers was especially highly valued. 'Whenever we were separated, even from his earliest childhood, he wrote to me every day', wrote Alice Lubbock, and during the war Eric continued to be 'very very good about writing'.[123]

But the affections of a mother sometimes had to vie with those of a sweetheart, and mothers were keen to establish that they still held pride of place in a son's heart. A memorial book might be used to help reclaim love that had felt threatened. Alice Lubbock disapproved of Eric's girlfriend, Winifred Martin Smith, who is never directly mentioned in the memorial book.[124] The readers within Alice Lubbock's social circle, however, no doubt knew for whom these stern words were intended: 'I believe it is always good for a boy to be friends with a girl, but there is a risk often that it may end in love. To a boy of Eric's character there could be no pretending or cheap imitation – love for him was a beautiful thing, delicate and sacred'.[125] Mothers were often suspicious of their sons' dalliances and the speed at which they pursued them. Marie Leighton, although circumspect about Vera Brittain, was withering about an earlier sweetheart, 'Queenie', whom she accused of trying to ensnare her son, as if Roland had been totally passive in the affair.[126]

References like this hinted at tensions which had sometimes been simmering during the last months of a son's life. John Middlebrook's growing affection for his later wife Dorothy worried his mother so much that he largely concealed it from her. When Dorothy got pneumonia in Christmas 1915, his mother accused him of 'deluging' his sweetheart with letters. 'I do hope Mother you will trust me', he wrote, 'I do not think I shall make a fool either of Dorothy or myself'.[127] At the end of January 1916 he sent Dorothy a silver brooch, which, Middlebrook excitedly explained to his sister Bessie, 'she has written saying she has worn . . . in bed. Great, isn't it?' Bessie must not, however, let their mother know anything of this.[128] Negotiations could be awkward when a man went on leave, and had to juggle spending time with a sweetheart and time at home. Cecil Christopher got his sister to break the news of his intention to visit his fiancée 'Bob': 'while talking of leave, Val, I think that when I do go it is only right that I should to [*sic*] spend at least a couple of days at Ryde. I think both you and mother will acknowledge that fact. I have told Bob that I shall probably do so.'[129] Christopher anticipated that the arrangements might disappoint his mother, but they were not negotiable. Other men sought to reassure mothers that their affections had not been lost to another woman. A twenty-year-old Canadian soldier serving in France, Philip Edward William, wrote:

> Yes Mother darling you are my best girl. I have had several so called flames but have no other girl I would call my best girl. There are three I am fond of at present in different ways. They are Evangelina, Tudor and Phylis. This isn't a list in order of seniority but I like them all as great friends and am not as the story books say "in love" with any of them. I have plenty of time to think about that when I get home. But now and always Mum dear you are my very best girl.[130]

When a son died, a mother's feeling that she had been displaced might become more intense. Even a mother whose son was married, and who had therefore formally given up her place as the principal loved one, might feel a lingering possessiveness. Isa Quarry mentioned herself first among the mourning family when writing to Mrs Stephens of her loss, although she had learned of her son's death from her daughter-in-law. Her self-correction shows the tension between social convention and how this mother actually *felt*: 'He was very dear to us, his Mother, Wife + Sister tho' I say it I [should] put his Wife first.'[131]

Memorial books enabled mothers to re-cast their sons in an image of undivided devotion, which the tributes from others confirmed. The recollections of Mary Charteris – Yvo's youngest sister – single out his loyalty to his mother:

> I loved him better than anyone else in the world, and I remember telling him so once and hoping he would say he loved me best too, but he said mamma must come first and then me. I think he minded having to tell me this as he thought it would hurt my feelings, but I had forced him to.[132]

Others wanted to assure mothers that the son had continued to cherish her love right up to his death. After Frank Merivale died from influenza in November 1918, the Battalion chaplain wrote to Mrs Merivale 'He spoke so simply and naturally of all that his mother's influence had been for him.'[133]

The intensity of emotion that mothers expressed towards their sons in memorial books was not just a function of their grief, but reflected how the relationship had actually been experienced. These families often did not draw sharp distinctions between maternal and romantic love in the way that we do now. Arnold Hooper was at pains to show that no other woman occupied his feelings as strongly as his mother Louisa. He called her 'My dear little Mother' or 'our little angel', and promised her that he and Kenneth would remain bachelors. Father and sons were on the same romantic footing:

> It seems to me that the Girls at home are getting married in great numbers. The khaki uniform seems to do a lot of damage. Mary [his sister] is silent. I hope she is not caught out. I am in love, but it is still the little thing I have been in love with for years. I share her with you and Kenneth. She has got 3 men in Khaki, showing her huge attraction to men. Get the dear little thing photographed.[134]

There was not a hint of embarrassment in Arnold's confession to his father, and indeed Arnold sang his mother's praise to his friends as well:

> I tell them we call you angel, and treat you like something more than a Mother. An angel in our midst. Whom we can even flirt with, what flirtations we shall have. My knees are much larger than ever, plenty of room for your dear little body. What proud knees. I expect they will feel rather shy as they have not supported a little woman for nearly 2 years. They are reserved for the angel when she needs them. I should like you to send me a very small flat little Bible . . .[135]

There is a sexual aspect to the scene that Arnold paints here, of taking his mother's 'little body' on his big and manly knees; the act, moreover, is explicitly understood by Arnold himself to be erotic, as he imagines Louisa to be 'something more than a Mother', and his attention towards her as 'flirtations'. What Arnold conjures here is nothing less than the Oedipal fantasy of seducing the mother, and the drama is not just in the sons' heads, but in their mothers' too. Louisa worried that she had aged in their absence, and that on returning from the war they would no longer find her attractive. Meanwhile her desire for them had grown, and she would be the more ready to give herself to them:

> Kenneth darling, I am afraid I am looking older and uglier every day, I sometimes fear it may be a shock when you see me, and that you will not be able to love me as before; and you will be in fuller manhood, and I shall be ready to love you ever so much more than before.[136]

Louisa's fears disclosed themselves in nightmares in which she had lost her looks and was unrecognisable to her sons. In a letter that described this nightmare, Louisa recalled the obvious pleasure that Kenneth had once felt in her beauty. She could not now expect to move him so powerfully by her appearance; mere 'looks of love' would have to suffice:

> the day before, I had a horrid dream, I thought I was greatly changed, (my dread often). I saw myself, with a few horrid black bits of hair hanging loosely, a purple-red complexion, and a huge mouth, a truly terrible face, I remember saying to Mary, 'I am altering, do you think they will know me?', and she had to confess, that I was indeed changed. It was quite a relief to go to the glass, to see my plain, old but same little face . . . I remember distinctly, when you came home once, I was standing by our gate, I half expected you, though not so early as you came, and had put on a fresh white dress. I could see by your dear face, that you were pleased with your little Mother's appearance, that cannot be again, but I know I shall see in your dear face, looks of love, thank God for that. I expect I shall see you and our darling Arnold greatly improved.[137]

To the modern reader, Louisa's anxieties about ageing sound more like a wife's confessions to a husband than to a son, while Arnold's words of praise sound more like a husband's than a son's. In an era when Freud's ideas were yet to become commonplace, however, it was not necessarily felt as shameful to confess physical desire for a mother. On the contrary, these mothers and sons revelled in the physical aspects of their adoration which, as far as they were concerned, could not have been more pure in its origins.

The Hoopers were an evangelical family and their religious beliefs probably encouraged these heightened professions of love. Piety and desire are linked in the letter quoted above where Arnold moves abruptly from the image of his 'larger than ever' legs, to ask for a 'very small flat little Bible', the Word here calming down his amorous stirrings. Louisa had not only brought them up as devout Christians, but had turned the hearth into the altar, as Arnold intimated in birthday wishes to his mother in 1915:

> How I should have loved to kiss and nurse the little thing. But how much more would I love to kiss and make a fuss of that dear little thing now she has grown up to be a charming cultured lady, and incidentally my mother. Many happy returns. This is a happy return of last year, for we are a year nearer the time when all the Hooper Clan will return to the Shrine of the angel Louie, to adore and worship, and admire her learning, wisdom, beauty, and charm. How we love her.[138]

Wilfred Owen's correspondence with his mother, who was also evangelical, has the same kind of intensity, and at times also borders on the erotic.[139] When he was working as a curate's assistant in 1912 and living away from home for the first time, Wilfred requested a photograph of Susan. After receiving it, he wrote of the strength of his desire for her:

> Oh how do I stand (yes and sit, kneel, & walk, too,) in need of some tangible caress from you.
>
> Ink-slung ones are all very well in their way, and no one appreciates them more than I do; but my affections are physical as well as abstract – intensely so – and confound 'em for that, it shouldn't be so.[140]

This intensity was a feature of other middle-class families, too. In her memorial book, Marie Leighton commented that mothers could feel their sons to be more than children or even friends, but as 'in a certain sense, adoring lovers.'[141] *Boy of My Heart* tells how Marie Leighton cultivated an appreciation of women's fashion in Roland, got him to advise her on her outfits, and dressed to please him. If she had been out for the evening, she would wake Roland and get him to help unfasten her dress.[142]

Roland's budding romance with Vera Brittain seemed to fuel Marie Leighton's need for her son's attention. On the Friday night in August 1915 when he arrived in Lowestoft on his last home leave, explained Marie, he did not get in touch with Vera: 'To-morrow will do. Oh, by the way, Big Yeogh Wough, have you got any new clothes to show me?' 'There was only Sunday for her', remarked Marie of Vera. At bedtime on the Friday Marie sat beside Roland, her head resting on his pillow, her hand in his, kissing his hair as he fell sleep. The following morning he came down to her bed and lay across it, reading her little French fairy stories as she dressed and tidied up.[143] Vera arrived on the Saturday evening and, after playing records together until late in the night, Roland went to bed without saying goodnight to her. Marie expected still to be able to retain her place as his closest intimate: after escorting Vera up to her bedroom, she announced that she was 'soon going to tuck him up in bed'.[144]

On the Sunday, Roland and Vera went for a long walk and declared their love for each other. Roland 'actually kissed me' Vera wrote excitedly in her diary; she had felt the 'silkiness of his fair moustache' for the first time.[145] But hers was not the last kiss that Roland planted that night, for it was nearly four in the morning when Marie Leighton went up to Roland's bedroom to say goodnight to him.[146]

In the wake of a son's death the sexual drama tended to submerge itself in the spiritual, and in memorial books, what remained was not a physical union but a metaphysical one, a communion of souls. Mary Charteris recalled going to see Yvo after the death of a relative, 'when I was very unhappy, and we sat under the ancient elms in the Old Ground and watched the peaceful, nibbling sheep, almost in silence; but Yvo's gentle sympathy was very touching, and more healing than any words could have been.'[147] When a son could empathise without even the necessity of speaking, it was the purest sign he could give of his devotion.

Dreams, synchronous thoughts and spiritual phenomena often figure in mothers' reminiscences. Louisa Hooper reported to Arnold that 'On Saturday, whch [*sic*] was June 23, at times I felt strangely happy, and I also felt strongly that the happiness had something to do with you. I wonder if you have any corresponding feeling, I should be delighted to hear you had, that the bond of union between us is very strong'.[148] Premonitions were common. Alice Lubbock knew on her son's last visit home 'that he was not coming back.'[149] On the day that Middlebrook was shot through the arm, he kept pleading with his Captain not to write to his home address, but to his father's work address, so his father could break the news gently to his mother. Unconscious communication, however, proved a better way altogether of letting his mother know:

> mother had gone to bed early that night, July 25th, and . . . next morning when she came downstairs, she startled the family by saying that when they saw John again he would be without a left arm. She said that I appeared to her in her bedroom and pointing to my left arm all shattered, had said 'Look, Mother'. That is to say, in the Providence of God, I had been allowed to tell my mother myself – an answer to most urgent prayer.[150]

Stories like these would become the stuff of family myths, myths which showed the special understanding and sympathy, consecrated by God, which existed between mothers and sons.

On the night of 22 April 1916 – significantly, Easter Saturday – Mary Charteris had a 'dream-vision' that her elder son Ego had been killed: 'The atmosphere of the room seemed to quiver with excitement – I felt the stress and strain and saw, as if thrown on a magic-lantern sheet, a confused mass of black smoke splashed with crimson flame: it was like a child's picture of a battle or explosion.' Amidst it, Ego was standing tall and pale with a golden banner around his chest, 'its colour very beautiful, it swathed his body in spiral folds and seemed to protect him as he stood there with his face set and stern.' The visitation, she thought, had conveyed Ego's death without her 'actually realising', so that in the following anxious weeks, when they had no firm news about him other than that he was missing, she felt 'outwardly calm', as she already knew 'below the threshold of consciousness' that he was dead.[151]

How must Mary Charteris have felt, still receiving details from Yvo's comrades about his death the previous October, and now facing the likelihood that her other son was dead? The vision of Ego resplendent in gold bears the hallmarks of a manic defence against loss. When despair about the potential loss of a loved one feels unbearable, Melanie Klein tells us, the mind sometimes reacts by constructing a 'beautiful and perfect' replacement. It creates a '*picture*' [italics Klein's] which is not the real object or person, to guard against the fact that the object is in pieces.[152] Against the probability that Ego's body actually lay dismembered somewhere in Egypt (and hence that Mary's own mind is in pieces),

Mary Charteris imagined her son enveloped in a 'beautiful' banner. This dazzling image makes the war fade to nothing more than a 'child's picture of a battle', the shelling a mere puff of smoke, the blood a splash of red paint.

Ego is not just unimpaired in body, but wrapped in the banner of salvation, as if like Christ he is risen again. Manic defences are mobilised when the anxiety about a loved object feels intolerable, as it had for Mary Charteris as she waited for news of Ego. The premonition released her from worry and afterwards, she says, 'I was not anxious nor worried, but stunned.'[153] Wonderment took the place of grief. This kind of reaction differs from the depressive anxieties which are also experienced by bereaved people but which are characterised by feelings of guilt and remorse at the failure to put things right. The difference between these two kinds of states, manic and depressive, is poignantly conveyed in a nightmare reported by Mary's own daughter after Yvo's death. In Mary's dream, the loss is not made good, but felt even more acutely than in the conscious mind. Yvo is not dead, but out of his senses and wandering about; she should be able to help him but she cannot:

> For some years after his death I was haunted by the most terrible recurring nightmares that he had not been killed but was lost somewhere, insane and helpless, and that I could never reach him, though often he was near. These nightmares were always accompanied by that unearthly depth of sorrow, horror and freezing terror that one only experiences in dreams.[154]

The spiritualism so popular among middle-class mothers during the war might have had the same kind of emotional function as Mary Charteris' resurrection fantasy in helping to fend off the pain of loss. For, if a mother was so closely in tune with her son that it was possible to call him back, he was not totally lost to her. Communion promised release from despair.[155] The mother who proudly pinned her son's medals on her own chest on Armistice Day each year; Mrs Leighton, who ordered the destruction of her son's blood-soaked tunic so that it would not taint the glamour of his memory; those who quizzed the men in their son's platoon, eager to hear that he had been 'loved'; or who turned to spiritualism in the hope of contacting their sons, were trying to rescue something meaningful from the senseless carnage. The picture they constructed of the lost son was not always 'beautiful and 'perfect', a manic defence, but these mothers nevertheless felt compelled to distance and so preserve his memory from the bloody reality of the war.

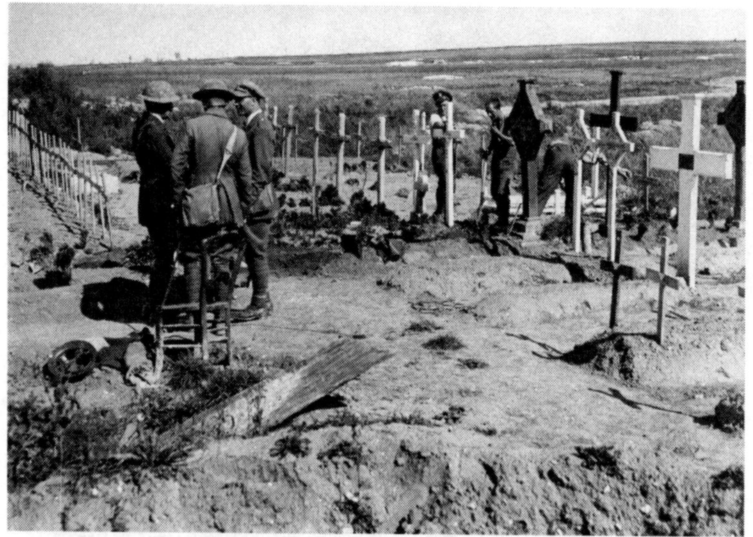

*23* Men tending graves in a war cemetery, September 1917

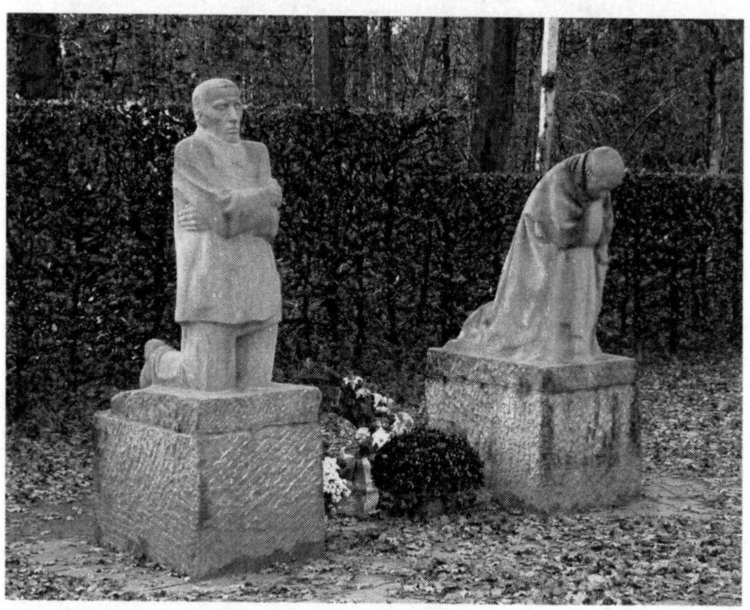

*24* 'The Grieving Parents', Kathe Kollwitz, Vladslo German War Cemetery, Belgium

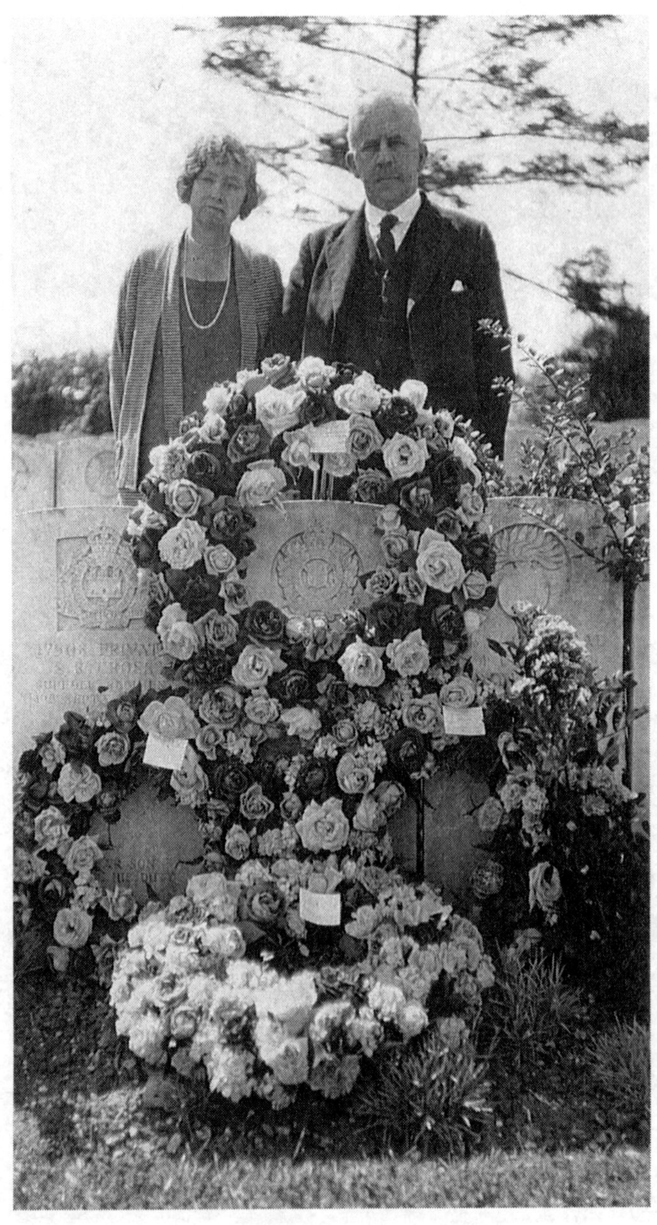

*25* A. G. Baker's parents visit his grave, 1925

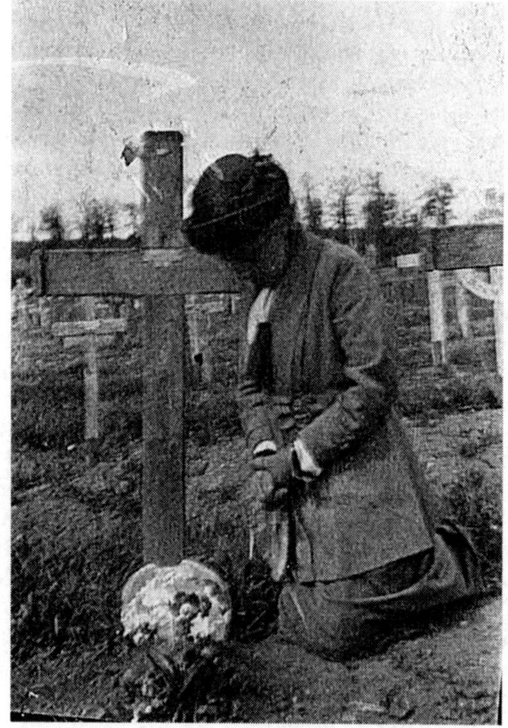

*26* Jim Tomlinson's mother kneels at his grave

## Notes

1 D.H. Fenton to Mrs Noone, nd, IWM 87/13/1. Information on James Joseph Noone's age, date of death and next-of-kin is from the Commonwealth War Graves Commission website, http://www.cwgc.org/search/casualty_details.aspx?casualty=291770. Accessed 19 July 2007.

2 Fenton to Mrs Noone, nd.

3 J. Keegan, *The Face of Battle* (London: Jonathan Cape, 1976), p. 268.

4 C. Acton, 'Bodies Do Count: American Nurses Mourn the Catastrophe of Vietnam', in P. Gray and K. Oliver, *The Memory of Catastrophe* (Manchester: Manchester University Press, 2004), p. 160; C. Acton, *Grief in Wartime. Private Pain, Public Discourse* (Basingstoke: Palgrave, 2007), pp. 1–17.

5 'The Long, Long Trail. The British Army in the Great War', http://www.1914-1918.net/dukes.htm. Accessed 16th April 2007.

6 S. Das, *Touch and Intimacy in First World War Literature* (Cambridge: Cambridge University Press, 2005), pp. 110–11.

7 Fenton, 'Inventory of kit', 11 September 1915.

8 See the discussion of the dying kiss and of Fenton's letter in Das, *Touch and Intimacy*. Das points to Fenton's use of the Pietà image as a means of 'deflecting' the erotic undertone of a kiss between two men 'to a maternal prerogative', pp. 122–3. The Fenton letter is also discussed by Joanna Bourke, *Dismembering the Male. Men's Bodies and the Great War* (London: Reaktion Books, 1996), p. 137.

9 See Julie-Marie Strange, '"She Cried a Very Little": Death, Grief and Mourning in Working-Class Culture c. 1880–1914', *Social History*, Vol. 27, No. 2 (May 2002), p. 160.

10 The Royal Welch Fusiliers buried nineteen men together on one occasion, and had to use the grave for cover when the Germans started shelling the plot. J. C. Dunn (ed.), *The War the Infantry Knew. A Chronicle of Service in France and Belgium* (London: Abacus, 1994), p. 80.

11 Quoted in R. Holmes, *Tommy. The British Soldier on the Western Front 1914–1918* (London: Harper Perennial, 2005), p. 298.

12 D. Winter, *Death's Men. Soldiers of the Great War* (London: Penguin, 1979), p. 259; A. Simpson, *Hot Blood and Cold Steel. Life and Death in the Trenches of the First World War* (London: Tom Donovan, 1993), p. 108; War Office. Directorate of Graves Registration and Enquiries, *The Care of the Dead. An Account of the Work of the Directorate of Graves Enquiries* (London: Eyre & Spottiswoode, 1916), pp. 10–11.

13 Directorate of Graves Registration and Enquiries, *Care of the Dead*, p. 11.

14 Winter, *Death's Men*, p. 259.

15 Dunn (ed.), *The War the Infantry Knew*, p. 417.

16 David Cannadine, 'War and Death, Grief and Mourning in Modern Britain', in J. Whaley (ed.), *Mirrors of Mortality. Studies in the Social History of Death* (London: Europa Publications, 1981), p. 207.

17 G. Talbot, *Gilbert Walter Lyttleton Talbot. Born September 1 1891. Killed in Action at Hooge, July 30 1915* (London: Chiswick Press, 1916), p. 84, p. 73.

18 W. B. P. Spencer to mother, 28 December 1914, IWM 87/56/1.

19 J. M. Winter, *Sites of Memory, Sites of Mourning. The Great War in European Cultural History* (Cambridge: Cambridge University Press, 1995), p. 31l.

20 The psychological impact on families of having a son listed as missing is discussed in Winter, *Sites of Memory, Sites of Mourning*, pp. 39–44; P. Jalland, *Death in the Victorian Family* (Oxford: Oxford University Press, 1996), p. 374, p. 377; Bruce Scates, *Return to Gallipoli. Walking the Battlefields of the Great War* (Cambridge: Cambridge University Press, 2006), pp. 52–60.

21 J. B. Middlebrook to father, 21 July 1916, IWM Con Shelf.

22 A. Simpson, *Hot Blood*, p. 109.

23 E. Blunden, *Undertones of War* (London: Penguin, 2000), p. 46.
24 Scates, *Return to Gallipoli*, p. 10.
25 Dunn (ed.), *The War the Infantry Knew*, p. 152.
26 C. Carrington, *Soldier From the Wars Returning* (London: Arrow Books, 1965), p. 219.
27 N. Gladden, *Ypres 1917* (London: William Kimber, 1967), p. 74.
28 R. Bickersteth to mother and father, 17 May 1915, The Bickersteth War Diaries and the Papers of John Burgon Bickersteth, Vol. 2, p. 582, Churchill Archives Centre, GBR/0014/BICK.
29 R. Bickersteth to mother and father, Bickersteth War Diaries, 17 May 1915.
30 Jalland, *Death in the Victorian Family*, p. 307.
31 Captain H. Campbell Ashenden to Mrs Hague, 11 July 1918, papers of H. W. Hague, IWM 98/33/1.
32 Letter from Second Lieut. O. C., 'D'. Coy to Frederic Spencer, 19 March 1915, papers of W. B. P. Spencer.
33 Rowland Hide to Mrs Dunning, 12 August 1917, papers of A. Higginson, IWM 95/1/1.
34 Rowland Hide to Mrs Dunning, 22 August 1917.
35 Second Lieutenant C. O. Tabberer to Mrs Tomlinson, 28 October 1915, papers of J. D. Tomlinson, IWM 87/51/1.
36 Captain Haley-Bell to Mrs Payne, 2 May 1919, papers of H. F. Payne, IWM 90/1/1.
37 Major A. R. Davis to Mrs Swettenham, nd but responding to her letter of 17 December 1918, papers of A. H. Swettenham, IWM 83/31/1.
38 A. H. Collart to Mr Carter, 7 April 1915, papers of H. Carter, IWM 86/8/1.
39 J. M. Scott, *In Memoriam. Poems and Letters, With Two Sermons by the Late John Millar Scott* (Alloa: Buchan Bros, 1917), p. 37.
40 Reverend C. E. G. Parry-Okeden, diary 7 April 1918, IWM 90/7/1.
41 J. H. Prowse and W. D. Warner to Mrs Tomlinson, 26 October 1915, papers of J. D. Tomlinson.
42 W. Gray to Mrs Dunning, 11 August 1917.
43 Gladden, *Ypres*, p. 42, p. 74.
44 Jalland, *Death in the Victorian Family*, p. 59, pp. 377–8.
45 Ella Bickersteth, 5 July 1916, quoted in J. Bickersteth (ed), *The Bickersteth Diaries 1914–1918* (London: Leo Cooper, 1995), p. 97.
46 Dorothy Etherston to Colonel Stephens, 16 May 1915, National Army Museum, 8902–201–1043 to 1396.
47 Second Lieutenant C. O. Tabberer to Mrs Tomlinson, 28 October 1915. J. M. Winter accurately gauges the tenor of officers' condolence letters: 'the man in question was loved by his comrades; he was a good soldier; he died painlessly.' *Sites of Memory, Sites of Mourning*, p. 35.
48 Keegan, *The Face of Battle*, p. 268.
49 W. Gray to Mrs Dunning, 11 August 1917.

50 W. H. R. Rivers, *Instinct and the Unconscious. A Contribution to a Biological Theory of the Psycho-Neuroses* (Cambridge: Cambridge University Press, 1920), pp. 190–1.

51 A. Wainwright to K. Tynan, 18 January 1915, Tynan/Hinkson Collection, John Rylands University Library of Manchester.

52 Scott, *In Memoriam*, p. 44.

53 Major Lawrence Jones to Mrs Payne, papers of H. F. Payne, 7 September 1919.

54 Douglas Finlay, Colonel RAMC to Rev. J. H. B. Wollocombe, 15 September 1916, papers of F. Wollocombe, p. 113, IWM 95/33/1.

55 V. Brittain, in A. Bishop, with T. Smart (eds.), *Vera Brittain. War Diary 1913–1917, Chronicle of Youth* (London: Victor Gollancz, 1981), p. 303.

56 Winter, *Sites of Memory, Sites of Mourning*, pp. 35–44; Scates, *Return to Gallipoli*, ch. 1.

57 Frederic Manning, in his novel *Her Privates We*, describes 'the painful way' a bereaved mother reaches out to her son's comrade Bourne, 'piecing him together out of her son's letters, as though he kept something of him which she had lost' (London: Serpent's Tail, 1999), p. 238. Joy Damousi regards the contact between bereaved families in Australia and the son's comrades as an attempt to 'revive a persona' of the dead man. *The Labour of Loss. Mourning, Memory and Wartime Bereavement in Australia* (Cambridge: Cambridge University Press, 1999), p. 9.

58 Owen Moorshead to Rev. J. H. B. Wollocombe, 14 September 1916; Douglas Finlay, Colonel RAMC to Rev. J. H. B. Wollocombe, 15 September 1916, both in papers of F. Wollocombe, pp. 112–13.

59 E. N. Makeham, *These to his Memory. A Selection in Prose and Verse from the Writings of Eric Noel Makeham* (London: Finden Brown, 1917), pp. xxv–xxvii.

60 R. S. Berkeley, W. W. Seymour, T. R. Eastwood and H. G. Parkyn, *The History of the Rifle Brigade in the War of 1914–1918*, 3 vols. (London: The Rifle Brigade Club, 1927–36), pp. 62–3.

61 Agnes Johnson to Mrs Stephens, 3 May 1915; Ruby Barber to Mrs Stephens, 24 March 1915, National Army Museum, 8902–201–1043 to 1396.

62 Mrs Willis to Mrs Stephens, 4 May 1916.

63 Rose Twomey to Mrs Stephens, 15 April, 18 April 1915.

64 Mrs M. Gilbey to Mrs Stephens, 19 March 1915.

65 On the significance for parents of returned clothing and personal effects see Jalland, *Death in the Victorian Family*, pp. 377–8.

66 R. Anderson to K. Tynan, 20 March 1915.

67 V. Brittain to E. Brittain, 23 February 1916, in A. Bishop and M. Bostridge (eds.), *Letters From a Lost Generation. First World War Letters of Vera Brittain and Four Friends* (london: Abacus, 1999), p. 234.

68 V. Brittain to E. Brittain, 14 January 1916, in Bishop and Bostridge (eds.), *Letters From a Lost Generation*, pp. 211–12; C. Leighton, Foreword in

A. Bishop, with T. Smart (eds.), *Vera Brittain. War Diary 1913–1917, Chronicle of Youth* (London: Victor Gollancz, 1981), p. 11.

69 Mrs Starky to Mrs Stephens, nd.

70 Isa Quarry to Mrs Stephens, 23 April 1918.

71 V. Brittain, *Testament of Youth. An Autobiographical Study of the Years 1900–1925* (London: Virago, 1978), pp. 421–2.

72 Ross, *Love and Loss*, p. 192.

73 Jalland, *Death in the Victorian Family*, p. 211.

74 J. M. Strange, *Death, Grief and Poverty in Britain 1870–1914* (Cambridge: Cambridge University Press, 2005), p. 75.

75 Strange, '"She Cried a Very Little"', p. 152.

76 Jalland, *Death in the Victorian Family*, p. 221.

77 Jalland, *Death in the Victorian Family*, pp. 300–1.

78 A. Gregory, *The Silence of Memory. Armistice Day 1919–1946* (Oxford: Berg, 1994), p. 40.

79 Personal communication with Mrs Marriott, Alf Swettenham's niece, June 2007.

80 Quoted in S. Collini, *Public Moralists. Political Thought and Intellectual Life in Modern Britain* (Oxford: Clarendon, 1993), p. 77. On the grief of widowers and the late Victorian assumption that 'strong men controlled their emotions', see Jalland, *Death in the Victorian Family*, p. 252.

81 Damousi, *The Labour of Loss*, p. 59.

82 Quoted in T. and V. Holt, *'My Boy Jack'. The Search for Kipling's Only Son* (London: Pen & Sword, 1998), p. 66.

83 Conan Doyle and Bonar Law were two other fathers whose grief was widely noted. Gregory, *The Silence of Memory*, p. 22. See also Cannadine, 'War and Death', pp. 213–17.

84 C. Asquith, *Diaries 1915–18* (London: Hutchinson, 1968), p. 92.

85 R. Anderson to K. Tynan, 17 March 1915.

86 Ellen Dickson to Mrs Stephens, 17 March 1915.

87 Ellen Dickson to Mrs Stephens, 28 March 1915.

88 R. Schulte, 'Käthe Kollwitz's Sacrifice', *History Workshop Journal*, Vol. 41 (Spring 1996), p. 199.

89 Makeham, *These to his memory*, p. xxx.

90 S. Grayzel, *Women's Identities at War. Gender, Motherhood and Politics in Britain and France during the First World War* (Chapel Hill, NC: University of North Carolina Press, 1999), p. 229–30.

91 Quoted in Gregory, *The Silence of Memory*, p. 33.

92 D. Lloyd, *Battlefield Tourism. Pilgrimage and the Commemoration of the Great War in Britain, Australia and Canada* (Oxford: Berg, 1998), p. 65.

93 Grayzel, *Women's Identities*, pp. 226–8.

94 Lloyd, *Battlefield Tourism*, p. 164, p. 169.

95 Lloyd, *Battlefield Tourism*, p. 135, p. 146.

96 Lloyd, *Battlefield Tourism*, p. 38.

97 P. Thompson and T. Lummis, 'Family Life and Work Experience Before 1918, 1870–1973' [computer file], 5th edition (Colchester: UK Data Archive [distributor], April 2005. SN: 2000), interview 364, pp. 25–6. The cost of pilgrimages fell in the 1920s partly due to organisations such as St Barnabas. Winter, *Sites of Memory, Sites of Mourning*, p. 52.

98 Lloyd, *Battlefield Tourism*, p. 169–70; John Pegum, '"The Old Front Line": Returning to the Battlefields in the Writings of Ex-Servicemen', paper given at First World War and Popular Culture conference, University of Newcastle, 2 April 2006.

99 Gregory, *The Silence of Memory*, p. 40.

100 Scates, *Return to Gallipoli*, p. 48.

101 T. Holt, *Major and Mrs Holt's Battlefield Guide to the Somme* (London: Leo Cooper, 1996), p. 224.

102 Scates, *Return to Gallipoli*, p. 49.

103 All inscriptions cited here are from Ljissenthoek Cemetery.

104 Of twelve examples used here, six were written by mothers, one by a father (dedicated to the mother), and one by a father and mother. In four cases the author is unknown but all these memorial books cite widely from sons' letters to their mothers.

105 Vera Brittain to Edward, 6 April 1916, *Letters From a Lost Generation*, p. 246.

106 Jalland, *Death in the Victorian Family*, p. 379.

107 As Jalland herself notes, a death in which the child preceded its parents was particularly shocking. Jalland, *Death in the Victorian Family*, p. 141.

108 Annotating letters, copying them out, or editing them for publication, families re-traced the son's experience in the trenches and his last moments, placing themselves at the scene. Damousi, *The Labour of Loss*, p. 60.

109 Talbot, *Gilbert Walter Lyttleton Talbot*, pp. 43–4.

110 Anon., *Boy of My Heart* (London: Hodder & Stoughton, 1916), p. 28.

111 I. Small to K. Tynan, 10 January 1915. Damousi also notes the tendency of bereaved mothers to create an exalted image of the dead son. *The Labour of Loss*, p. 131.

112 Janet Watson has done much to elaborate the idea of service, and to show how its meanings varied according to social class, rank and gender. But for Watson service is assumed to be for a national cause. *Fighting Different Wars. Experience, Memory and the First World War in Britain* (Cambridge: Cambridge University Press, 2004), pp. 41–52.

113 Grayzel, *Women's Identities*, p. 86; N. Gullace, *The Blood of Our Sons. Men, Women and the Renegotiation of British Citizenship in the Great War* (Basingstoke: Palgrave, 2002), p. 3.

114 W. C. Mayo, *In Memoriam. William Charles Mayo* (Sherborne: Sawtell, 1916), p. 35.

115 Makeham, *These to his Memory*, p. xxv.

116 R. Anderson to K. Tynan, 28 May 1915. For other examples, see Talbot, *Gilbert Walter Lyttleton Talbot*, letter from Major Ross, 5 August 1915: 'All the men of his company were very much attached to him', pp. 43–4; letter from Captain C. H. Rowe to Mr Spencer, 12 March 1915: 'The NCOs and men, believe me, had good reason to love him.' Papers of W. B. P. Spencer.

117 A. A. Lubbock, *Eric Fox Pitt Lubbock, born 16th May 1893. Killed in Aerial Fight Near Ypres, 11th March 1917. A Memoir by his Mother* (London: A. L. Humphries, 1918), p. 241.

118 Anon., *Boy of My Heart*, p. 32.

119 Talbot, *Gilbert Walter Lyttleton Talbot*, pp. 48–9.

120 Lavinia Talbot also included one of Gilbert's school essays in which he had quoted Browning on the soldierly ideal of mortal sacrifice: 'O lover of my life, O Soldier saint/Who put his breast between the spears and me.' Talbot, *Gilbert Walter Lyttleton Talbot*, pp. 47–9.

121 H. Parry, *In Memoriam: Harold Parry, Second Lieutenant, K.R.R.C.: Born at Bloxwich – December 13th 1896. Fell in Flanders – May 6th 1917* (London: W.H. Smith, nd), p. vii.

122 M. C. W. Charteris, *A Family Record* (London: Curwen Press, 1932), pp. 310–12.

123 Lubbock, *Eric Fox Pitt Lubbock*, p. 2, p. 214.

124 IWM Catalogue entry, Capt. The Hon E. F. P. Lubbock, IWM PP/MCR/406.

125 Lubbock, *Eric Fox Pitt Lubbock*, pp. 9-10.

126 Anon., *Boy of My Heart*, p. 62.

127 Middlebrook to mother and father, 31 December 1915.

128 Middlebrook to Bessie, 31 January 1916.

129 W. C. Christopher to Val, 16 December 1916, IWM 88/11/1.

130 P. E. William to mother, 22 May 1917, quoted with permission of Philip C. Gunyon.

131 Isa Quarry to Mrs Stephens, 23 April 1918.

132 Mary Charteris (daughter) quoted in Charteris, *A Family Record*, p. 336.

133 Reverend J. Aglionby to Mrs Merivale, 22 November 1918, papers of J. H. Merivale, IWM P471.

134 A. Hooper to L. Hooper, quoted in L. Hooper to K. Hooper, 15 July 1915, Liddle Collection, DF066.

135 A. Hooper to L. Hooper, quoted in L. Hooper to K. Hooper, 9 April 1916.

136 L. Hooper to K. Hooper, 22 November 1915; 3 April 1917.

137 L. Hooper to K. Hooper, 6 October 1916.

138 A. Hooper to L. Hooper, quoted in L. Hooper to K. Hooper, 30 September 1915.

139 Owen sometimes writes to his mother 'almost as a lover', remarks his biographer Dominic Hibberd. *Wilfred Owen. A New Biography* (London: Weidenfeld & Nicolson, 2002), p. 23.

140 W. Owen to mother, 20 May 1912, in J. Bell (ed.), *Wilfred Owen. Selected Letters* (Oxford: Oxford University Press, 1985), p. 52.
141 Anon., *Boy of My Heart*, p. 18.
142 Anon., *Boy of My Heart*, p. 57, p. 84, p. 136.
143 Anon., *Boy of My Heart*, pp. 210–12.
144 *Chronicle of Youth*, pp. 248–9.
145 *Chronicle of Youth*, p. 259.
146 Anon., *Boy of My Heart*, p. 215.
147 Charteris, *A Family Record*, p. 309.
148 L. Hooper to A. Hooper, 25 June 1917.
149 Lubbock, *Eric Fox Pitt Lubbock*, p. 239. Premonitions could also be experienced by fathers: shortly before his actual death, Roland Leighton's father dreamt four times in one week that his son was dead and walking arm-in-arm with a dead comrade. Anon., *Boy of My Heart*, p. 68.
150 J. B. Middlebrook memoir, IWM Con Shelf, p. 126.
151 Charteris, *A Family Record*, p. 372.
152 M. Klein, *Love, Guilt and Reparation and Other Works 1921–1945* (London: Virago, 1994), p. 270.
153 Charteris, *A Family Record*, p. 372.
154 Charteris, *A Family Record*, p. 336.
155 Siegfried Sassoon's poem, 'Supreme Sacrifice', composed in June 1917, comments on the psychological function of spiritualist beliefs:

> Her tired eyes half-confessed she'd felt the shock
> Of ugly war brought home. And then a slow
> Spiritual brightness stole across her face . . .
> 'But *they* are safe and happy now', she said.
> (*Siegfried Sassoon. The War Poems*, London: Faber & Faber, 1983, p. 81)

# 6

# 'Nameless dread'

> In war, as in air accidents, 'insides' are much more visible than it is normally well to imagine. (Paul Fussell, 1989[1])

When Lance Corporal Roland Mountfort was wounded on the Somme and hospitalised in Rouen, he scrawled a note to his mother. He had 'seen in 3 days more wonderful, more pitiful + more horrible sights than would suffice any ordinary mortal for 3 lifetimes'.[2] He was then moved to the Mile End Military Hospital in London, from where, four days later, he wrote again. He apologised for keeping his family in suspense but he had only just settled down and did not yet feel 'at home here.' There was 'a tremendous lot to tell you – so much in fact that at present I am not going to start on any of it.' He mainly described his trip back on the hospital ship Asturia, and his 'nice clean flesh wound', which caused him no pain.[3]

It was another three days before Mountfort felt able to write at more length, this time penning a twenty-page description of the days leading up to his wounding.[4] This, combined with the Battalion Diary, allow us to construct a detailed account of his part in the Battle of the Somme. His Battalion, the 10th Royal Fusiliers (Mountfort had joined the so-called 'Stockbrokers' Battalion', a 'Pals' unit, early in the war) went into trenches at 8pm on the evening of 9 July 1916, acting in support for the 13th Rifle Brigade, who were preparing to attack Contalmaison. The dead, caught by machine-gun fire, 'lay about in great numbers' as they made their way forwards.[5] German snipers' rifles, grey blankets, Prussian helmets, clips of dum dum cartridges, and a postcard to '"mein lieber, lieber Hans" from "Deine Elise"' lay scattered about, but Mountfort took nothing, for '[a]fter I had seen dead bodies lying on all sides in the weird attitudes of sudden death, souvenirs seemed a bit paltry.'

They huddled that night in first support-line trenches which had been badly battered by shelling. The next two days were spent, as the Battalion Diary put it bluntly, 'digging night and day to get some kind of cover', and suffering 'considerably' from enfilade fire (which came side-on to their trenches).[6] Mountfort reported that they were 'shelled often + had a good few casualties'. On 10 July they were put to burying the German and British dead around La Boisselle, who in Mountfort's words 'were lying all over the road + in the open square. They had been there some little while, + some were embedded in the mud or half buried in rubbish.' One had to be dragged up from a store shed, another from a dug-out. The Battalion buried around fifty bodies that day.[7]

On the evening of 10 July, already exhausted from their digging, they were pushed up to front-line trenches to relieve the 13th Rifle Brigade, which had lost four officers and around 400 men.[8] They ended up taking part in a confused attack, rushing over their own front line and almost to the German trenches amid machine gun fire: 'Men were going down every minute, + since there had previously been bodies lying all the way the place began to look a bit rotten.' Just as Mountfort became 'sure that there was nobody leading us + we should just go running on till there was no one left', an order came to retire. They spent the rest of the night holding a section of front-line trenches under heavy shelling. Mountfort was in a bay with a wounded Rifle Brigade man lying on the trench floor and another 'wounded in the throat + making gurgling noises, sitting on the fire step. Then a shell burst on the parapet + half buried us all.' Five men among the two sections crowded into the bay were hit, including Fredericks, in whom his sister 'Gwyneth was always interested. I saw him go down just in front of me.' When it became light the following morning (11 July) they were ordered to dig down but in the bay there was 'a German trouser + boot protruding in one place', which 'rather put us off making it as deep as we should have liked'.

On their second morning holding the front line (12 July) Mountfort was sent to carry rations up to twenty men who had been holding an advanced trench:

> For 500 yards it is paved with English dead. I don't know what happened, but they were evidently caught there by an awful shell fire – some say our own. In places you must walk upon them, for they lie in heaps. I went up with rations, + again to help carry down a casualty on a stretcher. I won't describe that trench until I have forgotten it a little.

On the evening of 12 July the Battalion was moved back to the support line, having lost thirty-six men from shelling in 48 hours.[9] Mountfort and his comrades dug 'little cubby holes in the side + curled up like hedgehogs' to sleep. The man in the funk hole next to Mountfort tried to deepen it, struck some sacking, and 'went on + got as far as a blood-stained cap; + then he went to dig a new hole.' Mountfort found sacking in his hole too, but 'didn't trouble to move. What the eye doesn't see etc.'

At 9 a.m. on 15 July, after resting for three nights in the support trenches, they were ordered back to the front line for an attack on Pozières. Mountfort went over the top into what the Battalion Diary described as 'heavy machine gun fire'.[10] He ran with his head down for 200 yards or so before he felt a punch on the shoulder. He lay down in a shell hole with two other men, one wounded in the leg, the other with a 'bad wound' in the back. After an hour and a half, worried by the crumps that were falling around him, he made his way back through trenches 'full of dead' – this time German – to the aid post, and to the hospital at Albért where his wound was dressed before he was taken by hospital train to Rouen.

Mountfort's letter ended with a description of the wound on his shoulder:

> My wound is dressed twice a day, + is more painful every time – a sign, as I am assured, that it is healing up nicely. It has to be 'packed' at the lower entrance, which means that a few yards of bandage are poked up with a knitting needle, to keep it open + allow it to discharge. It consists of a little blue mark on the top of my shoulder where the bullet went in, + a long deep slit a few inches down my back where it came out. Possibly it turned a little in its course. The official diagnosis on my sheet is 'Gun shot. Small entry wound above right clavicle; large furrowed wound on scapular muscles at exit.'

For Mountfort, the most upsetting part of the battle was not his own wounding. It was a classic 'Blighty' and had got him back home without a permanent disability, unlike most of the 237 other casualties in the Battalion that day.[11] Nor was his distress wholly due to the scale of death and wounding he had seen. What affected him just as much was the way in which bodies had been mangled. There was the man who gurgled as his breath expired through the bullet wound to his throat. There were the German soldiers on the first night who lay 'on all sides in the weird attitudes of sudden death', and the English soldiers whose bodies, smashed by shell-fire, lay thick on the floor of the advanced trench. Mountfort was not even insulated from horror when asleep, for body parts lay just beneath the funk holes. There was his own wound, with its neat hole on entry, flaring out beneath his skin into a cavity large enough to take yards of bandage to fill, and its furrowed exit. It could (with the aid of a mirror) be inspected close up, and described in detail, unlike the shell-blasted bodies he had walked over, about which he could say nothing 'until I have forgotten it a little'.

Despite the terrors he experienced at the Somme, Mountfort was well enough by October 1916 to be sent to train with the 6th Royal Fusiliers, a Reserve Battalion. In February 1917 he rejoined the war, this time in East Africa although, like many, he was hospitalised on numerous occasions with dysentery and malaria. After the war he worked in the legal department of the Prudential Insurance Company, and died of cancer in 1930 when he was just forty years old.[12]

Mountfort's wound may have been quick to heal but he did not escape unscathed from the Somme. He often felt low during his two-month stay in hospital. In early August he reported that he hadn't much to say; it was an hour to bed-time and he had been 'perseveringly [*sic*] doing nothing all day; with the result that I feel very limp + vacant.' Having fallen 'into a reverie till bed-time' that evening, he spent the next day 'in much the same way.' He grieved for his friends, a 'little fellow, a most delightful companion' and a solicitor from Yorkshire. 'I don't think the selection a good one', he stated bluntly, as both of them were 'much cleverer and more useful individuals' than he.[13] Shortly before joining the 6th Royal Fusiliers in Dover, he went on holidays to Llangollen with his mother: 'I wasn't being exactly brilliant, but I didn't seem to be able to help it.' He was dreading the prospect of return to Army life, which 'I still loathe with all the hatred of which I am capable.'[14] This was something he had not found it possible to declare until after he was back in Blighty. His half-brother recalls the veteran Mountfort as 'a most fastidious man particularly in regard to personal appearance and cleanliness'.[15] Army life tended to encourage fastidiousness such as this, but it may also have helped Mountfort hold himself together.

Mountfort was not alone in finding it difficult to convey the scenes of war that affected him most. Robert Graves claimed that his 'emotion-recording apparatus' failed after the battle of Loos, but horrific images played on his mind long afterwards. While recuperating at Harlech at the end of the war, shells 'used to come bursting above my bed at midnight.'[16] Sometimes a battle-stressed soldier might become deaf, mute, experience temporary blindness or lose his memory.[17] The psychologist

William McDougall described a shell-shock victim who 'showed no trace of comprehension of spoken or written language'.[18] The assault of violent experiences caused the mind to seal itself off from the world: it could no longer take things in. The emotional residues of violent experiences nevertheless gnawed away within the unconscious, unthought.

This chapter examines states of mind that felt beyond comprehension, and whose effects remained within the unconscious long after battle. It asks: what kinds of experiences brought men to the edge of madness? And what was it about the nature of trench warfare that could do this? Many soldiers suffered from periods of what has been called 'battle stress', although never becoming incapacitated to the point where they were withdrawn from the line. The frequency with which soldiers reported cases of war nerves among comrades, and the morally neutral tone some adopted, suggests how little they felt separated them from the victims. The subaltern Graham Greenwell, although remaining staunchly positive about the war throughout, did not judge men who broke down. In letters home to his mother in 1915 he noted one man 'gone a bit off his head'; and how, after a violent bombardment in their front lines shortly afterwards, a signaller was 'mortally wounded and one bomber broke down.'[19] During the battle of the Somme he was similarly uncensorious towards 'a poor chap who has suddenly gone groggy with shell-shock.'[20] As far as Greenwell and many other soldiers with long experience of trench warfare were concerned, men wounded mentally or physically were equally casualties.[21]

In its very genesis, the term 'shell-shock' related to soldiers whose mental functioning was so impaired as to 'incapacitate a man from the performance of his military duties.'[22] Studies of shell-shock have little to say about the majority who continued to carry out their military duties with at least a minimum of competence, but who suffered from periodic or even chronic emotional disturbances. The emphasis in the literature on shell-shock, moreover, has been on the aftermath of symptoms and treatment, rather than on the events that brought men into Casualty Clearing Stations and military hospitals in the first place. Ben Shephard, in his history of shell-shock, *A War of Nerves*, mentions how 'extreme and sudden horror and fright' could lead to its onset.[23] But this still begs the question: what sorts of experiences were most frightful?

In part, this focus on treatment rather than genesis reflects the practical concerns of contemporaries. W. H. R. Rivers, for example, charged in his capacity as a military psychiatrist with getting soldiers back to the front, said little about the events that had caused them to break down.

Lack of preparation was as much the problem as trench warfare itself. One of the 'chief causes' of 'nervous disorders', he believed, was that soldiers had been forced to endure 'hardships and dangers of unprecedented severity with a quite insufficient training'.[24] In treating these soldiers, Rivers concentrated on their tendency to repress their memories. His emphasis on the secondary mechanism of repression reflected the tension that military doctors sometimes experienced between humane impulses and military duty: Rivers could do something about how the memory of the event was handled, but not about the way the war itself was waged.[25] Freud's pre-war ideas did not help him much, for they also bypassed the traumatic event. Locked as psychoanalysis was into explanations founded on the sexual dramas of the infant, it seemed to have little to say about the shocking scenes being witnessed by grown men.

Military historians tend to adopt a rationalistic perspective when discussing the impact of violent deaths and injuries, assuming that they were frightful because they brought men face to face with their own mortality. Denis Winter argues that the sight of dead men occasioned horror because, 'at the back of the mind was the knowledge that the corpse was once a living man like oneself, in the same situation and therefore initially no more likely to meet death than oneself.'[26] There is truth in this. As Robert J. Lifton argues in *The Broken Connection*, contact with death is a central feature of trauma among survivors of war.[27] But more is at stake emotionally than a simple recognition that the body shattered on the trench floor could be one's own, an anxiety that is derived from the prospect of a premature end. Powerful irrational feelings were stirred by such sights. Certain types of death could threaten psychic disintegration, and hence it is important to understand what it was about the *manner* of death and violence, that made it disturbing.

So also, Joanna Bourke's *Fear. A Cultural History*, which is centrally concerned with the nature of trauma, tries to decentre the privileged place that 'psycho-history' has in the history of fear. Modern combat, she argues, is terrifying because it often immobilises the soldier, and in so doing frustrates his basic fight/flight instinct. He must passively take what comes at him; he cannot escape or adequately resist. Bourke is right to emphasise the effect of immobility. W. H. R. Rivers felt that the prolonged experience of danger without an 'ability to manipulate the world' was a principal factor in the onset of war neuroses, and soldiers in their letters and memoirs often commented on the stress caused by having to passively endure shelling.[28] Bourke argues that fear is compounded by a further factor, the fear of fear itself. Men, and especially military commanders who had to show an example to the men, were afraid of being thought cowards and the need to keep a stiff upper lip added to the strain. But the kinds of symptoms presented by battle-stressed soldiers suggest that there was more to battle stress than neural reactions or the burden of manly performance. Bourke describes an American soldier who presented himself to his Battalion surgeon explaining that 'I can't stand them shells. My stomach hurts. They tear my stomach to pieces'.[29] His mental organisation had broken down. Although not physically injured, he was so profoundly disturbed by the violence around him that his anxieties were experienced, not as akin to, but actually *as*, flesh-and-blood wounds. Men often felt that the mental pressure of trench warfare was literally tearing their bodies to pieces. Lieutenant A. B. Scott wrote in his diary that he was 'going all to pieces'; a month later, he was 'slowly and surely . . . breaking up.'[30] Such states cannot be wholly comprehended as a matter of linguistic convention, social pressure or physiological reflexes.

Like many others, Mountfort was unable to describe mutilated bodies, the advanced trench littered with dead men upon whom he had trodden to bring rations to the living. As these men were the victims of shell-fire, Mountfort might have seen limbs rent from torsos, faces smashed in and bodies gaping open. In his memoirs of the Somme, Norman Gladden intimates what Mountford could not; not just the sight, but the stench which brought him to the point of fainting:

> The dead man lay amidst earth and broken timber. It seemed like a sacrilege to step over him but there was no evading the issue. Never before had I seen a man who had just been killed. A glance was enough. His face and body were terribly gashed as though some terrific force had pressed him down, and blood flowed from a dozen fearful wounds. The smell of blood mixed with the fumes of the shell filled me with nausea. Only a great effort saved my limbs from giving way beneath me. I could see from the sick grey faces of the file that these feelings were generally shared.[31]

Imagine this body multiplied by the dozen, the smell the more pungent because of 'very warm' weather, and we can begin to sense what Mountfort could not tell his mother.[32] Sometimes it was not the obliteration of bodies but their life-like pose that caused distress. The Scots Grenadier Stephen Graham remembered two fellows in a shell-hole with frightened looks on their faces, crouched together as if one had been saying to the other "'keep your head down." Now in both men's heads there was a dent, the sort of dent that appears in the side of a rubber ball when not fully expanded by air.'[33]

Wilfred Bion's memoir of his time as a tank commander, written in 1919, describes the cumulative impact of experiences like this. It recounts one horrific incident after another in forensic detail. By late September 1918 'I had lost my nerve. Everything I did was difficult; in action I had to force myself to do my mere job. I became more or less paralysed by the thought of action, and my brain would not work'.[34] His comment about patients in psychoanalysis: 'I say they *are* regressed' [italics his], had a point of reference in his own war. Though he was called up as an Army psychiatrist in the Second World War and worked at the Northfield Hospital with veterans who had broken down, Bion rarely wrote about war. When he did, comments his daughter Parthenope Bion Talamo, 'it was almost as though he were forced into doing so by external circumstances.'[35] Nevertheless, the distinctive psychoanalytic ideas that Bion developed during the 1950s speak to the extreme disturbances of battle-stressed soldiers.[36] War, says Bion Talamo 'formed part of the real personal emotional experience on which his theories lie.'[37]

Central to these theories is the concept of 'containing', which relates to the infant's anxieties and the mother's way of dealing with them. For Bion these anxieties at the most primitive level have to do with death, the infant's 'feeling, say, that it is dying'.[38] The baby finds these feelings unbearable and projects them into the mother for her to deal with, and to give back shorn of their terror. However, the mother often finds herself unable to take in the baby's distress. She might empathise so much that she becomes upset herself, or she may feel frightened and project anxiety straight back. A baby whose distress cannot be contained by the mother might experience what Bion calls 'nameless dread', a feeling that its anxieties are not only intolerable, but cannot be made sense of. Its anxieties fragment within the psyche, and are then felt to attack it, much like the American soldier who experiences his fear as splinters which are tearing apart his stomach.

Terror was a feature of trench warfare, even more than it is in the daily care of infants, where the mother is often able to soothe the baby by showing that the threat it perceives is not as great as it supposes. But on the Western Front, fear was a rational response: there really were splinters of metal flying about which would kill and maim. This fact taxed every soldier and most – even those who professed to enjoy battle – experienced moments of extreme distress. Charles Carrington is sometimes cited by military historians as a counter-example to the 'horror' school of memoir-writing. At Ovillers-la-Boiselle, however, he came across a signaller in the cubby-hole of a trench wall. Carrington asked for directions but the man 'slowly raised his head and looked at me with blank appealing eyes. I saw that two rivulets of blood were running slowly from his throat into the collar of his tunic.' Carrington had to leave the man behind, but 'his face remained with me.'[39] The failures of containing described by the psychoanalyst Bion in the 1950s not only chimed with his own war experience, but with the experiences of many veterans.

## Regression and containing

The stresses of battle affected men of the war generation particularly deeply because they were between childhood and adulthood. Their identities were divided between the image of soldierly prowess and manly responsibility, and the memory of home and childhood. They were, in Ben Shephard's apposite phrase, 'half men half boys'.[40] It was after battle that the trench soldier appeared most childlike. The Australian journalist C. E. W. Bean described men returning from battle as being 'like boys emerging from a long illness.'[41] Frederic Manning wrote of how men hid away in the 'warm smelly darkness of the tent', seeking through sleep the 'healing of oblivion'.[42] As soon as Mountfort and his comrades got back to the relative safety of the support trenches they curled up 'like hedgehogs', and slept. The tendency towards regression could be long-lasting: ten years after the war, Charles Carrington commented, he was still 'retarded and adolescent.'[43]

Regression was pronounced among the most serious cases of battle stress. The psychologist William McDougall noted a patient who had lost the ability to feed himself, and who insisted on the nurse tasting his food before accepting it from her spoon.[44] The behaviour of the soldier suffering from war strain, wrote G. E. Smith and T. H. Pear, having observed shell-shocked men at Maghull Military Hospital, 'presents a considerable resemblance to that of the child'; while the physician's approach should be 'precisely that which the sensible mother exhibits towards a child who exhibits sudden and unreasonable fear'.[45]

When men were in regressed states, they needed containing. This could show itself in the reports they gave of their difficulties in sleeping. We saw in Chapter 4 how Ernest Smith related his bad dreams to his mother just before settling down to sleep, as if he might stave off their reappearance by telling her. Erich Maria Remarque describes Paul Bäumer falling into a deep sleep after laying out barbed wire during the night. He awakens disorientated and distressed, thinking he has fallen asleep in the garden at home: 'I don't know whether it is morning or evening, and I lie there in the pale cradle of dawn waiting for the gentle words which surely must come, gentle and comforting – am I crying? I put my hand to my face; it is baffling, am I a child?'[46] What Remarque describes – and it is a refrain in the book – is a situation where men are thrown back into a child-like state of unbearable distress, yet where there is no mother to assuage their pain: the man who hovers above Bäumer as he awakens is not his mother, but his comrade Katczinsky. Men under stress might bring to mind times when they had been nursed by their mothers. In Edward Chapman's letter home from the Somme, he recalled that 'This time last year I was in bed with typhoid; what a very happy time that was for me, at all events'.[47] What had at the time been a serious illness was now, in the aftermath of battle, a treasured memory of maternal care.

Because conditions on the Western Front were so unsanitary, men often suffered from stomach problems. These made them miserable and in need of looking after, often when they were already feeling fearful or demoralised. Matt Webb attributed his diarrhoea to the long stint he had served on the Western Front without leave, and to the stress of shelling: 'I am feeling very run-down having shooting pains in the head + weak + still suffering from diarrhoea all of which is doubtless the result on the nervous system of the recent bad shelling we have had so much of + the shock of which affects you in all kinds of ways.'[48] An upset tummy could be a telling sign of feelings otherwise suppressed, as Webb himself realised.[49]

When men had upset stomachs they remembered earlier bouts of sickness. The 'Gastroenteritis' that Eric Marchant contracted after an exhausting spell in the trenches was a long-standing complaint. He hinted at the relationship between anxiety and his stomach problems: 'I have been overtaken by an attack of my old gastric trouble together with a little nervous trouble'; it had occurred while 'we are very close to some big guns which I find rather trying.'[50] Second Lieutenant Lyndall Urwick had been forced to withdraw from the front line with violent diarrhoea just prior to a battle which decimated his platoon. His letter to his mother from hospital intimated the roots of his complaint, explaining how 'I suddenly found myself curled up with a stomach-ache that put the best efforts of my childhood to naught.' Elsewhere in the letter Urwick described his stomach as his 'Little Mary', presumably the pet-name that his family had used when referring to his childhood tummy aches.[51] Not only were there similarities between the emotional situation of the child and of the battle-stressed soldier, but the experience of the front was sometimes felt to have *recapitulated* childhood states.

'Clothing and its part in the psychology of war', remarked the veteran Wyndham-Lewis, 'is a neglected subject.'[52] Men's descriptions of their clothing, like their accounts of their health, provided telling indications of their emotional state. Mothers had often chosen their sons' underwear, coats and other articles, so descriptions of what men were wearing served to bring them close. Edward Chapman wrote to his mother about how 'with your leather jerkin under my tunic, and the thick gray cardigan Father used to wear as well . . . I keep perfectly warm'.[53] The fact that his father had died the previous year added poignancy to the cardigan; it was a kind of talisman. He called the jerkin sent by his mother 'your . . . jerkin', as if he was being enveloped by a part of her. Chapman kept it after the war, complete with bloodstains from a wound in May 1917 which blinded him in the left eye. He loaned it to his son in the 1950s, but asked for it back soon afterwards. The jerkin connected him to a memory that he needed to hold on to even in peace time and middle age.[54]

In response to his mother's 'entreaties', Wilfred Owen bought a trench coat shortly before his departure for France, and wore it during his final visit from his mother.[55] Like Chapman, he occasionally mentioned it in letters as a means of conjuring a maternal presence. At Serre he survived the freezing cold because 'I had my Trench Coat (without lining but with a Jerkin underneath)'. The reference was a way of bringing his mother close, of showing how, as he put it later in the letter, 'the intensity of your Love reached me and kept me living'.[56]

But clothing could just as easily convey anxiety. When Owen returned from the line at St Quintin, the fate of his trench coat served as a means of communicating, not safety, but mortal peril. At one point he hung it on a bush, and seconds later, just as he dived for cover, 'a splinter ripped a hole through the chest & back'. Owen brings his mother close up against this threat to his life: the coat, he tells her, is the one 'which you used to button up for me at Southport'.[57] Like the distressed infant who seeks to disturb its mother's state of mind, Owen's mention of his overcoat, previously a source of comfort and warmth, serves to impress upon her just how narrow his escape from death has been.

The significance that a damaged coat might have for a mother is shown in Louisa Hooper's reaction to her son Kenneth. He had sent his overcoat back home after being wounded and becoming a POW. On receiving the coat, Louisa described it as 'the dear Coat, which you were evidently wearing when wounded. We were all deeply moved, you may be quite sure, at the sight of that dear precious Coat. Mary and I hugged it at once, I felt as if I must fondle it the whole day.' She told him she would send him out a new coat if necessary, as she 'cannot part' from this one.[58] Edward Chapman wrote to his twelve-year-old sister Hilda about the officer beside him who had been killed, and how soon afterwards he had discovered that his own tunic had 'two holes in it, where two pieces of shell went through. One is in the right arm, the other up by the collar'.[59] Chapman's letters home were – as he knew full well – usually read aloud, so it was highly unlikely that in writing to his sister, his mother would actually be spared the news of his narrow escape. The holes in clothing, imagined or actual, made those at home appreciate the damage that could be done to a son's body.

Esther Bick, who played a pioneering role in the development of infant observation in Britain, took Bion's concept of maternal containing back to an even more primitive stage of development, when the baby does not yet have a sense of its physical boundaries. At birth, she proposed, he feels that he is in danger 'of falling to pieces or liquefying. One can see this in the new-born baby trembling and quivering when the nipple is taken out of his mouth, but also when his clothes are taken off'.[60] Physical and psychic integration, Bick argued, go hand in hand. Skin is the primary way in which the baby recognises the boundary between itself and others. Holding by the mother reinforces its sense of physical boundaries, a process that, in turn, allows it to recognise that it has an internal psychic space.

## The containing objects of trench warfare

Something like the sensation of falling apart that Bick detects in the new-born baby is apparent in the descriptions men gave of the damage done by trench warfare. Memoirs tend to contain more graphic accounts of such sights than letters do, partly because the veteran was able to write without the constraints of military censorship, but also because many had simply been unable to take in these events at the time, and so they stuck in the mind, animating later recollections. One of the most fearful sights was a direct hit on a dug-out. Dug-outs were greatly valued in the line as they afforded some protection from shelling and rifle fire, and were relatively dry and warm. As Ilana Bet-El observes in her book

*Conscripts*, quoting from a ranker's letter, '"there was always something warm and welcoming about a dug-out"'.[61] Their significance as a haven is indicated by the frequent resentment that rankers felt because their officers had first right to dug-outs.

The domestic refuge, however, could easily become a tomb. After a direct hit men might be trapped inside, and the effect of an explosion in such a confined space would likely be catastrophic. After describing one such scene in which a dozen or so men had died, Guy Chapman wrote 'The day passed, leaving scarcely a trace in our memories.'[62] These events were too horrific to process at the time, though they remained within Chapman's mind, being, in W. H. R. Rivers' apt phrase, 'forgotten yet active'.[63] It was only in the early 1930s, when Chapman wrote his memoirs, that their 'trace' finally furnished a full description. Although they thanked God for their dug-outs, commented Graham Greenwell to his mother, it was always with an 'undercurrent of anxiety as to the strength of the lusty beams and boards above us.'[64] Eric Marchant gave the merest hints of his battle experience in May 1915, but the events he chose to narrate signalled his feelings well enough. Describing the aftermath of a direct hit on a dug-out, he focused not on the dead but on domestic upheaval. The shell 'fell on a dug-out near us, killing one or two men, and completely burying all the officers knives, spoons, forks, plates, dishes, utensils, some food, and also the equipment and rifle of one of the cooks.'[65] Edwin Campion Vaughan recalls the horrified fascination felt by him and his fellow officers when a shell burst next to their dug-out, peppering all the walls with shrapnel: 'Three separate chunks must have missed my head by inches, for the biscuit tin, tobacco tin, whisky bottles and a Tommy's cooker on the table were all smashed to bits . . .'[66] It was not only Vaughan's own miraculous survival that stuck in memory, but the smashing of so many carapaces, including the dug-out itself and the household items within.

The thought of a blown-up dug-out could produce extreme fear. Being buried in a bunker by shelling was the 'most common' theme in the dreams of soldiers, according to one account, and was frequently a cause of breakdown.[67] Captain J. C. Dunn, the medical officer of the 2nd Royal Welch Fusiliers, was one who had a phobia about being under fire in a dug-out.[68] Likewise, the terror felt by Wilfred Owen in his first experience of battle – holding a flooded German dug-out forward of the line for five days and being subjected to constant bombardment – stemmed partly from his and his men's conviction that it would be blown in.[69] Charles Myers noted an incident in which a dug-out was hit by a shell.

Two of the occupants were killed and the other two were blown against the far wall. One of the survivors, after being taken to the Aid Post, was found 'a little later wandering into the open, taking off his clothes, and explaining that he was going to bed.'[70] His reaction to the obliteration of his shelter had been to remove all bodily protection, and to seek out comfort in sleep. The mental capacity for containing his anxiety, we might conclude, had been destroyed along with the dug-out.[71] At one stage in the war, breakdowns caused by burial from shells were even given a distinctive pathological label: 'burial alive neuroses'. The rescued victims were initially 'unable to either convey or receive impressions.'[72] Their minds had become sealed off from the external world which had intruded so violently upon them.[73]

A tank penetrated by a 'direct hit' was another sight that could threaten psychic integration.[74] The shell would often ignite the tank's ammunition and fuel on impact, resulting in intense fires that could burn alive the crew within. As Bion's tank company passed by the Steenbeck on their way to the Third Battle of Ypres, they saw a 'terrible sight. There would be one or more holes where shells had entered and the blackened ruin of the tanks itself.'[75] Beneath a photo of one such tank, sunk into the mud with one track 'torn off' and looping wildly in the air, Bion's caption ensured that his parents would realise the full horror of what had occurred: '. . . The holes are very small as the shell has gone in and burst inside.'[76] Whilst reconnoitring after action near Amiens, Bion came upon five tanks, some from his own section, burnt out and 'left there looking like burst toads – the roofs lifted off, the sides bulging out.'[77] Death was 'brought home to me' during the Third Battle of Ypres, remarked the infantry subaltern Edwin Vaughan, 'not so much by the numerous corpses, as by the stranded and battered tanks'. The protective carapace had been obliterated: 'here a caterpillar belt blown away, there a great gaping hole in the side – all with the appearance of dead, abandoned giants'.[78]

There is an affinity between Bion's description of the mental state of the schizophrenic, and his 1919 memoirs of action at Cambrai, when his tank came under heavy machine-gun fire and shards of armour plating were flung around the cabin, peppering the crew. The schizophrenic, Bion later wrote, splits off his perceptual apparatus, which might allow him to distinguish between the internal and external reality, and expels it. These fragments of the ego are then felt as external, but they possess a persecutory quality. They are 'bizarre objects'.[79] Terms such as 'cut up' or 'split into minute fragments' to describe the ego of the schizophrenic, and of words such as 'violent intrusion', and 'assault' to describe the schizophrenic's perception of his fragmented ego, are unmistakably linked to Bion's war experience. At the conclusion of battle at Cambrai, Bion found his face was covered in blood, a result of the 'small pieces of tank that had stuck in my face'.[80] Others have speculated about what the violent language of Kleinian thought owed to the First World War, but in Bion the relation was more than a matter of cultural *Zeitgeist*; it was one of direct personal experience.[81]

## The terror of shell wounds

Not all wounds and not all deaths were equally distressing to the onlooker. Those most likely to be recounted in the memoirs and novels of veterans were the result of shelling.[82] In part, the prominence of shell-wounds in memory was a reflection of the statistical odds, since the majority (around 70 per cent) of casualties were due to shelling. Shelling, however, disturbed the soldier not just because of the scale of destruction it wrought, but because of the *kinds* of wounds it inflicted.[83] A shell wound could not count as a 'Blighty', commented the machine gunner George Coppard, since it usually involved extensive surface damage to the body.[84]

Two kinds of shell injury were regarded with particular horror. Men remembered cases where the boundary of the skin or skull was ruptured, exposing bodily matter. Thomas Hope saw a bloated corpse whose poisonous contents were held together only by the uniform: 'A limbless body here, the tunic fitting the swollen body like a glove'.[85] Edwin Vaughan wrote of similar deaths at Ypres in 1917. Whilst he was out walking at camp, prior to moving up to the frontline, there had been a sudden outbreak of shelling. Hearing screams he had rushed to help his men, but stumbled over a body. He 'stopped to raise the head, but my hand sank into the open skull and I recoiled in horror'.[86] During battle he had lain for some hours in a crater hole with numerous bodies, but one stood out. It was a corpse with 'a diamond-shaped hole in his forehead through which a little pouch of brains was hanging, and his eyes were hanging down; he was very horrible but I soon got used to him'.[87] From the mass of deaths, memory selected those where a man's insides were no longer enclosed and protected within the carapace.

Evisceration was among the most feared of all wounds. Anthony Eden recalls a conversation among his fellow officers about the ways they would prefer to be hit. Although each man had different preferences, 'we all agreed that the stomach was the one to be feared'.[88] Writing to his parents of intense shelling the previous day, Burgon Bickersteth conveyed his dread of a stomach wound. 'I always want some of the never-sheathe the sword type out here', he wrote, so that he might 'hear the crump coming and lie flat on the ground wondering whether a great jagged bit will tear your stomach out.'[89] Men before battle, noted Major-General J. F. C. Fuller, were known to deliberately avoid eating 'for fear of being shot through a full stomach'; they probably worried too that they might soil themselves.[90] Frederic Manning, early in *Her Privates We*, states that 'it is infinitely more horrible and revolting to see a man shattered and eviscerated, than to see him shot. And one sees such things; and one suffers vicariously, with the inalienable sympathy of man for man. One forgets quickly . . . One forgets, but he will remember again later, if only in his sleep.'[91] The experience is too painful to take in, so quickly slips from consciousness. Inaccessible to the conscious mind, it shows itself in troubling dreams.

Such fears had a rational basis. John Keegan estimates that, during the Somme, around a quarter of all 'intermediate' injuries – that is, wounds which did not kill a man immediately – would have been to the lungs or stomach.[92] And as Mountfort's account of the Somme indicates, soldiers were often in close proximity to the victims. Stomach wounds, if not treated quickly, were likely to be fatal: in a sample of 1,000 English cases of wounds to the abdomen, only eight survived.[93] Men suffering from stomach wounds were sometimes reported to have walked back to the aid post before dying. They suffered from intense pain and could actually see themselves dying.[94] At the same time, evisceration, whilst especially distressing to the bystander, was not the most common form of mortal wound. Men were more likely to die of head wounds, not all of which occasioned quite this degree of distress.[95]

Evisceration was not only feared because it might bring a lingering death, but because of the unconscious reaction it provoked. It was the presence of a man's insides on the outside that made it horrific. One occasion when W. H. R. Rivers was forced to pause and consider at more length the originating events of war neurosis, rather than the secondary effect of repression, concerned a case of evisceration. The victim had been flung by the force of a shell-blast into the distended stomach of a dead German, and his mouth was filled with the entrails. Rivers felt that for this man, the trauma was of such a magnitude that he should not be encouraged to recollect it; walks in the countryside were as much as could be done for him.[96]

The bayonet was an object of fascinated horror among soldiers in the First World War, although most never had to use it, and on one reckoning it accounted for less than 0.5 per cent of wounds.[97] Much of the fascination lay in its intended use, for the bayonet was meant to be aimed at the abdomen. The 'best place' to get a German in retreat, wrote Greenwell after attending a lecture on bayonet fighting, was in the kidneys.[98] A man might feel it in his own guts after bayoneting an enemy: the psychoanalyst Sándor Ferenczi reported violent abdominal contractions among soldiers who had taken part in such attacks.[99] Bayonet drill was used to 'awaken savage instincts' of hatred in the soldier, but it aroused equally primitive fears too.[100]

Melanie Klein's ideas about internal objects, the experience of which constitutes the very basis of emotional life, resonate with fears like these. The psychoanalyst Bob Hinshelwood has shown how, for Klein, internal objects were experienced within the deepest layers of the unconscious as physical entities. They were felt to be located, not within the mind, like Freud's super-ego, but in Klein's words, 'inside one's body, particularly inside the abdomen.'[101] Damage to the stomach, we might surmise, had the capacity to strike terror because this was the most primitive site of internal objects, and the boundary between these most inside parts, and the outside, had been obliterated.

Dismemberment was another form of death or wounding that men found especially disturbing. The most violent shell impacts could virtually obliterate the body, leaving little recognisable trace. Captain J. C. Dunn recalled how a signaller had just emerged from his dug-out on the Somme 'when a shell burst on him, leaving not a vestige that could be seen anywhere near.'[102] Men recalled body parts that were exposed when trenches were being deepened or re-built, such as the German trouser and boot which put Mountfort off from deepening his trench.[103] Horror lay in body parts grossly out of place, with only the man-made shell intact, striking poses that a living being never could. When Guy Chapman's shelter suffered from a direct hit, two stood out among the dozen or so dead. One was an orderly who had been 'half scythed in two by a piece of shell which had cleft him through the buttocks.' The 'most conspicuous body' was the one 'mixed up with the crushed wireless set; the head, one shoulder and an arm had been sliced clean away, leaving a raw trunk.'[104]

Shelling created terror because of the way it ripped bodies apart. George Coppard particularly disliked 'Minnies', mortar shells filled with scrap iron, whose concussion, he remarked, 'threatened to tear one apart.' In some cases, 'Men just disappeared and no one saw them go. His own personal fear was of 'flying shell fragments rending me apart.'[105] When Wilfred Owen succumbed to shell-shock in late April 1917, it was after having spent four days sheltering in a hole opposite a dismembered fellow officer from the Manchesters. The smell and sight of a body which was (as Owen put it) 'in various places around and about', could destroy psychic organisation, dependent as it was upon the experience of an integral body.[106] One of W. H. R. Rivers' cases concerned an officer who had found his friend's body blown to pieces, the head and limbs detached from the torso. The officer suffered afterwards from terrifying nightmares in which he would picture his dead friend as he had found him, or with his features and limbs eaten away by leprosy.[107]

The observations of Klein and Bick point towards the psychic roots of the terror surrounding wounds such as dismemberment. Klein comments that the ego of the very young infant is constantly moving between states of integration and disintegration. When anxious, the ego tends towards disintegration, and in this state (which Klein termed the paranoid–schizoid position) the baby feels that it is 'falling into bits'.[108] In Bick's formulation, nothing is felt to hold together the most primitive internal parts.

Certain kinds of death and mutilation had the capacity to recapitulate the most primitive and profound anxiety of the baby, that it had no secure physical boundary to differentiate its 'inside' from 'outside'. Bick's description of the new-born baby's emotional experience could stand for that of the soldier in the line. Looking onto a body that was in bits, he might be confronted with 'catastrophic anxieties of the dead-end, falling through space, liquefying, life spilling-out variety'.[109] Feelings of psychic disintegration found plentiful representation in the trenches, in the form of mutilated bodies. Gladden's memory of what it felt like to lose one's nerve under bombardment reveals the difficulty of insulating the mind from external assault: 'With every approaching scream, every cry for stretcher-bearers, I seemed to be torn apart.'[110] Reactions like this did not hark entirely from rational calculation about the end that might await the onlooker. Dismemberment and evisceration were external manifestations of what the frontline soldier *felt* emotionally, that his personality was leaking away or disintegrating.

## The psychic geography of trench warfare

The environment and routines of the trenches contributed to deep anxieties of this kind. Trench warfare distorted perception.[111] Sight, which was usually curtailed when men were in trenches, became over-loaded when they were out on top. During a bombardment at Ypres, Gladden was transfixed by a wave of fire that seemed to be 'pouring over the edge of the world towards us'. It was a liquid fire attack but 'I could no longer believe the evidence of my eyes, or my senses. It was all too incredible.'[112] Smell and hearing were distorted by over-stimulation. 'I have to not seen any dead', wrote Owen after his first experience of the trenches, 'I have done worse. In the dank air I have perceived it.'[113] Captain Leland wrote to his wife of smells so bad that 'I am inclined to be sick.'[114] The constant sound of shelling threatened to drive men mad; they could not get it out of their heads.[115] They were often reduced to crawling so as to minimise exposure to fire, their faces pressed to the primordial earth.[116] Their circadian rhythms were reversed and as a result they were not only tired but frequently became disoriented, as their tendency to mis-date letters attests. Will Hate's first diary entry after action in France reads 'Lose count of days + dates.'[117] At Wytschaete, Bion explains, 'I had lost all sense of time.'[118]

At zero hour, John Keegan comments, a 'cloud of unknowing' would descend on the First World War battlefield, the effect of the haze sent up by the barrage, the violence of high explosives and severed communications.[119] For the ordinary soldier, for whom the larger geography of No Man's Land was largely unknown apart from what he could spy through a periscope, it was not possible to piece together the wider situation. He could not survey the battlefield before going over the top. Huddled in trenches amid shelling, unable to see much or to move, men might become fixated on particular objects. Caught up in violent shelling, Private Bourne's 'vision seemed narrowed to a point immediately in front of him', writes Frederic Manning in *Her Privates We.*[120] In trenches at Wytschaete, Bion found himself staring for hours on end at a small piece of mud that hung from the low roof of his dug-out by a blade of grass.[121] As Esther Bick has noted of distressed infants, the intense focus on a nearby object helped, by 'momentarily at least . . . holding the parts of the personality together.'[122]

The soldier's inability to rely much on his senses contributed to regression, for it is through the senses, Bion and Bick argue, that the infant develops an ability to gauge reality and lessen anxiety. When hearing, vision, touch and smell are overwhelmed, the capacity to distinguish between the internal and external reality can be eroded, so that the external environment is felt to possess the qualities of damaging internal objects. When perception had failed and the risk of death was not a fantasy but a reality, the war-torn scene might become, not a representation of failed containing, but actually felt as a part of the mind. The disembodied and fragmented objects of the mind, now felt as real and external, would attack it, as Bion conveys in both his descriptions of tank warfare, and his psychoanalytic concept of bizarre objects.

Exhaustion and sensory disorientation struck at the capacity to distinguish between fantasy and reality. During Bion's stint in the trenches at Wytschaete when he would perform his duties at night and sleep in the day, he began to feel 'intolerably persecuted by unknown powers'. His dreams affirmed the reality of horror:

> I used to lie, tired out after the night, in a kind of stupor, which served instead of sleep. It was a weird business – the heat, and the nightmares out of which one started up suddenly in a kind of horror to find the sweat pouring down one's face. It was almost impossible to distinguish dream from reality. The tat-tat-tat of the German machine guns would chime in with your dream with uncanny effect, so that when you awoke you wondered whether you were dreaming. The machine-gun made you think everything was genuine, and only by degrees you recovered yourself to fall into uneasy sleep again.[123]

Nearly a decade after the war, when Bion was undergoing his medical training, he used to dream of clinging to the slimy bank of the Steenbeck: he would dig his fingernails in to stop himself slipping but with each movement would slither further towards the 'raging torrent'. He would wake up not knowing what was real and what he had imagined, and the prospect of these nightmares made him anxious about going to sleep.[124] Donald Hankey had experienced the same kind of confusion in 1916 while recovering from a wound:

> The absurd thing was that I couldn't wake up properly. I came on duty at midnight, was roused, got to my feet, and started to walk along the trench. And then the Nameless Terror, that lurks in dark corners when one is a small boy, gripped me . . . I must try to get more sleep somehow; but it is jolly difficult.[125]

The words that W. H. R. Rivers used to describe the war dreams of soldiers were like those used by Bion and Hankey, and he understood their origins in a similar way. The element of profound terror, Rivers argued, made these dreams comparable with the nightmares of children. Addressing the Royal Society of Medicine in December 1917, he called the sufferer's state one of 'reasonless dread.'[126] Later, in *Conflict and Dream*, he described it as 'unreasoning terror'.[127] In these dreams the sufferer *felt* as if he had actually re-experienced a distressing event, and he was put off from further sleep lest 'reasonless dread' returned. In his psychoanalytic writings of the 1950s and 1960s Bion would give a powerful explanation of such dreams, based on the idea that some emotional experiences were incapable of digestion. When the mind cannot process sense impressions in a manner that makes them capable of being thought, he states in *Learning From Experience*, then the patient 'cannot go to sleep and he cannot wake up.'[128]

Equally telling are the parallels between Bion's description of failed containing and wartime reports of the mental effects of bombardment. Bion remarks on how, when the mother cannot mediate the infant's terror, it not only feels that its terror is intolerable, but that it cannot be made sense of. As a result the baby comes to feel, Hinshelwood explains, as if it is living in a 'mysterious meaningless world.'[129] 'Nameless dread', the term that Bion used to evoke this state of mind, was not just similar to Rivers' 'reasonless dread' or 'Nameless Terror', it was the *very same* term that Hankey had used in 1916 to describe the irrational fears of men during battle.

What Hankey meant by 'nameless dread' was not unlike what Bion the psychoanalyst, writing in the 1950s, meant. For Hankey it was more than 'the fear of death rationally considered', and more than 'fear of hurt as hurt.' The soldier's situation amidst bombardment was more intense than this, it was 'an infinitely intensified dislike of suspense and uncertainty, sudden noise and shock.' The 'sensation of nameless dread' occurred when a man was cooped up in a trench, in the dark, amidst 'deafening noise and shock', watching high-explosive shells explode about him, in perpetual suspense but able to 'do nothing'. Hankey groped for phrases adequate to describe the mental effects of the violent assault, but he, like Bion, insisted on its *'irrational'* (italics mine) basis.[130]

A further element that contributed to 'nameless dread' was the tension that soldiers in battle experienced between others' distress and their own. When a man nursed a dying comrade, he faced a double trauma. All his senses were assaulted. He was close up to the broken carapace; he could hear and perhaps even smell the dying. He must touch the wound itself if he was to try and stem the blood, and hold the man's hand or cradle his head if he was to comfort him. Experiencing the infant's terror of falling apart himself, he must nurse another; and in a situation where his care, no matter how conscientious or tender, could often do little to ease the victim's pain, let alone save his life. Battle stress could stem from both elements; from, that is, a close-up encounter with an uncontained body, and from the despair of being unable to sustain another's life.[131]

George Coppard discovered his friend Jock Hershell lying in a latrine sap at Arras, badly wounded. He helped carry Hershell into the dug-out:

> At a glance I saw that his broad back had caught a blast of shrapnel. I slit his tunic and underclothes with a jack-knife and separated them. I winced at the sight. Jock's back was full of punctures, and blood bubbles were wheezing out of the holes as he breathed . . . The backs of his powerful upper arms hung in shreds. He appeared to be in no pain, though he was anxious and kept asking the extent of the injuries he could not see. We lied like hell and gave him first-aid, using nearly all our bandages, and iodine in the process. "You've got a Blighty one for sure," I cried.[132]

Bion gives a very similar description in his 1919 account of the Battle of Amiens. As he and his runner Sweeting (the runner was a messenger, usually a young man) crouched side-by-side in a ditch amid a fierce bombardment, a shell burst above them and severely wounded the 'young boy', whose 'left side had been torn away so that the inside of the trunk lay exposed.' Bion tried to bind Sweeting's wounds but the bandage 'simply didn't come near to covering the cavity . . . He kept trying to cough, but of course the wind only came out of his side. He kept asking me why he couldn't cough'. He 'kept on saying "I'm done for, sir! I'm done for!", hoping against hope I would contradict him.' As Bion tried to comfort the man and assure him that his wounds were 'nothing', the man 'gave me his mother's address, and I promised to write.'[133]

If Bion's experience of awaiting battle at Amiens, when he had sought comfort by nestling in the grass, stands as a prototype of what he would later call containing, this experience, shortly afterwards, stands for its failure. The child-like figure of the runner, his urgent desire to be in touch with his mother and the gaping hole in his side, convey not just the runner's demise, but Bion's own struggle to hold together. We might reflect, too, on the manner in which, during the Summer of 1919 as he waited to commence a History degree at Oxford, Bion sought to make sense of his war. Dedicating his war memoirs to his parents, he included photographs of dismembered bodies, as if his written account of the carnage was not itself sufficiently forceful.[134] When containing does not occur, Bion would explain forty years later, the child reacts by ever greater and more violent projections, in the effort to force its mother to recognise its distress. Wartime failures of containing produced veterans who, as the next chapter shows, felt compelled to impress their pain on loved ones.

* * *

In Paul Fussell's classic account *The Great War and Modern Memory*, he observes how difficult it was for trench soldiers to describe what they had been through. They could not find in the elevated and chivalric vocabulary of Edwardian Britain a means direct enough to convey the horror of the war. The ironic mode of description, Fussell argued, was one of the trench soldier's responses to this difficulty. Death was commonplace and irony served to make it memorable.[135]

Fussell cites Joseph Heller's Second World War novel, *Catch 22*, and its 'primal scene' of a bomber's evisceration, to illustrate the central place of irony in modern memory. The novel, comments Fussell, is notable because of the way it retains all the 'Great War irony' surrounding death. Yossarian works feverishly to dress the wounds of the aircraft gunner Snowden, not realising the full extent of Snowden's injuries. On unfastening his flak jacket, however, Snowden's intestines 'slithered down to the floor in a soggy pile'. Yossarian sees that his mission is hopeless but continues to mumble in a mechanical way, 'There there'. Commenting on this passage, Fussell concludes that irony, the difference between Yossarian's perception of what is happening (the wound is not mortal) and the reality (the man is dying), gives the account its imaginative power. These kinds of images haunt memory, however, not principally because they convey 'hope abridged', but because they bring us up against the primal horror of a body whose contents are spilling out.[136]

The scenes described by Coppard and Bion, where a man suffers from a catastrophic wound and his comrades are left helpless, are identical to Heller's, even down to the hollow reassurance given to the dying man. Yet almost half a century separates these accounts. While Coppard's *With A Machine Gun to Cambrai* was published in 1968, Bion's *War Memoirs* were written in 1919, more than a decade before the boom in war literature, and before (according to Fussell) any kind of collective script emerged among veterans about how to depict the war. The body spilling out its contents was not just a literary trope, and the similarities between veterans who recalled this scene cannot be wholly explained in terms of a new 'modern' language of direct description.

Rather, the similarities between these accounts, like the similarities between Hankey, Bion and Rivers as they seek to define 'nameless dread', tell us about the very deepest relationships between human emotions and words. As the repeated linkage of terms such as 'nameless' or 'reasonless' with 'terror' or 'dread' suggests, these men were struggling to assimilate deeply traumatic emotional sensations. They searched for words to express horror, not because their *language* was inadequate but because the actual emotional experience was not then, and perhaps never would be, capable of being thought.

Historians of the First World War have sometimes preferred to analyse personal accounts of horror as if they were little more than cultural forms, artefacts with a semantic history, rather than emotions carried through words, and thus the emotional experience of trench warfare has tended to be viewed at one remove. Yet the buttoned-up codes of Edwardian society did not stop men from describing the mass horror of trench warfare, any more than the emergence among the literary elite of a 'literature of horror' in the 1920s and 1930s permitted them to do so. Perhaps the reality of 'nameless dread', a mind falling apart under the pressure of trench warfare, remains too uncomfortable even for later generations to contemplate. Faced with scenes of psychic dissolution, it is safer for the historian to stay in the realms of the rational: to study collective memories of the war and their cultural genesis; the contrasts and continuities between 'traditional' and 'modern' ways of representing war; or the social expectations surrounding death and emotions. These are the ways in which we try to make safe the unconscious residues of violence and terror, dispatching them to a kind of cultural strongbox from which they cannot burst out. If the emotional history of the war is to be about more than cultural conventions, historians need – as Bion did in developing his psychoanalytic ideas – to take seriously the sensation of 'nameless dread'; in the process, not locking away the pain of the past, but trying to digest and contain it.

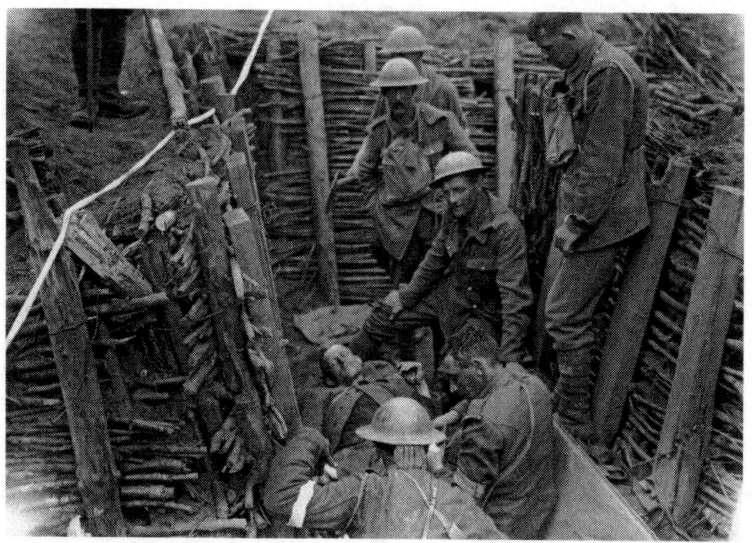

*27* An Irish Guardsman attends to a wounded German soldier, July 1917

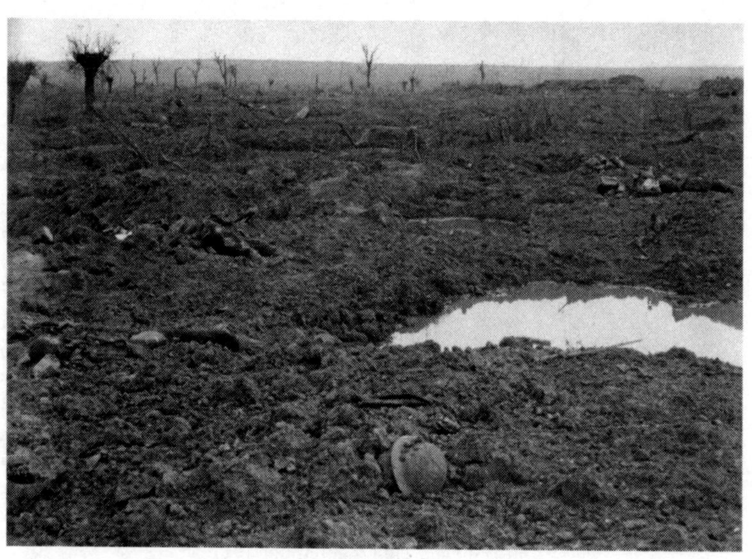

*28* Tin hat and body parts in mud, Third Ypres, September 1917

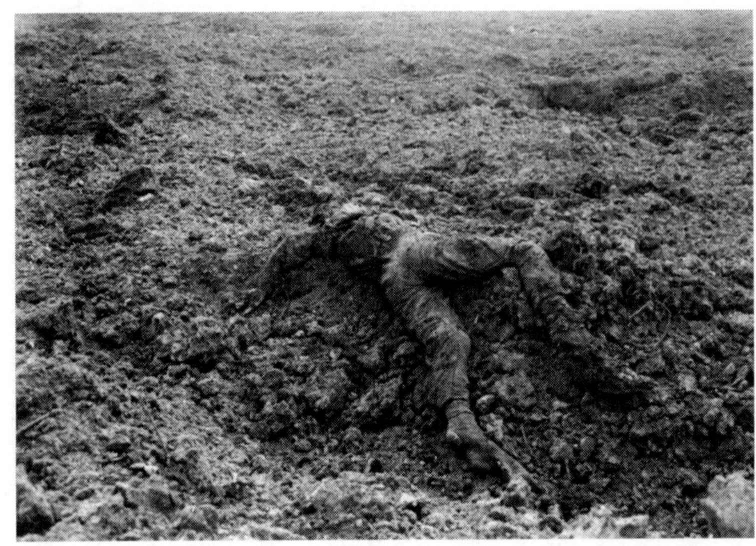

*29* Corpse in mud, Third Ypres, September 1917

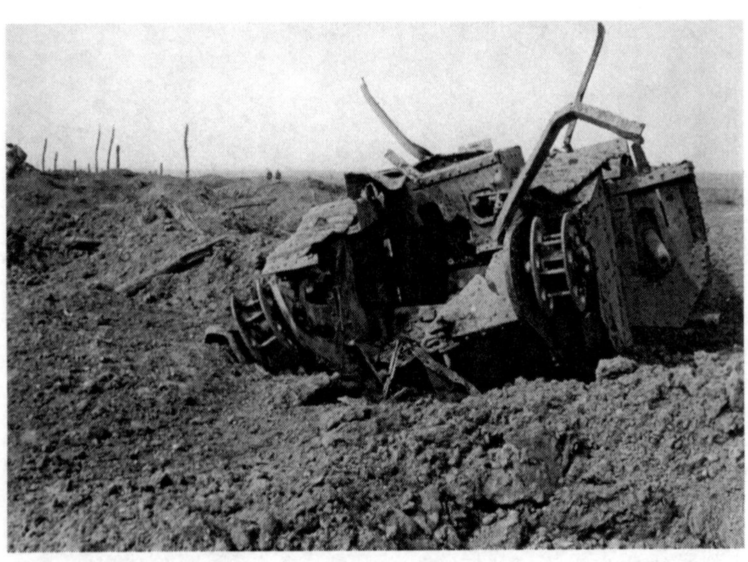

*30* Shelled tank, September 1917

## Notes

1 P. Fussell quoted in S. Audoin-Rouzeau and A. Becker, *1914–1918. Understanding the Great War* (London: Profile Books, 2002), p. 24.
2 R. D. Mountfort to mother 16 July 1916, IWM Con Shelf.
3 Mountfort to mother, 20 July 1916.
4 Mountfort to mother, 23 July 1916. Subsequent details of Mountfort's experience on the Somme are from this letter unless noted otherwise.
5 War Diary of 10th Battalion Royal Fusiliers, 8 July 1916, National Archives WO 95/ 2532.
6 War Diary, 9 July 1916.
7 War Diary, 10 July 1916.
8 War Diary, 10 July 1916.
9 War Diary, 11 July 1916.
10 War Diary, 15 July 1916.
11 War Diary, 15 July 1916.
12 IWM catalogue notes, 'The First World War Letters of R. D. Mountfort', p. 5.
13 Mountfort to mother, 2 August 1916.
14 Mountfort to mother, 22 October 1916.
15 IWM catalogue notes, Mountfort, p. 2.
16 R. Graves, *Goodbye to All That* (Harmondsworth: Penguin, 1960), p. 240, p. 235.
17 On loss of hearing and sight see G.E. Smith and T. H. Pear, *Shell Shock and its Lessons* (Manchester: Manchester University Press, 1917), p. 11. Amnesia, comments William McDougall, was 'very common among soldiers during the war'. 'Four Cases of "Regression" in Soldiers', *Journal of Abnormal Psychology*, Vol. 15 (1920–21), p. 153.
18 McDougall, 'Four Cases', p. 137.
19 G. Greenwell, *An Infant in Arms. War Letters of a Company Commander 1914–1918* (London: Allen Lane, The Penguin Press, 1972), p. 56, p. 63.
20 Greenwell, *An Infant in Arms*, p. 129.
21 Samuel Hynes notes the sympathy of First World War soldiers towards frightened men. *The Soldier's Tale. Bearing Witness to Modern War* (London: Pimlico, 1998), pp. 60–5. This was not always the case. Norman Gladden 'despised rather than pitied the actual victims who gave way to such weakness.' *Ypres 1917* (London: William Kimber, 1967), pp. 167–8. On fear see M. Roper, 'Between Manliness and Masculinity: The "War Generation" and the Psychology of Fear in Britain, 1914–1970', *Journal of British Studies*, Vol. 44, No. 2 (2005), pp. 343–63, and Helen Peters, '"Unmanned Men": In What Ways Did the Experience of Shell Shock Challenge Early Twentieth Century Notions of Masculinity?', unpublished MA Dissertation, Department of History, University of Essex, 2004.
22 Smith and Pear, *Shell Shock and its Lessons*, p. 1.

23 B. Shephard, *A War of Nerves. Soldiers and Psychiatrists 1914–1994* (London: Jonathan Cape, 2000), p. 31.

24 W. H. R. Rivers, *Instinct and the Unconscious. A Contribution to a Biological Theory of the Psycho-Neuroses* (Cambridge: Cambridge University Press, 1920), p. 206.

25 Shephard, discussing Freud, highlights the tensions within military psychiatry between helping the patient and getting him back into war service. *A War of Nerves*, p. 137.

26 D. Winter, *Death's Men. Soldiers of the Great War* (London: Penguin, 1979), p. 132.

27 R. J. Lifton, *The Broken Connection. On Death and the Continuity of Life* (New York: Simon & Schuster, 1979), p. 170.

28 Rivers quoted in E. Leed, *No Man's Land. Combat and Identity in World War I* (Cambridge: Cambridge University Press, 1979), p. 182. E. K. Smith described having to 'just . . . sit tight during the attack', as 'a passive part which was rather trying.' Smith to mother, 13 August 1915, *Letters Sent From France. Service with the Artists' Rifles and the Buffs, December 1914–December 1915* (London: J. Cobb, 1994), p. 79. See also Niall Ferguson, *The Pity of War* (London: Penguin, 1998), p. 341.

29 J. Bourke, *Fear. A Cultural History* (London: Virago, 2005), p. 203.

30 Bourke, *Fear*, p. 216. Bourke describes Scott as suffering from 'psychic numbing', but his mental pain is sharply conveyed in the diary entries quoted.

31 N. Gladden, quoted in Winter, *Death's Men*, p. 133.

32 War Diary of 10th Battalion Royal Fusiliers, 10 July 1916.

33 S. Graham, quoted in Winter, *Death's Men*, p. 207.

34 W. R. Bion, *War Memoirs 1917–19* (London: H. Karnac, 1997), p. 156.

35 P. Bion Talamo, 'Aftermath', in Bion, *War Memoirs*, p. 310. Bion published a paper on civilian morale in 1940 with the arresting title 'The War of Nerves'. In it, he argued that the worker on the home front needed to 'feel the care of a good parental image that feeds and clothes.' In a sense, his 1919 memoir could be said to enact the breakdown of a mental image of care such as this. '"The War of Nerves": Civilian Reaction, Morale and Prophylaxis', in E. Miller (ed.), *The Neuroses in War* (London: Macmillan, 1940), p. 190.

36 For brief details on Bion's experience at Northfield hospital see R. E. López-Corvo, *The Dictionary of the Work of W. R. Bion* (London, H. Karnac, 2003), p. 10; R. M. Young, 'Bion and Experiences in Groups', http://human-nature.com/rmyoung/papers/pap148h.html. Accessed 7 May 2007; and T. Harrison, *Bion, Rickman, Foulkes and the Northfield Experiments* (London: Jessica Kingsley, 2000).

37 Bion Talamo, 'Aftermath', in Bion, *War Memoirs*, p. 311. James Grotstein remarks in passing that Bion's war experiences 'must certainly have

contributed to the concepts of "nameless dread", "catastrophic change", and "mental turbulence"'. J. Grotstein, 'Towards the Concept of the Transcendent Position: Reflections on some of "The Unborns" in Bion's "Cogitations'", *The Journal of Melanie Klein and Object Relations*, Vol. 11, No. 2, 1993, p. 58. Other events in Bion's life apart from the war and his group work with veterans should be considered as well, not least the loss of his first wife Betty in childbirth during the Second World War, when Bion was serving in Brussels; and then the experience of bringing up his daughter Parthenope on his own. During this time – 1945 to 1953 – he also underwent an analysis with Melanie Klein. See W. R. Bion, *All My Sins Remembered. Another Part of a Life and the Other Side of Genius. Family Letters* (London: H. Karnac, 1991), pp. 1–70.

38 W. R. Bion, 'A Theory of Thinking', in W. R. Bion, *Second Thoughts. Selected Papers on Psychoanalysis* (London: H. Karnac, 1987), p. 116.
39 C. Edmonds, *A Subaltern's War* (London: Anthony Mott, 1984), pp. 86–7.
40 The term 'infantry', notes Shephard, originally denoted 'a collection of youths.' *A War of Nerves*, p. 118.
41 C. E. W. Bean, quoted in Winter, *Death's Men*, p. 187.
42 F. Manning, *Her Privates We* (London: Serpent's Tail, 1999), p. 11.
43 C. Carrington, *Soldier From the Wars Returning* (London: Arrow Books, 1965), p. 280.
44 McDougall, 'Four Cases', p. 138.
45 Smith and Pear, *Shell Shock and its Lessons*, pp. 71–2.
46 E. M. Remarque, *All Quiet on the Western Front* (London: Vintage, 1996), p. 42.
47 E. F. Chapman to mother, 27 August 1916, IWM Con Shelf.
48 M. Webb to mother and father, 1 September 1915, IWM 90/28/1.
49 See M. Roper, 'Re-remembering the Soldier Hero: The Composure and Re-Composure of Masculinity in Memories of the Great War', *History Workshop Journal*, Vol. 50 (Spring 2000), pp. 181–205.
50 E. Marchant to father, 14 June 1915, IWM DS/MISC/26.
51 L. Urwick to mother, 25 September 1914, private collection.
52 P. Wyndham-Lewis, quoted in S. Das, *Touch and Intimacy in First World War Literature* (Cambridge: Cambridge University Press, 2005), p. 83.
53 E. F. Chapman to mother, 5 February 1917.
54 'Letters From France', catalogue notes by Richard Chapman, p. iii, papers of E. F. Chapman, IWM Con Shelf.
55 W. Owen to mother, 23 November 1916, in J. Bell (ed.), *Wilfred Owen. Selected Letters* (Oxford: Oxford University Press, 1985), p. 202.
56 Owen to mother, 4 February 1917, in Bell (ed.), *Wilfred Owen. Selected Letters*, p. 216.
57 Owen to mother, 6 April 1917, in Bell (ed.), *Wilfred Owen. Selected Letters*, p. 236.

58 L. Hooper to K. Hooper, 4 September 1916, LC DF066.
59 E. F. Chapman to Hilda, 28 October 1916.
60 E. Bick, 'Further Considerations on the Function of the Skin in Early Object Relations', in A. Briggs (ed.), *Surviving Space. Papers on Infant Observation* (London: H. Karnac, 2002), p. 66.
61 I. Bet-El, *Conscripts. Forgotten Men of the Great War* (Stroud: Sutton Publishing, 2003), p. 102.
62 G. Chapman, *A Passionate Prodigality. Fragments of Autobiography* (New York: Holt, Rinehart & Winston, 1966), p. 202.
63 Rivers, *Instinct and the Unconscious*, p. 196.
64 Greenwell, *An Infant in Arms*, p. 53.
65 Marchant to 'Everybody', 21 May 1915.
66 E. C. Vaughan, *Some Desperate Glory. The Diary of a Young Officer 1917* (London: Leo Cooper, 1987), p. 192.
67 Leed, *No Man's Land*, p. 22; Smith and Pear, *Shell Shock and its Lessons*, p. 2.
68 K. Simpson, 'Dr James Dunn and Shell-Shock', in H. Cecil and P. Liddle, *Facing Armageddon. The First World War Experienced* (London: Pen & Sword, 1996), pp. 506–10.
69 Owen to mother, 16 January 1917, in Bell (ed.), *Wilfred Owen. Selected Letters*, pp. 213–14.
70 C. E. Myers, *Shell Shock in France 1914–18* (Cambridge: Cambridge University Press, 1940), p. 42.
71 The fragile protection afforded by the dug-out is captured by R. C. Sherriff in his play *Journey's End.* It is set within a dug-out and centres on domestic routines of eating, resting and the comings and goings of the officers. At the end of the play the dug-out entrance is blown in, sealing the young and mortally wounded volunteer Raleigh within. The space of survival has become a tomb.
72 Leed, *No Man's Land*, pp. 22–3.
73 This was helpfully pointed out to me by Andrew Briggs.
74 In her work on the psychic resonance of the tank, Trudi Tate notes the terror men experienced when the carapace failed. *Modernism, History and the First World War* (Manchester: Manchester University Press, 1998), esp. p. 139.
75 Bion, *War Memoirs*, p. 25.
76 Bion, *War Memoirs*, opp. p. 35.
77 Bion, *War Memoirs*, p. 133.
78 Vaughan, *Some Desperate Glory*, pp. 207–8.
79 W. R. Bion, 'Development of Schizophrenic Thought', in W. R. Bion, *Second Thoughts. Selected Papers on Psychoanalysis* (London: H. Karnac, 1987), p. 38.
80 Bion, *War Memoirs*, p. 52.
81 Tate, *Modernism, History*, pp. 90–4. Patrick Wright observes in his study of the tank, that 'Bion did go on to elaborate a theory of the self in which the

idea of "the container" featured prominently'. P. Wright, *Tank. The Progress of a Monstrous War Machine* (London: Faber & Faber, 2000), p. 118.

82 The descriptions of shelling in memoirs and novels often serve, in Robert J. Lifton's words, as images of 'ultimate horror'. They condense the experience of death and destruction, forcing the reader to take it in. Lifton, *The Broken Connection*, p. 172.

83 J. Keegan, *The Face of Battle* (London: Jonathan Cape, 1976), p. 264. For an account of the effects of shrapnel and high explosives see R. Holmes, *Tommy. The British Soldier on the Western Front 1914–1918* (London: Harper Perennial, 2005), pp. 399–404.

84 G. Coppard, *With A Machine Gun to Cambrai. A Story of the First World War* (London: Cassell, 1980, first published in 1968), p. 54.

85 T. Hope quoted in Winter, *Death's Men*, p. 132.

86 Vaughan, *Some Desperate Glory*, p. 191.

87 Vaughan, *Some Desperate Glory*, p. 201.

88 A. Eden, *Another World 1897–1917* (London: Allen Lane, 1976), p. 111.

89 J. Bickersteth (ed.), *The Bickersteth Diaries 1914–1918* (London: Leo Cooper, 1995), p. 266.

90 J. F. C. Fuller, quoted in Keegan, *The Face of Battle*, p. 241. Warwick Deeping, in his fictional memoir of 1936, *No Hero – This* (London: Cassell. 1936), has the new Medical Officer Stephen Brent confess his worst fears to a battle-hardened comrade: 'I suppose one's interior can be a bit of a surprise packet. I don't want to dirty my breeches.' Deeping, p. 205.

91 Manning, *Her Privates We*, p. 11.

92 Keegan, *The Face of Battle*, p. 268.

93 Winter, *Death's Men*, p. 193.

94 Remarque depicts a man arriving at the dressing-station holding his guts in his hands, while Fussell, writing about his support for the dropping of the Atomic bomb, invokes the horror of dying this way: 'Why delay and allow one more American high school kid to see his own intestines blown out of his body and spread before him in the dirt while he screams and screams when with the new bomb we can end the whole thing just like that?' *All Quiet*, p. 97; 'Thank God for the Atomic Bomb', *The New Republic*, 26 August 1981, quoted in L. Smith, 'Paul Fussell's *The Great War and Modern Memory*: Twenty-Five Years Later', *History and Theory*, Vol. 40, No. 2 (May 2001), p. 251.

95 Winter, *Death's Men*, p. 193.

96 Rivers, *Instinct and the Unconscious*, p. 192. Pat Barker draws on this case in her novel *Regeneration* (Harmondsworth: Penguin, 1992), p. 173.

97 J. Bourke, 'In the Presence of Mine Enemies: Face-to-Face Killing in Twentieth Century Warfare', www.history.ac.uk/eseminars/sem21.html. Accessed 2 October 2006, p. 2.

98 Greenwell, *An Infant in Arms*, p. 142.

99 S. Ferenczi, cited in Leed, *No Man's Land*, p. 179.

100 Captain H. Meredith Logan, quoted in J. Bourke, *An Intimate History of Killing. Face-To-Face Killing in Twentieth-Century Warfare* (London: Granta Books, 1999), p. 153.

101 R. W. Hinshelwood, 'The Elusive Concept of "Internal Objects" (1934–1943). Its Role in the Formation of the Klein Group', *International Journal of Psychoanalysis*, Vol. 78 (1997), p. 884.

102 J. C. Dunn quoted in Keegan, *The Face of Battle*, p. 264.

103 Mountfort to mother, 23 July 1916. Remarque described a near identical sight, a 'leg that has been torn off, with the boot on it still completely undamaged'. Remarque, *All Quiet*, pp. 49–50.

104 G. Chapman, *A Passionate Prodigality*, pp. 201-2.

105 Coppard, *With A Machine Gun*, p. 39.

106 W. Owen to M. Owen, 8 May 1917, in Bell (ed.), *Wilfred Owen. Selected Letters*, p. 242.

107 Rivers, *Instinct and the Unconscious*, pp. 190–1.

108 M. Klein, 'Notes on Some Schizoid Mechanisms', in M. Klein, *Envy and Gratitude and Other Works 1946–1963* (London: Vintage 1997), pp. 4–5.

109 Bick, 'Further Considerations', p. 70.

110 Gladden, *Ypres*, p. 65.

111 On distortion of perception see Leed, *No Man's Land*, pp. 124–31.

112 Gladden, *Ypres*, p. 143.

113 Owen to mother, 19 January 1917, in Bell (ed.), *Wilfred Owen. Selected Letters*, p. 215.

114 H. J. C. Leland to wife, 13 August 1917, IWM 96/51/1.

115 'I have never been so absolutely cowed before as I was when sitting in my dug-out, which I knew was no good against a direct hit, listening the whole time to the whistle of shells, a noise which I couldn't get out of my ears', wrote Graham Greenwell. *An Infant in Arms*, p. 64.

116 See the discussion of crawling in Das, *Touch and Intimacy*, pp. 43–4.

117 W. T. Hate diary, 23 August 1914, IWM 86/51/1. See also Wilfred Owen to mother, 6 April 1917, in Bell (ed.), *Wilfred Owen. Selected Letters*, p. 235.

118 Bion, *War Memoirs*, p. 95.

119 Keegan, *The Face of Battle*, p. 260.

120 Manning, *Her Privates We*, p. 174.

121 Bion, *War Memoirs*, p. 94. The experience is recalled again, almost word-for-word, in Bion's memoir of the late 1970s: 'I lay beneath a tin roof watching a piece of mud swinging rhythmically at the end of a straw each time a shell burst.' *All My Sins Remembered*, pp. 59–60.

122 E. Bick, 'The Experience of the Skin in Early Object Relations', in Briggs (ed.), *Surviving Space*, p. 56. I am grateful to Bob Hinshelwood for pointing this out.

123 Bion, *War Memoirs*, p. 94. Paulo Sandler sees this passage of the memoirs as an instance of what Bion would later describe as the 'psychotic personality',

where animate and inanimate are confused. P. Sandler, 'Bion's War Memoirs: A Psychoanalytical Commentary.' http://psychematters.com/papers/psandler2.htm, p. 6. Accessed 21 January 2005.

124 Bion, *War Memoirs*, 'Commentary', p. 208; Bion, *All My Sins Remembered*, p. 16, p. 38.

125 D. Hankey, *A Student in Arms* (London: Andrew Melrose, 1917), p. 91.

126 Rivers, *Instinct and the Unconscious*, p. 196.

127 Rivers, *Conflict and Dream* (New York: Harcourt, Brace & Co., 1923), p. 74.

128 W. R. Bion, *Learning From Experience* (London: H. Karnac, 1991), p. 7.

129 R. W. Hinshelwood, *A Dictionary of Kleinian Thought* (London: Free Association, 1991), p. 354.

130 Hankey, *A Student in Arms*, pp. 126–31.

131 On the self-blame of survivors see Robert J. Lifton. 'What is extremely important in addition to the ultimate threat', he argues, 'is the limited capacity to respond to the threat and the self-blame for that inadequate response.' *The Broken Connection*, p. 170.

132 Coppard, *With A Machine Gun*, pp. 119–20.

133 Bion, *War Memoirs*, pp. 124–7.

134 Bion, *War Memoirs*, p. 3. Parthenope Bion Talamo is surely right to describe the 1919 memoirs as 'almost raw material, with hardly any emotional or intellectual elaboration'. The 'unchewed and almost undigested' bloody episodes contained therein were repeated in Bion's later writings such as *All My Sins Remembered*; as if, comments Talamo Bion, 'no further working-through were possible'. 'Aftermath', in Bion, *War Memoirs*, p. 309.

135 P. Fussell, *The Great War and Modern Memory* (Oxford: Oxford University Press, 1975), p. 31.

136 Fussell, *The Great War*, pp. 34–5.

# 7

# The return of the soldier

Around the evening of 16 August 1917, with home leave looking increasingly likely, Captain Herbert Leland had a 'singular dream':

> I dreamt that someone threw a bomb at me and it smashed the glass of my watch. I was furious, as I remember your telling me that the glass was unbreakable. It was a very real dream. When I woke up, I looked at my watch – the glass was all right, but the watch, fully wound up, had stopped, and refused to go, although I tried every shaking and thumping I could give it without actually breaking it, so I gave the matter up as a bad job, and put it away, being very inconvenienced all day without a watch, I borrowed one from one of the men. This morning I happened to look at mine and found the uncanny thing ticking away merrily and nearly run down. I wound it up and it is going as well as ever. How can you account for this?[1]

Leland here asks his wife Lena to ponder his 'uncanny' watch, whose behaviour – stopping in sync with his dream, only to mysteriously right itself afterwards – seemed more fantastical than his 'very real' dream. But Leland is surely also asking himself in the letter, as well we might too, what the experience tells us about his state of mind; appreciating that the confusion between dream and reality was characteristic of battle-stressed soldiers.

Leland was certainly battle-stressed. His position as Divisional Staff Officer for musketry meant that he was often roving around the back areas amid bombardments from the German big guns. Leland's letters to Lena in Edinburgh between late June when he arrived in France, and his dream in mid-August, are dominated by the shelling: 'Two more shells have just burst overhead with a tremendous crash', he writes on

21 June, while in early July 'The air never seems to be free of shells, and the ground fairly shakes'. On 13 July, six pieces of shrapnel fell within 'a yard or two' of his dug-out, any one of which might have given him a '"kingdom Come"'. Three shells fell within a dozen yards in late July, showering him with earth and stones; the closest, which fell 'a yard or two from me', was a dud and failed to explode. 'We are daily bombed and battered', he reported on 30 July.[2]

By early August he was 'just DEAD BEAT'. All he wanted to do was to 'get home . . . and tumble into bed, and sleep for a month, or a year.' Among his own men, camped for much of the time in leaky tents, the constant shelling was taking its toll and some had become '"windy"'.[3] The fetid smells were making him sick, and he was finding it difficult to sleep.

Leland's dream presages his admission in December 1917 to the Special Hospital for Officers in Palace Green London, suffering from a racing heart, inability to sleep, headache and loss of vision. In 'Beyond the Pleasure Principle' Freud argued that the mind was normally protected by a kind of shield which, with the help of the senses, filtered stimuli from the external environment and allowed it to be stored or 'bound'. 'Mechanical violence' however – and though Freud does not actually say so, shelling provides such a case – could break through this shield and overwhelm the mind.[4] Leland's dream seems to picture this very moment, when an explosion smashes the face of his watch. The watch, as Leland discovers on waking, though its face is not cracked, has actually stopped, and this also points to traumatic neurosis, for as Freud notes, at the moment of trauma, the ego, which operates with a linear sense of time, is overwhelmed by the excess of sensation. The intruded-upon unconscious – which knows no sense of time – cannot 'bind' the experience without the ego. The watch, 'wound up' but temporarily frozen, anticipates Leland's own cracking up.

His dream must have been unsettling, for this was not the first time that Leland had suffered from mental problems. A Regular soldier aged forty-four in 1917, he had served in India, the South African war, west Africa and Ireland. In 1913 he returned to Britain on sick leave from Southern Nigeria. According to the medical report compiled in Calabar, Leland had been suffering from prolonged insomnia, which led him to 'throw himself excessively into the duties and physical activities of his profession' so as to exhaust himself. He had 'secretly . . . indulged in alcohol' to help him sleep.[5] While the medical report was not wholly unsympathetic to Leland, the War Office back in London lighted on the phrase 'delerium tremens', an anonymous Army official underlining it in thick pencil. Consequently in August 1914 Leland was told that he would be put on the half-pay list for a year, but deprived of all income as 'your disability was due to circumstances over which you had control.'[6] In response, Leland wrote a letter of protest asking that the decision be re-considered. He would be happy to train junior officers or NCOs, or indeed to 'serve in any capacity' in either the New Army or the Territorial Forces. He genuinely wanted to do his bit, but his letter ended with a pointed remark about his personal circumstances: 'I may add that I am without any private means, that I am married, and have three children.'[7] It is unclear when Leland found his way back into the Army, but in late 1916 a Court Martial acquitted him of the charge of 'conduct to the prejudice of good order and military discipline'.[8] 'Category 'A' he might have been, but Leland was never likely to get through the onslaught he found himself amid in 1917.[9]

Leland was undoubtedly vulnerable because of his history, but at the same time, his situation as he felt himself to be falling apart, was not unusual. Life in the line placed his marriage under stress, as it did many. The longer the war went on, the further apart he and Lena seemed to grow in their attitudes to the war. In late June he had remarked that 'I don't think you quite realise [w]hat this kind of warfare is like', as 'Practically every casualty you see is from shell fire.' 'There is no romance in this war', he wrote on 10 July, 'It is nothing but murder, pure and simple . . .' On 4 August 1917, the third anniversary of the declaration of war, he marvelled at how anxious he had been in 1914 to get to the Front, and how frustrating it had felt to have to 'remain inactive.' He continued: 'Now. Well; I don't know what to think.' His division was about to be moved up North (towards Ypres) and was 'for the line again'. He sharply disputed Lena's view: 'I am glad you think things are going on well up North. There is nothing like being optimistic. I wish you could spend 24 hours in this spot. You would be very optimistic then ! I don't think !!'[10]

Frustrated as Leland was by Lena's enthusiasm for the war, he also worried that her feelings towards him might have changed. After all, she had married a professional soldier and had certain expectations of him. The week before his dream Leland had 'rather damaged my features' when, travelling on horseback through a wood, he struck a tree. A thorn had entered his left eye, completely closing it up: 'I fear that you will be very disappointed in me this time, for I am really worn out and very war worn . . . It is just pouring with rain, and I am soaking . . .'[11] He would not return home on leave looking like the war hero she perhaps wished him to be.

The dream of the watch records these ambivalent feelings. It seems probable that Lena had given him the wristwatch, for in the dream it is she who tells him about its unbreakable glass. Perhaps she had even bought it as a good-bye present before he left for France, as relatives commonly did.[12] On the one hand the dream seems to value the watch as a token of Lena's love, and express sadness that it is now damaged. On the other hand Leland is angry because Lena insists that the watch-face is unbreakable, just as she continues to think that the war is 'romantic' and that he is a hero. Leland, significantly, is not just recording the dream in a private record such as a diary, but telling his wife about it in a letter. Lena must be made to understand how disturbed he felt. The dream seems to say something like: 'you boosted me up so that I seemed invulnerable, but how will you help me now that I am breaking down?'

Leland's behaviour after his dream, his leave now immanent, bears out his ambivalence towards Lena. Having just lunched on Bully beef, he relished the thought of home-cooked food. 'All I want', he said, was fish, fowl and milk, 'No beef.' But he was far from positive about the souvenirs she had asked for. German shells 'are so very bulky, and weigh very heavily'; 'Goodness only knows how I am going to get them home', he grumbled. We do not know how Leland spent the reunion with his wife and children, but he was filled with despair on his return. Home felt more remote than ever; if the dream of his broken watch had been remarkable because so 'very real', leave was 'nothing more than a dream.' 'How I hate leave', he wrote as he made his way through France to his Division, 'The returning is just too damnable. You cannot come down to my present state of misery (no not misery – melancholy)'.[13] Leland was missing her sorely: the pain of his return, as his careful substitution of the word 'melancholy' for 'misery' suggests, felt something like a death.[14] She must never be allowed to suffer like he had and yet perhaps he was also resentful that she, safe at home, would never be brought as low as he.

Leland became more distressed in the months after his leave. Around him men continued to be killed, one of them 'a few minutes ago'. 'I am very muddled' he writes after being under heavy shellfire 'all night'. Leland did not confess to drinking, but his batman Hilton certainly was, and had gone to ground – 'nothing can unearth him' – so Leland was often hungry.[15] He had become convinced that he was going blind, his hands were shaking, he was having 'awful dreams', and taking morphine to help him sleep. Meanwhile Lena continued to find his letters 'thrilling and make your heart stand still!' He simply could not get through to her: 'I have told you nothing, nor can I describe what it is like'.[16]

It was not only Leland's marriage that the war put under pressure, but his batman's as well. Having put his unreliability down to nerves, Leland eventually discovered that Hilton's wife had written saying that she 'wants to have nothing more to do with him.' Hilton had asked Leland to intercede on his behalf, so Leland had written 'telling her that as I had an affectionate interest in Hilton and as we had gone through some very rough times together lately, would she write and relieve his mind.' He thought no good would come of it; Hilton's wife was one of many women who were incapable of realising how they had made their husbands suffer by their conduct.[17] The message about unsympathetic and disloyal wives, couched conspicuously in the plural, would not have escaped Leland's wife.

When Leland was finally withdrawn from the front in late November he worried because 'I don't know how you will take it'. He felt 'disgusted with myself' that he had gone off sick, but he wanted to assure Lena that he was no coward: 'It is not my fault. I have fought against it for a long time.' In fact, he explained, one of the doctors had told him the breakdown was only as severe as it was because he had hung on for so long. [18] Leland's letters reach an abrupt conclusion once he was back in Britain and in the Special Hospital for Officers. Here he was likely – this being the first of Lord Knutsford's small and lavishly provided private hospitals – to have received sympathetic treatment, including a period of convalescence in the countryside.[19]

There is a pointed similarity between the last letter in the collection and Leland's own pleading letter to the wife of his batman just three weeks earlier. The letter is from Major James Woods, RAMC and informs Mrs Leland that her husband has 'slight mental confusion and profound exhaustion.' Woods notes that Leland has suffered similar attacks before. The letter ends with a request: 'I know he will be very glad if you could come to London so as to be able to see him occasionally.'[20] The Medical Officer Woods was now petitioning Leland's wife, just as Leland had petitioned his batman's wife. These soldiers were acting on each others' behalf to try and ensure that women were kept constant in their support; but for Lena, the journey to London might not have been feasible given Leland's periods without income and the three children she was looking after on her own.

We cannot say how Leland's marriage fared after his recuperation, but from the Army Records it is clear that the fervent wish he had expressed as he went sick in October 1917, never to 'stray again' from home, was unfulfilled.[21] In early February 1918 he was admitted again to a convalescent hospital, location unknown, and he drifted in and out of convalescent hospitals until September 1918 when he rejoined a Reserve Battalion.[22] 1920 saw him stationed in Singapore, from where he was sent back to Britain due to 'sickness on military duty', and deemed unfit for general service.[23] He was living in Edinburgh in 1920 and he served during the state of emergency in spring 1921 when the miners went out on strike, no doubt putting him at loggerheads with some of his fellow veterans. In 1923 he is listed as living in Gloucestershire; then in 1924, just outside Colchester, from where he put in a final application for promotion to Major, which he had been trying to do since 1920, presumably in the hope of increasing his pension.[24] That application was refused and between 1924 and his death in 1931, Leland lived on retired pay of around £237 a year. A professional soldier he may have been, but he conformed to the stereotype of the financially straightened ex-officer as the 'damaged man' that would appear widely in post-war literature.[25]

* * *

Leland's yearning to be home, coupled with occasional exasperation and anger towards his wife, was not unusual among battle-stressed veterans. These volatile feelings, though they were expressed in relationships with lovers, wives and families afterwards, originated in the soldier's experience of the war itself. In the initial stages of their service on the Western Front, marching mile after mile in the heat, or suffering from the wet and cold, eating indifferent food and missing their families, the idea of home was an antidote. They not only imagined their loved ones but beds, home-cooked food, toilets and baths. The thought of coming back home helped them endure the privations of Army life. As the men liked to sing as they marched in heavy and ill-fitting boots, three miles in every fifty minutes, with up to 60lb of kit on their backs: 'When this blasted war is over/Oh how happy I shall be!/When I get my civvy clothes on,/No more soldiering for me.'[26]

Yet the longer they served and the longer the war went on, the more far-removed the prospect of return became. We can see this in Leland's pessimism that the developments around Ypres in Autumn 1917 that his wife had such high hopes for, might actually resolve the deadlock. In the event Leland was proved right and it took a further year before the dénouement, by which time the total number of dead from battles on the Western Front stood at around 4 million.[27] The war threatened to become a way of life, and indeed for younger men soldiering was the only adult life they knew. When the men from the Toc H rest-hut voted in January 1918 on the motion 'This House is decidedly convinced that the war will be over this year', the tally was 80 for and 80 against, and the motion was passed only on the Chairman's casting vote. In January 1916 it had been passed by 150 votes to 8.[28] Two of the most famous marching songs of the war convey respectively the soldier's feeling that he had no idea how he had landed up in such a hell-hole ('We're here/ Because/ We're here/Because/We're here,/Because we're here.'); and his longing to get back: 'I want to go home/ I want to go home'.[29]

The soldier's existence was split. The less likely it was that he would make it back, the more precious the refuge of home became. The more he witnessed of war's horror, the less he could tell people back home. Men tried to keep the violence of trench warfare from their mothers, not only to spare them, but because they needed to preserve a part of themselves undamaged by the madness. Parthenope Talamo Bion, herself a psychoanalyst, speculated about why her father Wilfred did not write to his mother during the war. It was, she thinks, 'an unconscious attempt to preserve her in his own mind as a container as undamaged as possible by hideous news.'[30] Try as they might to preserve the good maternal objects within their minds from violent attack, these young men often found it impossible to do so, and their envy of the civilian's safety, and anger at having to do the dirty work of a whole society, muddied the ideal.

At some point in a man's Army service – often precipitated by battle – this fragile psychic structure was pressed to the point of collapse. It happened to Norman Gladden when he lost his helmet during a heavy bombardment at Messines Ridge in 1917. He 'felt like a crab without its shell' and was paralysed by anxiety, unable to think about anything else other than his bare head, although of course a helmet gave no guarantee of safety.[31] With their mental and physical defences broken through, men like Gladden and Leland came to envy women their apparent safety, and to doubt the ability of those at home to bear their distress. The many stories of men calling for their mothers in death are not just sentimental tributes, they also register women's absence at a critical moment of need.

When Wilfred Bion visited Amiens in 1958 with his wife, he recalled the opening of battle there on 8 August 1918, when his runner Sweeting was fatally wounded in the chest and stomach.[32] For Bion, Sweeting's death seemed to have become (to use Robert J. Lifton's apt phrase), an 'image of ultimate horror', a memory that crystallised the human destruction and its emotional impact on the survivor.[33] Bion began to write an account of the battle, but was right in the middle of *Learning From Experience*, which would further develop his ideas about containing, so the memoir lay unfinished.[34] This 1958 account of Amiens, when compared with the memoir of battle he had composed for his parents in 1919, shows how death and destruction had become linked in his mind with the absence of the mother and with the failure of containing maternal objects. In the 1919 account Sweeting passes on his address to Bion, and Bion promises to write to the man's mother, but when he recollected the event forty years later, Sweeting pleads desperately, 'Write to my mother, mother, mother', and Bion tells him 'Oh, for Christ's sake shut up'.[35] Bion's revision of the scene sharpened its point: the dying man could not reach the one who had given him life and Bion was too terrified himself to deal with the man's distress.

The inaccessibility of women to the suffering soldier is captured by Siegfried Sassoon in his poem *The Road*, which describes men trudging up to Mametz village before a night attack in August 1916. The sides of the road are 'thronged with women' but they are consumed by their own worries, 'worn out with waiting, sick with fear.' In any case the men, 'Half dazed for want of sleep', are beyond care; they 'never see them.' 'Jock' slumps on the roadside:

> . . . No dream would mock
> Your reeling brain with comforts lost and gone.
> You did not feel her arms about your knees,
> Her blind caress, her lips upon your head.
> Too tired for thoughts of home and love and ease,
> The road would serve you well enough for bed.[36]

The state of mind that Sassoon evokes is not only one in which men are beyond women's containing, but in which the feminine potentially takes on a more sinister overtone. The 'lips upon your head' might even be the kiss of death.[37] In the early years of the war, amid the patriotic rush to join up, it was hard to voice dark sentiments like this, but by 1917, when men like Sassoon and Leland had begun to feel that the war would never end, anger began to crystallise as a public sentiment among some soldiers.[38] The notion that it was a mother's duty to sacrifice her son to the nation was now up for question; a sentiment that would develop in some quarters into 'mocking disapproval' of mothers.[39]

What also began to emerge, given women's absence from the scene of horror, was a new appreciation of how men had nursed each other. Comrades seemed to have supplanted mothers. When a man is injured, noted Wedgewood, he is 'in one moment a little baby and all the rest become the tenderest of mothers. One holds his hand; another lights his cigarette'.[40] When a severely wounded soldier stumbled against Leland as he slept, Leland wrapped the man in his blanket and the new – now 'very bloody' – overcoat given him by his aunt.[41] Deep feelings of comradeship could arise from this rough care of one man for another. 'It will be very hard to leave the Battalion after so many years', wrote Greenwell in his last letter to his mother in December 1918.[42] Charles Carrington, looking back on his life in the 1920s, concluded that 'I could not escape from the comradeship of the trenches which had become a mental internment camp, or should I say a soldier's home'.[43] Home lives after the war would be conditioned by the fact that women had been off-stage when they were needed most, and men had tried to stand in for them as carers.

## Coming home

In the best-known studies of the cultural impact of war, the story of the soldier's return is largely about the tensions between men, and how these played out in post-war public life and politics. It is a story about the anger of young men towards the old – Sassoon's fat and puffing generals – who had sent them to their deaths. Anthony Wohl, for example, concludes that the war 'taught an unforgettable lesson in generationalism', pitting the young men who had risked their lives against 'those directing the war from the rear and providing reasons for the slaughter'.[44] For Paul Fussell, the 'adversary' mentality of 'them' and 'us' had its roots in the hostility between the front-line soldier and the Staff behind the lines, the latter's mis-conceptions about the war being carried into civilian consciousness through journalists like Hilaire Belloc and the owner of the *Times*, Lord Northcliffe.[45] Samuel Hynes, in *A War Imagined*, also regards the soldier's resentment towards the 'Old Men', the profiteers and politicians, as a central myth of the war, though he extends the veteran's targets to include 'ignorant, patriotic women'.[46]

This literature does not suggest it, but the soldier's return was as much about women as men. Its most immediate emotional impact was felt, not within the sphere of public debate and popular culture, but among families. Men imagined coming back to the arms of a mother or wife. C. W. Taylor, half-starved and suffering from dysentery, lay hidden in a railway carriage after escaping from the POW camp in Langensalza, convinced that he would die, and 'dreaming of Old England and my mother.' Among his papers at the IWM is a cherished letter from the King, trusting that on his return he would be 'able once again to enjoy the happiness of home.'[47]

Amid these heightened expectations, the actual return was often slow and frustrating. Ten months after the Armistice there were still a million men in uniform and many of them complained bitterly in letters home about being unable to get back.[48] Once they had been demobilised, however, the transition to civilian could be abrupt and disorientating. Uniforms could be exchanged for a demob suit. R. W. Brierley thought he had been 'unwise' to opt for the suit while H. Clegg's poorly dyed cast-off was 'several times too small'. Clegg's collar was 'size 14½" to fit a 17" neck', and his multi-coloured necktie 'came adrift while when tying it'.[49] In memoirs the ill-fitting suit serves as a metaphor of the awkward adjustment to the identity of civilian, and of the war hero's shoddy treatment.

Though many had chafed under the arcane structures of Army life, they were at the same time habituated to them. Noakes could not visualise permanent return as the Army had become a way of life; the nearest he could think of was leave. For Noakes, as for Leland, the war was where he belonged and home was nothing more than a dream. Younger men – and half the troops in France in 1918 when the armistice was declared were eighteen – found it all the more disorienting because they had no other adult identity than as a soldier.[50] So used was C. R. Hennessey to being fed and provisioned by the Army, that even after being demobilised, he and his mates hung around the Army canteen in Dover waiting for their pocket ration.[51] He was sad to leave his pal Percy Eels at Victoria Station, having been together since 1916. He boarded a number 16 bus for Kilburn, 'with only a small parcel of personal effects and a tin hat. When I reached the house I found my Mother and Sister there, having no idea that I was about to descend on them at that particular time.' They ran him a bath and prepared a hot meal while he rested up. He completely divested himself of his military identity next day, building a bonfire in the back garden and flinging his louse-ridden uniform, underclothes and socks onto it.[52] What he would do next was not so clear.

Taylor's return lacked the element of surprise, for as he walked down his street he was spotted by the neighbours, who were crowding around by the time he reached his house, so he could not have time alone with his mother. His desire for his mother's undivided attention was perhaps all the greater as he was still visibly under-weight after the POW camp; while she, being illiterate, had been unable to communicate with him for many months. Taylor quickly settled into to his pre-war habits, sleeping on the old sofa in the front room, fourteen people crammed into a six-room house.[53]

Some were unable to return to their families. Brierley's mother and father had died during the war. After demobilising he took the train to Leeds and headed for his uncle's house, but found them away on holidays and was put up by his best mate's mother. He later lodged and had to go on the dole.[54] William Breakspeare's mother also died during the war, due to worry, he believed, about her seven sons in the Army. William returned to find his father dissolute, unemployed and cadging from his sisters. He set up house with his younger brother, their father having pretty much abandoned the family home to the two veterans. William was concerned for his brother, who had lost so much weight in a POW camp that 'I didn't recognise him.' William had his own worries. He had contracted malaria in the war and continued to suffer from bouts of dysentery, eventually having a breakdown which affected his memory. He was unable to work, 'I just – idled around'. The doctor said to him, '"Breakespeare", he says, "you're all to pieces – you're starved." He says, "you'll have to pull yourself together."' The two brothers managed to get by but it was a piteous situation. They just 'existed, I can't say we lived because it was too difficult at that time.'[55]

Many returned soldiers suffered from poor health. The most serious cases were often permanently institutionalised, while hundreds of thousands of others – including some whose letters are quoted in this book – carried lesser injuries. The clerk Tom Corless was invalided out of the Army after gas damaged his eyes. He was able to return to clerking, and retired as Chief Cashier at Oldham Transport, but he needed a magnifying glass to read.[56] Arthur Gibbs, the well-heeled young subaltern whose mother lavished parcels on him, was gassed and grew a moustache to cover the shrapnel wound to his mouth. His daughter Jennifer, born in 1929, does not remember him ever being fully well, and he died of emphysema in 1945 aged fifty-one.[57] All three Nugee sons served in the war and survived, but all were wounded. George was gassed and had a spot on his lung, and bits of shrapnel were still working their way of

Francis' body in the 1950s. Andy, who had almost died of injuries to his face, neck, leg and arm, became a priest and lived to eighty-two, though by then he could barely see in his good eye.[58]

These veterans often felt angry about what had happened to them. Their memoirs sometimes record a moment of confrontation with a man who had stayed at home while they were defending their country. The ruddy health of the home man, when they had been brought low by their military service, was a cause of aggravation. R. Gwinnell got a job in a factory making shells after he was wounded, but he couldn't stand the moaning of the war workers, especially when one fellow complained about the pay awarded to his mate Taff, a veteran who 'had a piece out of his skull'. After two years Gwinnell was laid off. He vowed he would not go back to the estate where he had worked before the war. Life in the ranks had probably made him fed up with taking orders, but perhaps too he was a bit more confident of himself. In any event it proved impossible to find another job, and he was soon back on the estate driving pheasants. It was wet and miserable, and his resentment burned through:

> One thing will always stick in my mind. A big pompous man, a hopeless shot, had managed, by luck, to bring down a hen pheasant. It dropped into a great heap of thorns. I could just see it, and was trying to get my arm down to reach it. Before I could grab it, it ran away. I was wearing my old Army trousers at the time. All day long I heard him telling the other guests 'I got a bird, and all that b . . . fool had to do was to bend down and pick it up. I think he had been in the Army. No wonder the war lasted so long. . . .' Why I didn't bash him over the head, I'll never know.[59]

Taylor had a not dissimilar experience. He was building a beach hut in Bournemouth with his mate Bill Pendray, who had been wounded on the same day as he. The owner of the beach hut kept asking for changes that did not need doing, and Taylor, sick of being bossed around, decided to put him straight:

> This annoyed him and he turned on me like a wild beast. He was about 4 stone over-weight and looked as though he had made a fortune out of the War. My thoughts went back to the days when I was a prisoner and I saw red. I could hardly keep my hands off him.[60]

It is striking that Gwinnell and Taylor recall the offending figure as fat. These men were a source of envy for their prosperity, and they reminded the veteran of how fragile was his own health and how ephemeral his standing in civilian society.

* * *

If the 'fat cat' was the butt of unalloyed anger the same could not be said of women. These relationships were more deeply ambivalent, because veterans depended on women to nurture them back to health. Women's role in the veteran's recuperation is conveyed in Rebecca West's novel of 1918, *The Return of the Soldier.* The fact that West was a woman gave her a certain freedom to explore the dependence of the returned soldier, a dependence that veterans themselves could resent. In West's novel Chris Baldry has lost his memory after being concussed by a shell blast. His pretty, bourgeois wife Kitty is by turns frightened and impatient at his condition, but his ex-sweetheart, the down-at-heel Margaret, is moved to help him. Margaret's love has a strongly maternal aspect. When Chris sees her for the first time after his breakdown, he runs towards Margaret and collapses on his knees:

> I saw her arms brace him under the armpits with a gesture that was not passionate, but rather the movement of one carrying a wounded man from under fire. But even when she had raised his head to the level of her lips, the central issue was not decided . . . although it was a long time before I looked again they were still clinging breast to breast. It was as though her embrace fed him, he looked so strong as he broke away.[61]

Significantly, the physical contact involves, not a kiss, but the holding of the damaged soldier. Margaret's embrace is a life-giving force, and that embrace is seen as a repetition of the care between comrades at the front. The veteran's recovery depends on women's ability to go back with the veteran to the moment of the traumatic break and mediate his uncontained distress.

In a later scene of West's novel the narrator comes across the two figures in a woodland:

> He lay there in the confiding relaxation of a sleeping child, his hands unclenched and his head thrown back so that the bare throat showed defencelessly. Now he was asleep and his face undarkened by thought one saw how very fair he really was. And she, her mournfully vigilant face pinkened by the cold river of air sent by the advancing evening through the screen of rusted gold bracken was sitting beside him, just watching.[62]

'Just watching'. This is what Bion describes as 'reverie', where the mother is attuned to the baby's emotional state, and, through her cradling and soothing words, makes its anxieties tolerable. But the modern tone of psychological acuity is not the only thing that makes West's image emotionally powerful, for she also draws here on the traditional vehicle of the Pietà nursing the wounded Christ.

Giovanna Rita Di Ceglie, in a commentary on Bion's theories, notes how the idea of mothering, and its physical embodiment in the home, are linked to containing. 'To go back to the house metaphor', she says, 'Bion's model tells us why we need to rest in our maternal home before we can have our own.'[63] What Rebecca West gives us in *The Return of the Soldier* is a narrative of rest in the maternal home. It is Margaret's capacity for reverie that enables Chris to pass through his mental paralysis and resume his adult life and responsibilities as a husband and soldier.

Historians have noted the popularity of marriage and domesticity among veterans, and perhaps the deep appeal of home as a space of recuperation is an explanation for this.[64] Leland's comment just as he was about to go on leave, imagining that he will fall into bed and sleep for a month or a year, shows how much he longed for home as a refuge. So too does the comment of Stephen Brent, the protagonist of Warwick Deeping's novel *No Hero – This*, as he spends his last night of leave in bed with his wife. She 'strokes my head, and I feel like a child in the arms of its mother.' They do not make love, for 'Crude sex does not enter into a relationship that is built up of understanding and profound compassion.'[65] Seth Koven is right to note the 'representational convergence' between the damaged veteran and the child within post-war society, but the link was more than a matter of public discourse; it was felt in the most intimate relationships.[66]

Women were drawn into relationships with men who had been wounded physically and emotionally, and who wanted comforting, and there were many such men among veterans. In 1929, over a decade after the war's end, 40 per cent of all serving soldiers were in receipt of a pension and 200,000 were officially recognised as suffering from war-related nervous conditions.[67] Among casualties like these, found the American ex-military doctor Norman Fenton in a study carried out in the mid-1920s, the extent of emotional and financial support from families was an important element in the degree of recovery.[68]

Many men were never medically diagnosed with a war-related condition, but still needed looking after by wives and families. They wanted to put the war behind them but were ill at ease in the homes to which they returned. In the memoir of the miner Rowland Luther, written when he was an old man, it is striking how the events that spanned from the war's end to the mid-1920s – unemployment, his breakdown, being nursed back to health, marriage and family life, and the loss of comrades – fold back into the moment of return to his village in South Wales. He tried to find work at his old pit, but was told he was not fit for heavy work, 'as my muscles had become soft':

> I found this to be true. Eventually I obtained a pension of 17/6 a week. I had cracked up, and had just become skin and bone. My life had even been in despair, but by good attention, I picked up again, after being delirious and re-living my life as a soldier.
>
> I was now married, and starting a family. The war had become a thing of the past, until the War Memorial was erected, and I stood and gazed at the names of so many of the men I knew – there were over 400, and I pictured my own name there – to what purpose, I do not know. Everything had changed so much – everyone was miserable, food was dear and scarce, and I sold my Army coat back to the Army for £1, payable at any railway station.[69]

The elite did not face Luther's financial hardships but could be equally dependent on the 'good attention' of a woman. Herbert Asquith – 'Beb' to his wife Cynthia – was 'very, very tired' after returning from France with shell-shock. Cynthia sat at his bedside, reading and talking to him, and doling out cigarettes in an effort to stop him chain smoking. His step-mother, Margot, was concerned about his drinking. On one occasion he fainted and Cynthia 'had to feed him like a baby.'[70]

The veteran's demands for nursing taxed relationships with wives and lovers. Cynthia Asquith sometimes thought that Beb had become a grumpy old man, but at other times – as her comment about feeding him suggests – he seemed like a child.[71] If the returned soldier needed rest in the maternal home, he also wanted to be restored as a man and to feel desired. Food and sleep were not enough for Leland; he also wanted his wife's admiration. The different demands for mothering and sexual attention were difficult to juggle.[72]

The appeal of home as a place of recuperation, and of women as carers, is shown in the romantic attachments that became promises of marriage to wounded veterans. Robert Graves had a 'sickbed attraction' to a nurse while recovering from shell-shock in mid-1917, and shortly afterwards fell in love with his future wife Nancy Nicolson.[73] They were married in December 1917 after a four-month courtship and their first child was born in January 1919. Nancy had to endure alongside Graves the shells that burst in his dreams at night. He slept a lot, suffered from bouts of influenza and worried that he was a drag on Nancy.[74]

John Middlebrook had been interested in Dorothy, a family friend, for some months before he was shot climbing out of a trench in No Man's Land and had his left arm amputated. 'Dorothy and myself are getting fairly well on the way to intimacy now, but I am really trying to mark time', he wrote to his father just before he was wounded, his caution about proceeding too quickly compounded by the disapproval of his mother and the outcome of hasty wartime matches.[75] Once Middlebrook returned disabled to England, however, the pace of the relationship quickened. As Middlebrook described it in old age, 'When I was wounded, I had a letter from her in my breast pocket – it got bloodstained – and her letter to me in hospital after my sister had given her the news, gave the game away to both of us and to go forward was the only way. She herself had a bout of the worst kind of pneumonia earlier in 1916 and this also had drawn us together.'[76] In Middlebrook's mind, the moment of his wounding was also the moment in which Dorothy touched his heart.[77] Dorothy had decided to devote herself to the disabled veteran.

Charles Templer met his future wife Dais on the day war was declared. He visited her on every home leave and carried a Christmas card in his pocket with her photograph on it. Templer proposed to Dais in October 1918. His timing was significant, for earlier that year he had come close to death during a patrol when his platoon got stranded in forward trenches. Their commanding officer was wounded, and Templer took charge, firing away at German soldiers with such ferocity that his rifle blew up in his hand. Templer looked on helpless as one of his men panicked, ran towards the Germans, and was hit by a hand grenade: 'I got to him and found he had a terrible wound in the throat and when I tried to raise him, his blood gushed all over my tunic. It was impossible to bind the wound as he would have strangled.' It was the prospect of a future with Dais that stopped him from losing his head as his comrade had done. He was urged on by the thought that 'Dais was something I would not know, especially if I got a bayonet through my gut.' His lust for life, however, revealed the very violence he thought to escape from. After he proposed to Dais, they had walked to her uncle's house, where Charles kissed and held her so violently that 'Suddenly she collapsed in my arms'. Dais was left with bruises down her front from the buttons of his tunic. Taken aback by the vehemence of his embrace, the following day she told him 'In future you must be more gentle with me Charles.'[78]

Stuart Cloete also hoped that Eros would help dull the pain of war. He was hit in the back and groin on 27 August 1918, all but severing his femoral artery, and would almost certainly have bled to death if it was not for a Guardsman who – defying orders to leave all wounded – fetched field-dressings from the dead to patch him. But he was also helped to live by a sudden vision that the 'two most important things in a man's life were love and war. War I had. Love I must get if I ever got out of this.' On the hospital ship he heard the doctors discussing his case; one said '"If his mother breastfed him he might pull through."' Even among these professionals, though it seems for physiological rather than psychological reasons, the quality of the original relationship with a mother was seen as crucial. Cloete found the comment interesting as he had been wet-nursed, and might therefore have owed his life to his nurse Elsa rather than his mother. Certainly he had not cried out for his mother when in pain, as men were known to do; he only 'wanted my girl', Eileen.'[79]

In the early weeks of his recovery Cloete underwent five operations and was in severe pain. Eileen, who was working as a nurse at the time, visited him every day and so did his mother, but it was Eileen he pined for. Day in, day out, he 'just lay there waiting for her', and when she arrived he would hold her hand and cry.[80] After he began to recover he got Eileen to lay her hand on his genitals: he needed to know that his manhood was intact. Cloete proposed to Eileen in mid-October 1918 and they were married secretly at a registry office at the end of that month, just two months after Cloete's wounding. For all the urgency of Cloete's desire and their avid reading of Marie Stopes' new book *Married Love*, sex was not a success. Cloete, who was used to the 'relatively uninhibited' customs of the French, found Eileen rather reticent. This was the first time she had made love, and it cannot have been easy given Cloete's injuries. The sight of Cloete naked would hardly have been alluring, for both his buttocks had been 'blown half off', and he had other wounds at the base of his spine and in his groin, while the practicalities of trying to avoid aggravating his wounds must have made intercourse more than usually awkward.[81]

After the war he and Eileen moved to a remote village in France, where Cloete, physically and mentally exhausted from the war, finally 'let go'. He avoided people, cried a lot, and had 'terrible nightmares'. One night, on waking from a bad dream, he almost stabbed Eileen. Cloete wanted Eileen's exclusive company; he was 'Living on a kind of emotional island with the girl I loved', in a 'private bubble out of time.' Cut adrift from her friends and family, caring for Cloete through his breakdown, Eileen must have been at her wits' end on occasion.[82]

Eighteen years later they broke up. Though fond of each other, Cloete believed that their 'sexual incompatibility' was the cause. The difficulties lay primarily with Eileen, who, he discovered later, had been assaulted at the age of twelve by a friend of her father's. Perhaps Cloete could not afford to consider how far the demands he had made on Eileen to make him whole again might have contributed to the break-up. His dependence was perhaps just as much the 'rock on which the ship of our romance was to founder' as Eileen's supposed frigidity.[83]

Men like Cloete were anxious to set up their own homes. C. W. Taylor's life turned out better than he could ever have expected, although his ordeal as a POW left him with stomach pains for the rest of his life. He married in 1922 and had two children, a daughter in 1923 and a son in 1928. After living with his mother-in-law they managed in 1923 to get their own flat near the London docks where Taylor worked. Eventually he became Clerk of Works at the docks and was given accommodation on site, but he longed for the space and quiet of the countryside, so they bought an acre of ground out in the Essex village of Wickford which Taylor cleared and on which he built his own home. They kept chickens and grew fruit trees. His stomach pains were a cause of 'more work for my wife', and on one occasion during the Second World War they became so bad that he had to be hospitalised. While in hospital there was a bombing raid, and Taylor lay in his bed with bombs going off while the casualties were brought in around him. The violence of the scene, familiar as it probably was, would hardly have settled his stomach.

Charles Templer's successes gave him even more opportunity than Taylor to realise the dream of a home in the country. He had set up his own company in the 1920s and, having initially lived above the premises in Acton with Dais and his two sons, by 1934 he had saved enough to buy a house near Dorking on eleven acres of land. It had a tennis court, garden, greenhouses and orchard, and three acres of copse. They kept animals, grew their own vegetables and cultivated flowers. [84] Military service in rural France and Belgium had shown these urban Londoners what could be gleaned from the land, but nothing could be further from the churned-up mud of the trenches than the grounds they nurtured.

Many veterans, unlike their fathers, were keen to be involved in bringing up their children. John T, married in 1913, had a daughter after he returned from France. He liked to 'push her out in the pram, that was my delight, that was . . . I was never too proud to push a pram.' He reckoned that after the war, 'the man took over duties . . . including pushing the pram . . . [that] they didn't attempt to do before 1914.'[85] Veterans could identify with the vulnerability of children, and, often having more adult experience of sickness than others, could empathise with their ailments. Templer had a very clear memory of the birth at home of his son Phil in 1924, and Charles Edward in 1930. Phil got diphtheria shortly after his brother's birth and had to go to hospital, and he remembers Phil pleading, 'Can't you come with me Dad?'[86]

Along with the capacity to nurture, many veterans were troubled by moodiness and flashes of temper towards their loved ones. Ruth Armstrong's father seemed to settle in quickly after his return, but his war stories showed how split his mind had become. He 'used to walk around with me on his shoulder, and he told me nice stories. The nasty stories, he told my mother.' Ruth's father eventually became clinically paranoid, convinced that his wife had had an affair in his absence.[87]

Another daughter of a veteran, born just after the Second World War, recalled her father's graphic descriptions of his war forty years earlier. These included picking lice out of his socks, enduring the miseries of a diet of dry biscuits and bully beef, and suffering from dysentery which had produced blood and green slime, but which he believed had saved his life by necessitating his despatch to a field hospital behind the lines. Like many other veterans, he was subject to frightening outbursts of verbal rage, but he also showed great tenderness, particularly to very young children, and his daughter felt that his anxiety about his children's health, which had had lasting effects on them, was directly connected to his war and particularly the dysentery.[88]

Not all veterans were able to keep their tempers in check. As Peter Barham shows in his study of traumatised veterans, when a man was admitted to an asylum it was often because domestic violence had made life unbearable for his wife and children. Frederick Bull locked his wife up in a room, Charles Davies had been beating his wife and Richard H attempted to strangle his.[89] These were men whose disturbances were too great for families to manage, but who also suffered because they had lost the support of their loved ones. It is interesting that A. P. Herbert, whose 1919 novel *The Secret Battle* related the mental turmoil of the conscientious officer Harry Penrose, was later to sponsor the 1937 Matrimonial Causes Act which made lunacy grounds for divorce.

Many veterans wanted women around them to help support their recovery. The 'saving grace' for some of the cases who passed through war hospitals, says Peter Barham, was the fact of having been married. He describes the extraordinary account of Mrs H, who in 1926 took her husband William out of Middlewood Asylum where he had been diagnosed with delusional insanity, and looked after him until his death in 1970. William was 'like a child but also frightening at times', and watching over him had made her life a 'misery'.[90] The wives of disabled veterans were just as taxed, often working to supplement pensions, tending to their husbands' wounds and doing the jobs around the house that a husband normally would have done.[91]

Without a wife or other relative to care for them, men were likely to get stuck in institutions, and the longer a man was institutionalised, the weaker his family ties became. A report from Long Grove mental hospital in 1946 found that half its remaining First World War veterans did not receive letters or visits from relatives.[92] Deborah Cohen's study of disabled veterans reveals a similar picture of the hardships faced by those living outside families. Men who had been permanently hospitalised had poor life expectancy. A third of the 850 residents in the Star and Garter hospital died at the hospital, most before they were aged 35.[93] These men were too seriously injured to live in, and benefit from, a home life. Domesticity was good for veterans, but their loved ones bore the cost, a cost largely hidden from public view.

## Veterans and their mothers

While some yearned for marriage and a family on their return, others seemed unable to leave their mothers. The playwright R. C. Sherriff was one such. His mother accompanied him to Oxford when he decided to undertake a degree at the age of thirty-five, and she went with him to Hollywood when he was asked to write the screenplay of the spectacularly successful 1928 theatre production of *Journey's End*.[94] The 'extraordinary closeness' between Sherriff and his mother presents a stark contrast to *Journey's End*, which, as Robert Graves and Alan Hodge note in their portrait of inter-war Britain, contained not a single woman in the cast.[95]

Willis Brown was another who seemed unable to get away from his mother. His sister Margaret recalled that as a small child he was often ill, suffering from whooping cough, measles, chicken-pox and scarlet fever. Yet Willis could not bear his mother fussing over him. She was a demonstrative woman, and liked to cuddle Willis, but he 'detested it'.[96] When Willis was nineteen he enlisted in the Royal Marine Brigade, but shortly afterwards became critically ill with meningitis and had to be sent home. Just six weeks later he was thrilled to be given the medical clearance to join his unit in Gallipoli supervising the construction of trenches, but soon after reaching the peninsula he began to suffer from dysentery. The letter that he sent his mother from Gallipoli in June 1915 ends on a rather desperate note: 'p.s. I wish I could come home the same time as the letter'.[97] At some point later in June or July 1915 Willis went missing for several days, until a 'scarecrow figure' was seen staggering about in the moonlight above the trenches, exposed to the Turkish guns and delirious with hunger, dehydration and fever.[98] Willis was sent to hospital in Alexandria suffering from enteric fever, and was invalided home to Charing Cross Hospital in October 1915.[99]

Margaret would not forget her first sight of him, 'a long, emaciated creature, with great hollow eyes, a greenish-yellow skin and limbs that were all sticks and knobs.' Most extraordinary was his head, which after having been shaved, had grown a crop of 'soft golden baby-hair.' He would joke about the peculiarities of the Australian soldiers, but would not talk about 'anything else' that had occurred on the peninsula. The expression on his face was one of 'dumb horror'. On his regular visits to the family home in Sidcup, Kent, his mother, full of pride, could not resist getting her friends to 'accidentally' call in on the returned war hero. On one of these visits, recalled his sister, Willis lost his temper when the 'inevitable questions' from his mother's friends began:

> He told them, very quickly and calmly, but horrors such as none of them had ever dreamed of (that was before the days of brutally frank war-books) and once started, he couldn't stop. He gave them the lot, and then got up and walked out to the waiting car without saying goodbye to anyone. Mother was outraged and still more affronted by a note that arrived next morning saying that he'd rather not come home any more just yet.

Willis' mood of bold defiance did not last long, however, for after being moved to the Naval Hospital at Portland he sent a letter hinting that he was being poorly treated. His mother drove to the hospital and confronted the naval officials, saying '"I want to take him home, in my car, NOW."' 'I can't cope with all that emotion that Mother goes in for', Willis once exclaimed to his sister, yet he found it hard to break the tie.[100]

In some war memoirs the hostility towards mothers is explicit, and shocking given their veneration before the war. Robert Graves in *Goodbye to All That* famously quotes a letter supposedly published by a 'Little Mother' in *The Morning Post*, praising those who 'mother the men' as the true heroes of the war effort. As if to show that the Little Mother was not alone in her madness, Graves printed a string of replies in fervent agreement with her.[101] Although Graves did not comment on these letters, his subsequent account of being on home leave in Kent with a comrade's mother (actually at Weirleigh, the house of Siegried Sassoon's mother), who traipsed the corridors of the family home trying to make contact with her dead son, conveyed well enough Graves' view of mothers as ghoulish and out of touch with the front, where the real heroes were to be found.

Similarly, much of the satire in Richard Aldington's *Death of a Hero* is aimed at mothers. The first third of the novel, which depicts the middle-class upbringing of George Winterbourne, is mentioned less often than the book's account of trench warfare and Winterbourne's '*menage à trois*'. The book opens with Mrs Winterbourne's reaction on receiving the news of George's death on the Western Front. She 'liked drama', and 'uttered a most creditable shriek, clasped both hands to her rather soggy bosom, and pretended to faint.' As her lover – the twenty-second she had taken during her promiscuous life – consoles her, the pretence at a 'mother-heart' gives way to a 'wholly erotic' reaction. The narrator continues: 'The war did that to lots of women. All the dying and wounds and mud and bloodiness – at a safe distance – gave them a great kick, and excited them to an almost unbearable pitch of amorousness.'[102] Aldington regarded his novel as an attempt to unburden himself of 'poisonous stuff' from the war, and his friend Derek Patgrove recalled him crying as he remembered the trenches.[103] He wrote the book very quickly: part one was written in ten days on the island of Port Cros whilst D.H. Lawrence and Frieda were staying with him.[104] The fact that this is the part of the novel that deals with George Winterbourne's early life, suggests that the 'poisonous stuff' he was trying to exorcise was not just the war, but the malign influence of those women who had put their loved ones through it 'at a safe distance.'

Hostility to mothers was not confined to the literary avant-garde but could also be found in middlebrow literature. Warwick Deeping's bestseller *Sorrell and Son* is about the struggle of an officer who, living in reduced circumstances through no fault of his own, brings up his son alone. Most of the female characters in the novel are sexual predators. Sorrell's ex-wife walks out when her son is little, but reappears when he reaches late adolescence, and introduces him to two sexually voracious young women. As in the war, the men must look after each other and Sorrell manages – despite his wife – to keep his son on the path of purity and get him through a degree at Oxford University. D. H. Lawrence summed up such currents of hostility in a comment to Cynthia Asquith in 1918: 'I feel I am all the time rescuing my nephew and niece from their respective mothers, my two sisters; who have jaguars of wrath in their soul, however they purr to their offspring. The phenomenon of motherhood, in these days, is a strange and rather frightening phenomenon.'[105]

The overt anger towards mothers in Aldington, Graves and Deeping was exceptional, unlike the hostility directed towards the politicians, profiteers or puffy generals. By contrast with these 'Old Men', mothers were likely to be, in Malcolm Smith's apt words, 'indirectly but clearly' targets.[106] There were some, such as Siegfried Sassoon, who strenuously avoided making their mothers targets. Sassoon's relationship with his mother was perhaps more intense than some, his father having separated from Theresa when Siegfried was a small boy. At the end of the war Sassoon returned to Weirleigh, and though he found the atmosphere stultifying, particularly his mother's ardent patriotism, she was not among his list of detested civilians. In his *Memoirs of George Sherston*, though many of the characters are close approximates to real people, Sherston differs from Sassoon in being an orphan. Aunt Evelyn, Sassoon was keen to assure his mother, represented 'only a very faint portrait of a very small part of your character.'[107]

By replacing his mother with Aunt Evelyn, Sassoon was able to avoid having to deal with his ambivalent feelings towards Theresa. Nevertheless there were some parallels, as both women – real and fictional – were largely spared his wrath. The *Memoirs* describe George Sherston's recuperation in hospital in London, shortly before his protest against the war. He was angry towards those who 'couldn't understand': senior officers too strongly imbued with the spirit of the Regiment, elderly male civilians, the sisters of officers who suppressed 'all unpalatable facts about the War', and his hunting friends too old to have served. But when Aunt Evelyn came up to see him 'I felt properly touched by her reticent emotion; embitterment against civilians couldn't be applied to her.'[108] Sherston's love for his Aunt Evelyn could not be sullied, and the same applied to Sassoon's own mother: his anger was split off and projected onto the uncomprehending civilians with whom he was less intimate.

Sassoon was outraged when in the autumn of 1929 he learned of the description of Theresa in Robert Graves' forthcoming memoir, and he tried to get the manuscript amended. He did not want Theresa dragged into the limelight and he warned her not to read the book.[109] For her seventieth birthday in 1928, he composed a poem in her honour. *To*

*My Mother* continues the Edwardian ideal of the mother as the angel of the home:

> I watch you on your constant way,
> In selfless duty long grown grey;
> And to myself I say
> That I have lived my life to learn
> How lives like yours unasking earn
> Aureoles that guide, and burn
> In heart's remembrance . . .[110]

The volume contains an intimate drawing of a mother holding her child, the two of them cheek-to-cheek, but perhaps all is not as it seems, for it was sketched by Sassoon's flamboyant lover Stephen Tennant, of whom Theresa was wary.[111] She was not the only one, Theresa would have concluded from the pamphlet, in Siegfried's thoughts.

Another covert way in which veterans expressed their anger was by rejecting the moral codes associated with their mothers. In *Goodbye to All That*, Graves claimed that his mother had influenced his character little apart from in matters of Christian morality, which the war had led Graves to dispute. Recalling his mother's moral tales, he explained how 'She kept off the subject of war as much as possible, always finding it difficult to explain how it was that God permitted wars.' Home leave in Easter 1916 was particularly trying because he felt obliged for his mother's sake to attend what turned out to be a three-hour church service.[112] Graves' attitude was one of passive protest, sitting through the service so as to 'please Mother'. Charles Miller did much the same thing. In a letter written to his daughters in 1938, he recalled the 'tremendously high standard' set by his mother in spiritual matters, and how saddened she used to be by their invariable failures to live up to those standards. He 'came to look on church as a bore, but not liking to sadden . . . mother adopted a good many subterfuges.'[113] When around their mothers, these sons went through the motions of dutifulness even although they had lost their faith.

In the private and published war memoirs written in the half-century between the 1920s and the 1970s, it is striking how little veterans have to say about their mothers. They appear to have coped on their own. Mothers are thought to have known little of the dangers sons faced. Charles Miller's comment was typical: 'I was her only son and the apple of her eye; one merciful thing was that I do not think that my mother was ever able to visualise fully the realities of war, and the horror of it.'[114]

Brady thought the formulaic prose of their letters home – 'I'm in the pink, hope you are the same' – was a reaction to censorship and the fact that families 'had their own problems of deprivation, poverty, grief and distress'. They did not wish to 'pile on the agony.'[115] Regardless of rank and class, mothers appear unable to bear the painful truth. The normal containing relationships between mother and child are reversed.

The reality was of course more complicated. The perceived fragility of mothers and the thought that they should be spared violence was an issue for correspondents during the war. John Middlebrook was unusally frank in complaining to his father about the anodyne letters he felt he must write: 'the everlasting note of optimism that I have to sound to mother seems to me to sound very hollow and unconvincing. Do you really think it serves its purpose, Father?'[116] The pretence was hollow indeed, for Middlebrook's letters to his father were far from optimistic, and as Middlebrook well knew, were read by his mother.

In memoirs, the tendency to think that sons had been successful in shielding mothers grew. Harold Owen thought their mother's war years, though anxious, were 'perhaps rewarding ones too' because the three brothers were 'meticulous in lessening these anxieties in every way possible'.[117] Wilfred's letters to his mother, however, were often quite graphic and the words and phrases that evoked horror would re-appear in his war poems.[118] Nor were Brady's letters as circumspect as he recalled. One – sent via a comrade on leave so as to escape censorship – describes the effects of whizzbangs, shrapnel and high explosive: 'terrible near shaves. Dead and wounded lying all over the place.' As with most letters home, it is animated as much by the need to convey as to protect mothers from what Brady called the '"horrors of war"'.[119]

Over time the idea that mothers had been spared the worst became one of the myths of the war. The myth did bear a relation to reality for, as this book has shown, mothers both did and did not want to know the worst, and sons may not have been wrong in thinking their mothers too fragile to bear the truth. In the myth, however, mothers never had to witness horror. A version of this myth appears in Clare Leighton's account, written in 1980, of the moment in early 1916 when her dead brother Roland's muddy and blood-soaked clothes were returned. According to Vera Brittain, Mrs Leighton had been so upset by the sight and smell of Roland's clothing that she had ordered them to be destroyed, but Clare's account, though not actually at odds with Brittain's, recalls the moment of concealment, rather than the moment of discovery. It is a cold morning in January:

> I carry two heavy kettles. They are filled with boiling water, for we are about to bury the tunic – blood-stained and bullet-riddled – in which Roland has been killed . . . Father watches the windows of the house, for my mother must not see this tunic that Father has hidden from the packages of Roland's effects returned from France. I am to thaw the frozen earth so that it may be buried out of sight.[120]

Notice here how strong is the impulse in Clare Leighton to keep the horrific sight from her mother, her repetition of 'bury', 'mother must not see'; 'buried out of sight.' Her own feelings about the loss of the brother she adored are eclipsed by the need to protect her mother. Mothers were sometimes forced to take in the horror of war, even when they preferred not to; but in the post-war myth created by the war generation it was the mother's shielding that was remembered, and it was the children who did the shielding.[121]

The notion that wives and especially mothers had been spared the worst, allowed men to maintain the Edwardian ideal of women as emotionally fragile, and of themselves as dutiful. Yet it had an aggressive undercurrent, for it discounted the anxieties that mothers had actually felt. It forgot the support that they had been given, the parcels lovingly assembled and the voluminous correspondence which had kept alive the memory of home. The veteran seems to complain: 'I not only had to contain myself, I had to concoct a tale for your benefit, so you would not break down!'

Paul Fussell, Samuel Hynes and others have described the emergence in war poetry and memoirs of a new language of direct description which expressed the horror of war in plain and powerful terms. We might ask, in the context of the myth of women's ignorance, who is this horror directed at? Part of the impulse in writing memoirs was to unveil civilian ignorance; as Stefan Audoin-Rouzeau and Annette Becker assert, they were not merely composed 'for the sake of the civilian population' but '*against* them.'[122] The veteran's violent descriptions broke the code that mothers should be kept ignorant, much as Willis Brown did when he angrily recounted to his mother's friends the gruesome sights of Gallipoli.

The desire to bring the horror of war home to mothers also seems to animate Aldington's *Death of a Hero*. The second part of the book is a graphic account of life in the line. George Winterbourne experiences a 'breach in the shield' of his mind, to use Freud's phrase, when he and his comrades try to deal with the aftermath of a direct hit on a sap.[123] Two men lie in the trench: 'The head of one man was smashed into his steel helmet and lay a sticky mess of blood and hair half-severed from his body.' The other was still alive, but suffering from massive injuries. Winterbourne looks on as his commanding officer tries to bind the man's wounds, and then sprints back to fetch the stretcher-bearers, but returns too late to save the man's life.[124] Scenes such as these explain the disparagement of Edwardian domesticity in the first part of the novel. Wives and mothers had feigned sympathy; they did not want to understand so must be forced to experience the breach themselves.

The horrific scenes in *Goodbye to All That* can also be seen as a riposte to uncomprehending women. A man whose brains are splattered all over his cap lies in the bottom of a trench 'making a snoring noise mixed with animal groans.'[125] A company commander is wounded in the lungs and stomach and crawls along the trenches towards the stretcher bearer's dug-out. His fellow officers cannot decide what to do with him; one becomes paralysed by the scene and keeps 'blubbering: "Poor old Boy, poor old Boy!"' A platoon sergeant is 'screaming from a stomach wound, begging for morphia.'[126] In between these scenes of horror, Graves snipes at patriotic war-mongers like the 'Little Mother' and her supporters. An emotional logic links the two elements of Graves' memoir, for the battle scenes disabuse women of their romantic notions of war.[127] War literature like *Goodbye to All That* attempts to project into women, to make *them* feel, the unbearable distress that men have suffered.

## Reconstructing manliness

Anger towards those who had been safe at home was one consequence of the war, but it could also foster sensibilities more usually associated with femininity than masculinity. Crisis encouraged some to appraise the ideals of manliness with which they had gone to war.[128] Peter Barham has suggested that, among men driven mad by the conflict and among those treating them, a softer, more feminine self sometimes emerged. In the work of people like Meyer in America, and Smith and Pears in Britain, there was a desire to identify with, rather than regard as pathological, the serviceman's suffering. In Smith and Pears' words, 'unless the sympathiser has a true appreciation of the patient's condition, he cannot really feel *with* the sufferer.'[129] This empathetic attitude was one that, through reflection on the transference and counter-transference, later psychoanalysts like D. W. Winnicott (and, although Barham does not mention him, Wilfred Bion) would make central to their therapeutic practice.[130]

For the battled-stressed soldier, the moment of breakdown could potentially also be a moment of liberation. This was something that the poet Ivor Gurney perceived; he oscillated, Peter Barham shows, between a sense of his neurasthenia as a weakness for which the toughness of Army life was an antidote, and as a 'creative capability that he wants to embrace.'[131] Gurney was not alone among traumatised veterans in feeling both damaged and regenerated by his experience. At around the time of his dream of the supposedly tough but actually broken wristwatch, Leland had a profoundly moving experience involving another timepiece. He had been to visit the Divisional Staff, who at this time were billeted in a spectacular chateau, with pepperbox spires, mosaic floors created in Rome, walls painted with fleur-de-lys, terraced gardens and fish ponds. It was said Leland, the 'most beautiful place I ever saw.' Although the Germans had ruined much of the interior, marking the parquet floor with their hobnailed boots, cutting all the pictures into pieces and pillaging books, lying across the library was 'the most beautiful clock I have ever seen . . . The dial is undamaged and the wooden framework is only just splintered.' Like Leland himself, here was another miraculous survivor of the German violence, slightly scratched on the exterior (you will recall that Leland had recently scraped his face on a tree branch) but with its essential workings still intact. If Leland's dream of a broken wristwatch conveyed his feelings of falling apart, here was a waking vision of holding together. And though Leland worried about what his wife would make of him, this delicate object was undeniably beautiful. Leland's admiration of the clock is at odds with the stoic ideal of the soldier, an image now, in Leland's own self-description, 'war worn'.[132]

Comradeship, though galvanised *against* the incomprehension of women, could encourage a softer conception of manliness. Many veterans continued to take an interest in the lives of the men they had served with, and memoirs like Templer's contain parallel stories about their mates. They missed the intimacy of comradeship. Jack Cornes found it hard to adjust to the 'jungle' of civilian life because in the Army everything had been shared, and 'most of us had one comrade with whom we shared everything.'[133] At the end of the war, Gwinnell was surprised to feel 'very depressed. After four years with all the troubles, I was going to miss my old comrades.'[134] Guy Chapman, in his 1933 memoir, *A Passionate Prodigality*, described how heart-rending it was to see the Regiment being diminished bit by bit through demobilisation. On their last march back through Belgium 'Looking back at those firm ranks as they marched back into billets, to the Fusilier's march, I found that this body of men had so much become part of me that its disintegration would tear away something I cared for more dearly than I could have believed. I was it, and it was I.'[135] Chapman's wife Storm Jameson astutely observed that the writing of memoirs by veterans was itself a way of preserving the exclusivity of the war time bond, an act of 'cultural piety.'[136]

This comradeship, though largely between men of the same rank, could cross divides of rank and class. It was not unknown for a ranker to look up his officer when passing through his home town, or to drop him a line at Christmas.[137] The IWM contains a letter, written two years after the war, by the batman J. James to his old officer, Stanley Wootton. Its tone is rather depressed. James mentions health problems, and resorting too freely to his old vices of drink and gambling. He had recently attended a Brigade reunion, and the experience had prompted him to contact Wootton: 'I was only wishing I could have seen you there an Officer and a gentleman.' His desire to communicate again with Wootton was not only sparked by nostalgia for the war, but by the whizz-bang which hit a tree above their platoon, 'leaving 'me + you untouched + the other poor lads killed such is fate.' James' remembering was involuntary: 'thoughts of the lot over there flash into my mind which sometimes one cannot help.'[138] The mutual witnessing of carnage, the miracle of their survival and his repeated disturbing recollections of the incident had encouraged James to contact his old officer again.

In the war men had become skilled in the domestic arts. They could rustle up meals with whatever was at hand, sew buttons on and wash clothes. Even Captain Leland, who could rely for most of the time on the services of his batman Hilton, had to fend for himself during the worst of the shelling. Many had seen men die, had passed by mangled bodies at close quarters, and comforted those who had no hope. They had lived closer to the stuff of life than most, and to sickness and death. They were inured to injuries that a civilian might shrink from. Hallie Miles describes how, at a patriotic tea that she had organised for returned soldiers during the war, a man with no arms asked one of the women serving to help feed him. Miles and the young waitress became upset at the sight and had to hide their tears, but another waitress 'asked if she might feed him. The soldier who sat next to this armless hero was so tender too and held the cup of tea to him to drink from and put bits of cake into his mouth.'[139] The experience of nursing each other could give men capacities for nurturing that outlived the war. Eric Leed rightly asserts that the trauma of war 'produced a body of men with an enormous need for care and reassurance, a need combined with anger and hostility towards the society that had placed them in the position of victims.'[140] But it also produced men who, having experienced the depths of human need, were practised carers.

Charles Templer's wife Dais died suddenly in 1982, two years before he set down his memoirs. Templer's account was both a testament of war and of his love for Dais. The concluding pages, which tell of her death, also reveal the long shadow of the war: 'I had lost the girl I had loved since our first meeting on August 4th 1914, through the years of war until our engagement on 2nd October 1918, demobilisation in 1919, waiting to re-establish myself in civilian life, finding somewhere we could live together, our marriage 3rd August 1922.'[141] For Templer the war was emphatically not 'in parentheses'.

Dais had been severely disabled in the final years of her life. She had had two hip operations and even getting about the house was difficult. 'She needed my care', Templer commented. He gave a detailed description of the crisis on the evening of Monday 11 January 1982 when Dais began to feel sharp pain in her lower back. They went ahead with preparations for their dinner, Templer making her usual cocktail, but she had no appetite. Templer took her upstairs to bed where she seemed more comfortable, and then went back to wash up and launder some of her clothes, as Dais was incontinent and there was always washing to do. On returning to the bedroom he found her lying unconscious across the bed. Templer covered her in their eiderdown and called the ambulance. The ambulance men arrived soon after and wrapped Dais up well with blankets. They put her on a stretcher on one side of the ambulance, and Templer sat opposite. During the journey to hospital, 'Dais kept raising herself up and looking at me with very frightened eyes, which made me jump up, only to be pushed back in my seat by the attendant while he gently lay her down again.' In the hospital he sat with her and held her hand:

> I told her that I had loved her since our first meeting all those years ago and that she was the only woman in my life. As she did not speak, I wondered if she understood what I was telling her. So I asked her if she would like me to take care of her rings. She moved her hands at once, taking off her engagement ring and the solitaire diamond ring I had given her in more recent years, putting them in my hands. I then said, 'Would you like me to kiss you'?, and immediately she put her lips up for me to kiss.

The next morning the Sister rang. She asked if Templer was sitting down, and then said that she was sorry to say Dais had died in the early hours of 12 January.[142]

As his wife's health declined Templer had taken on the household tasks and additional help that Dais needed. He knew what to do when she became seriously ill, and was able to comfort her on the journey to hospital. The fact that this was not the first time he had undertaken this kind of mission may have made it easier for Charles, despite his own distress, to help Dais. He had done much the same thing for Dais' brother John in the war, when John was wounded by shrapnel in both legs. Although Charles himself was wounded in the shoulder, he had gone looking for John, eventually finding him on a hand cart in trenches that risked being rushed by the Germans. John had said 'Get me out Charles', and Templer, after holding John's hand for a while, had guided him out of the trenches and towards a lorry which had taken them both to the base hospital.[143]

The war continued to exert its influence over matters of life and death in the half century after its end. Dais' trip to hospital was not the first time that Templer had seen the terror of the dying close up. It may not have been the first time he had saved the rings of a dying person for their loved one, or even the first time he had kissed the dying. These were men who had been called on to comfort others when terrified themselves. The experience of being beyond containing left lasting scars, but it could also foster a quality of empathy that the young Edwardian recruit, about to leave for France and keen to do his bit, would not have anticipated as a legacy of the war.

## Notes

1 H. J. C. Leland to Lena Leland, 17 August 1917, IWM 96/51/1.

2 Leland to wife, 21 June, 10 July, 13 July, 27 July, 28 July, 30 July 1917.

3 Leland to wife, 8 August, 27 July 1917.

4 In 'Beyond the Pleasure Principle' (1920) Freud seems to modify his earlier rejection of the idea that traumatic neurosis was due to the physical effect of violent concussion on the brain, and his advocacy of a wholly psychological explanation. The two positions, he now believed, were not irreconcilable. Traumatic neurosis could be caused by a 'breach in the shield against stimuli and by the problems that follow in its train', but Freud's concern was still with psychological factors, such as the lack of preparedness for anxiety, rather than molecular damage to the brain. S. Freud, 'Beyond the Pleasure

Principle', *The Standard Edition of the Complete Psychological Works of Sigmund Freud*, tr. J. Strachey, Vol. 18 (London: Vintage, 2001), p. 31.

5 Confidential Report on the Recent Illness of Captain H. J. C. Leland D. S. O., 19 August 1913. This and all subsequent references to official correspondence concerning Leland are from his military service records at the National Archives, WO 374/41657.

6 Lieutenant General E. E. Codrington, Military Secretary to H. J. C. Leland, 2 September 1914.

7 Leland to The Secretary, War Office, 6 September 1914.

8 Proceedings of Courts Martial Submitted For the Inspection of the Adjutant-General, 28 November 1916.

9 After conscription was introduced the following categories were introduced. Category 'A' meant fit for general service; Category B 1, 2 and 3 meant fit for garrison, labour and sedentary work abroad, respectively; and Category 'C' meant sedentary service at home camps.

10 Leland to wife, 25 June, 10 July, 4 August 1917.

11 Leland to wife, 8 August, 9 August 1917.

12 See for example D. Starrett memoir, p. 34, IWM 79/35/1.

13 Leland to wife, 21 August, 24 August, 7 September 1917.

14 Thanks to Christina Twomey for pointing this out.

15 Leland to wife, 3 October, 4 October, 5 October 1917.

16 Leland to wife, 2 November, 26 October, 21 October 1917.

17 Leland to wife, 14 November 1917.

18 Leland to wife, 28 November 1917.

19 Woods to Mrs Leland, 8 December 1917. On the Knutsford hospitals for officers see P. Barham, *Forgotten Lunatics of the Great War* (New Haven: Yale University Press, 2004), pp. 43–4.

20 J. Woods to Mrs Leland, 8 December 1917, IWM 96/51/1.

21 Leland to wife, 26 October 1917.

22 Leland military service record, register no. 97913/17, minute sheet 1.

23 Leland military service record, register no. 97913/21, minute sheet 3.

24 Letter from Captain Hawkesworth, Lieutenant General, Military Secretary, 13 March 1924; Letter from Major E. Parry, Lieutenant General, Military Secretary, 26 June 1920.

25 The term is used by Martin Petter, '"Temporary Gentlemen" in the Aftermath of the Great War: Rank, Status and the Ex-Officer Problem', *The Historical Journal*, Vol. 37, No. 1 (March, 1994), p. 129.

26 J. Brophy and E. Partridge (eds.), *The Long Trail. Soldiers' Songs & Slang 1914–18* (London: Sphere Books, 1969), p. 50.

27 H. Tooley, *The Western Front. Battle Ground and Home Front in the First World War* (Basingstoke: Palgrave, 2003), p. 263.

28 T. Wilson, *The Myriad Faces of War. Britain and the Great War, 1914–1918* (Cambridge: Polity, 1986), p. 545. Toc H or Talbot House was a rest house

opened in Poperinghe in December 1915 by the Reverend Tubby Clayton, and named after Gilbert Talbot.

29 Brophy and Partridge, *The Long Trail*, p. 32, p. 48.

30 W. R. Bion, *War Memoirs 1917–19* (London: H. Karnac, 1997), p. 310.

31 N. Gladden, *Ypres 1917* (London: William Kimber, 1967), p. 63.

32 See Chapter 6, on Sweeting's death, p. 264.

33 R. J. Lifton, *The Broken Connection. On Death and the Continuity of Life* (New York: Simon & Schuster, 1979), p. 172.

34 Bion's wife Francesca appended his unfinished 1958 account of Amiens to the *War Memoirs*, pp. 215–308.

35 Bion, *War Memoirs*, pp. 124–7, p. 255.

36 S. Sassoon, *Siegfried Sassoon. The War Poems* (London: Faber & Faber, 1983), p. 51.

37 I am grateful to my mother, Ailsa Roper, for pointing this out.

38 On the emergence of voices of protest against the war see S. Hynes, *A War Imagined. The First World War and English Culture* (London: Pimlico, 1992), chs. 7–10.

39 N. Gullace, *The Blood of Our Sons. Men, Women and the Renegotiation of British Citizenship in the Great War* (Basingstoke: Palgrave, 2002), p. 69.

40 J. Wedgewood quoted in D. Winter, *Death's Men. Soldiers of the Great War* (London: Penguin, 1979), p. 201.

41 Leland to wife, 3 October 1917.

42 G. Greenwell to mother, 26 December 1918, *An Infant in Arms. War Letters of a Company Commander 1914–1918* (London: Allen Lane, The Penguin Press, 1972), p. 251.

43 C. Carrington, *Soldier From the Wars Returning* (London: Arrow Books, 1965), p. 280.

44 A. Wohl, *The Generation of 1914* (Cambridge, MA: Harvard University Press, 1979), p. 222.

45 P. Fussell, *The Great War and Modern Memory* (Oxford: Oxford University Press, 1975), pp. 82–90.

46 S. Hynes, *A War Imagined*, pp. 243–6, p. 384, p. 439.

47 C. W. Taylor memoir, np, IWM 01/8/1.

48 R. Van Emden and S. Humphries, *All Quiet on the Home Front* (London: Headline Publishing, 2003), p. 300. Sarah Jane Dawson did her best to placate her son Sam, who was still waiting to be demobilised in August 1919: 'of course dear you been out there away from all your own, you feel and notice every little thing . . . I was pleased to hear you say you would content yourself the best you could until you did come home, that's the way to view things when you cannot alter them.' S. J. Dawson to son, 11 August 1919, private collection.

49 R. W. Brierley memoir, p. 123, IWM P191; H. Clegg memoir, p. 74, IWM 88/18/1.

50 R. Holmes, *Tommy. The British Soldier on the Western Front 1914–1918* (London: Harper Perennial, 2005), p. 617.
51 C. R. Hennessey memoir, p. 301, IWM 03/31/1. Gwinnell and Taylor tried to join the police after the war, comforted perhaps by the structure and routine, but Gwinnell was rejected due to ill-health and Taylor eventually lost his temper with the drill sergeant and had to resign. Gwinnell memoir, p. 134, IWM 01/38/1; Taylor memoir, np.
52 Hennesey memoir, p. 303.
53 Taylor memoir, n.p.
54 R. W. Brierley memoir, p. 123.
55 P. Thompson and T. Lummis, 'Family Life and Work Experience Before 1918, 1870-1973' [computer file], 5th edition (Colchester: UK Data Archive [distributor], April 2005. SN: 2000), interview 42, p. 79, pp. 3–4.
56 I am grateful to Tom Corless' niece, Mrs Sheila Roome, for this information.
57 I am grateful to Arthur Gibbs' daughter, Mrs Jennifer Keeling, for this information.
58 See Chapter 2, pp. 90–1 for details of Andy's wounding. I am grateful to Ted Nugee, George's son, for this information.
59 Gwinnell memoir, p. 132.
60 Taylor memoir, np. Jack Cornes, who worked for the Great Western Railway, recalled how 'my temper used to fly up' at his civilian workmates. He thought his reaction was typical, for the 'mood of the soldiers returning from the war zones was an angry one.' F. J. Cornes, p. 15, IWM 99/22/1. Anger, and in particular a sense of betrayal by a 'callous society', remarks Robert J. Lifton, is commonly felt by war veterans. He argues that, if not directly enacted as physical violence, anger can be beneficial for the traumatised veteran: it is turned outward, not inwards, in an effort to re-establish psychic integrity. *The Broken Connection*, p. 149.
61 R. West, *The Return of the Soldier* (London: Virago, 1980), pp. 122–3.
62 West, *The Return of the Soldier*, p. 142.
63 G. Di Ceglie, 'Symbol Formation and the Construction of the Inner World', in S. Budd and R. Rushbridger (eds.), *Introducing Psychoanalysis. Essential Themes and Topics* (London: Routledge, 2005), p. 103.
64 See Alison Light on the attractions of home as a retreat, *Forever England. Femininity, Literature and Conservatism Between the Wars* (London: Routledge, 1991), pp. 8–10, p. 211; J. Bourke, *Dismembering the Male. Men's Bodies and the Great War* (London: Reaktion Books, 1996), pp. 168–9.
65 W. Deeping, *No Hero – This* (London: Cassell, 1936), p. 288.
66 S. Koven, 'Remembering and Dismemberment: Crippled Children, Wounded Soldiers and the Great War in Great Britain', *The American Historical Review*, Vol. 99, No. 4 (October 1994), p. 1169. The war, Koven notes, 'bitterly reimposes on wounded male soldiers the dependence, but not the innocence, of childhood' (p. 1171).

67 Winter, *Death's Men*, p. 252; A. Young, 'W. H. R. Rivers and the War Neuroses', *Journal of the History of the Behavioural Sciences*, Vol. 35, No. 4 (Fall 1999), p. 359.
68 P. Leese, 'Problems Returning Home: the British Psychological Casualties of the Great War', *The Historical Journal*, Vol. 40, No. 4 (December 1997), pp. 1060–1.
69 R. M. Luther memoir, p. 46, IWM 87/8/1.
70 C. Asquith, *Diaries 1915–18* (London: Hutchinson, 1968), p. 81, p. 99.
71 Beb is 'just like a querulous old professional invalid complaining of his nurse', writes Cynthia on 9 December 1915. Asquith, *Diaries*, p. 109.
72 Depictions of disabled veterans in American post-war film, Sonia Michel observes, highlight their demands for 'sexual and maternal attention'. S. Michel, 'Danger on the Home Front: Motherhood, Sexuality and Disabled Veterans in American Postwar Films', in M. Cooke and A. Woollacott (eds.), *Gendering War Talk* (Princeton. NJ: Princeton University Press, 1993), p. 262.
73 R. P. Graves, 'Graves, Robert von Ranke', *Oxford Dictionary of National Biography*, http://www.oxforddnb.com/view/printable/3166. Accessed 20 September 2005, p. 2.
74 R. Graves, *Goodbye to All That* (Harmondsworth: Penguin, 1960), pp. 235–6.
75 J. B. Middlebrook to father, 21 July 1916, IWM Con Shelf.
76 Middlebrook memoir, p. 135, IWM Con Shelf.
77 Middlebrook's letters to his father from hospital make it clear that these feelings were mutual: 'She seems anxious to write and also for me to write and she confides in me pretty well.' Middlebrook to father, 5 October 1916.
78 C. G. Templer memoir, p. 25, p. 29, IWM 86/30/1.
79 S. Cloete, *A Victorian Son. An Autobiography* (London: Collins, 1972), p. 295, pp. 298–9.
80 Cloete, *A Victorian Son*, p. 301.
81 Cloete, *A Victorian Son*, pp. 304–7, p. 299.
82 Cloete, *A Victorian Son*, p. 317.
83 Cloete, *A Victorian Son*, p. 306.
84 Templer memoir, p. 43.
85 Thompson and Lummis, 'Family Life and Work', interview 5, p. 37, p. 39.
86 Templer memoir, p. 43.
87 Van Emden and Humphries, *All Quiet on the Home Front*, pp. 306–8.
88 This information was given to me by a participant during a seminar on Trauma and the First World War at the Psychoanalysis and History seminar series, Institute of Historical Research, Spring 2005.
89 Barham, *Forgotten Lunatics*, p. 204, p. 240.
90 Barham, *Forgotten Lunatics*, pp. 352–3, pp. 340–1.
91 These wives needed considerable stamina, notes Deborah Cohen. *The War Come Home: Disabled Veterans in Britain and Germany, 1914–1939* (Berkeley: University of California Press, 2001), p. 107.

92 Barham, *Forgotten Lunatics*, p. 421.
93 Cohen, *The War Come Home*, p. 130.
94 Rosa Maria Bracco, *Merchants of Hope. British Middlebrow Writers and the First World War* (Oxford: Berg, 1993), p. 166.
95 Bracco, *Merchants of Hope*, p. 174; R. Graves and A. Hodge, *The Long Weekend. A Social History of Great Britain 1918–1939* (London: Faber & Faber, 1940), p. 216. Stephen Garton notes that women were often absent from Australian veteran memoirs. The focus on mateship, he argues, was a way of disavowing the family, as if women had played no part in the support of men during the war or in their recuperation afterwards. 'Longing For War: Nostalgia and Australian Returned Soldiers after the First World War', in T. G. Ashplant, G. Dawson and M. Roper (eds.), *The Politics of War Memory and Commemoration* (London: Routledge, 2000), p. 231.
96 Margaret Brown to David Brown, 23 September 1964, pp. 1–3, in papers of J. W. Brown, IWM 01/52/1.
97 Willis Brown to mother, 15 June 1915, papers of J. W. Brown.
98 M. Brown to D. Brown, p. 10.
99 J. W. Brown military service record, 'Record of Services', National Archives, WO 339/13699.
100 M. Brown to D. Brown, pp. 11–12, p. 27. This pattern seems to have continued for much of the rest of Willis' life. After serving in Salonika, Suez and Palestine, he returned home at the end of the war, in his doctor's words, 'thoroughly run down and anaemic'. In the early 1920s he suffered from a bout of 'flu and pneumonia so serious that he had to be nursed at home. After Willis' wife died of TB in the mid-1920s, leaving him in debt, Willis moved back into the family home with his two children. M. Brown to D. Brown, pp. 13–14, p. 21, p. 24.
101 Graves, *Goodbye to All That*, pp. 188–91.
102 R. Aldington, *Death of a Hero* (London: Consul, 1965), p. 13, p. 18.
103 C. Tylee, *The Great War and Women's Consciousness. Images of Militarism and Womanhood in Women's Writings 1914–1964* (Iowa City: University of Iowa Press, 1990), p. 226.
104 Aldington, *Death of a Hero*, p. 5.
105 D. H. Lawrence quoted in J. Ruderman, *D. H. Lawrence and the Devouring Mother* (Durham, NC: Duke University Press, 1984), p. 10.
106 M. Smith, 'The War and British Culture', in S. Constantine, M. W. Kirby and M. B. Rose (eds.), *The First World War in British History* (London: Edward Arnold, 1995), p. 176.
107 Sassoon quoted in M. Egremont, *Siegfried Sassoon. A Biography* (London: Picador, 2005), p. 328.
108 S. Sassoon, *The Complete Memoirs of George Sherston* (London: Faber & Faber, 1972), pp. 450–2.
109 Egremont, *Siegfried Sassoon*, p. 347.

110 S. Sassoon, *To My Mother . . . Drawings by Stephen Tennant* (London: Faber & Gwyer, 1928).

111 Egremont, *Siegfried Sassoon*, p. 331, p. 363, p. 373.

112 Graves, *Goodbye to All That*, p. 31, p. 166.

113 C. C. Miller, 'A Letter from India to my Daughters in England', 1938, p. 2, IWM 83/3/1.

114 Miller to daughters, p. 27.

115 J. Brady memoir, p. 82, IWM 01/36/1.

116 Middlebrook to father, 7 July 1916.

117 H. Owen, *Journey From Obscurity. Wilfred Owen 1893–1918. Vol. III, The War* (Oxford: Oxford University Press, 1965), pp. 137–8.

118 In a letter to his mother after his first experience of battle, Owen writes of how he had to 'crawl, wade, climb and flounder over No Man's Land to visit my other post.' His poem 'The Sentry', begun a year and a half later when Own was at Craiglockhart war hospital, bears a close resemblance to these lines: it describes 'flound'ring about/To other posts under the shrieking air.'; Owen to mother, 16 January 1917, in J. Bell (ed.), *Wilfred Owen. Selected Letters* (Oxford: Oxford University Press, 1985), pp. 213–14; J. Stallworthy (ed.), *The Poems of Wilfred Owen* (London: Chatto & Windus, 1990), pp. 165–6.

119 J. Brady to father, 24 October 1916, IWM 01/36/1.

120 C. Leighton, 'Foreword', in A. Bishop with T. Smart (eds.), *Vera Brittain. War Diary 1913–1917, Chronicle of Youth* (London: Victor Gollancz, 1981), p. 11.

121 In this myth, it was not just the knowledge of horror among mothers on the home front that might be suppressed, but of the nurses who had tended to the wounded and dying at Casualty Clearing Stations and Base Hospitals. Despite the fact that these women had dealt with horrific wounds, they were not perceived to have suffered in the same way as the veteran. On the cultural work of screening mothers from the bloody body, see Carol Acton, 'Bodies Do Count: American Nurses Mourn the Catastrophe of Vietnam', in P. Gray and K. Oliver, *The Memory of Catastrophe* (Manchester: Manchester University Press, 2004), p. 160.

122 S. Audoin-Rouzeau and A. Becker, *1914–1918. Understanding the Great War* (London: Profile Books, 2002), p. 38.

123 Freud, 'Beyond the Pleasure Principle', p. 31.

124 Aldington, *Death of a Hero*, p. 291.

125 Graves, *Goodbye to All That*, p. 98.

126 Graves, *Goodbye to All That*, p. 132, p. 134.

127 Interestingly, it was a book written by a woman, and one who did not have any direct experience of the Western Front, that dared to mire mothers in horror. The journalist Evelyn Price, writing under the pseudonym Helen Zenna Smith, published *Not So Quiet on the Western Front* in the early

1930s. It was a sensationalist account of a woman ambulance driver, based on the diary of Winifred Young, and quickly became a bestseller. The fictional memoir begins with the central character explaining that the 'sordid reality' behind the propaganda of war must be shown to those mothers who, like her own, had publicly supported the war. Smith takes them on a tour of wounded men. These men's injuries, she insists, are not like the childhood illnesses that mothers imagined when they thought of wounded men: 'Let me show you the exhibits – lift your silken skirts aside – a man is spewing blood.' Quoted in C. Tylee, *The Great War and Women's Consciousness*, p. 198.

128 See M. Roper, 'Between Manliness and Masculinity: The "War Generation" and the Psychology of Fear in Britain, 1914–1970', *Journal of British Studies*, Vol. 44, No. 2 (2005) pp. 343–63.

129 Elliot-Smith and Pears quoted in Barham, *Forgotten Lunatics*, p. 153.

130 Barham, *Forgotten Lunatics*, p. 161.

131 Barham, *Forgotten Lunatics*, pp. 221–2.

132 Leland to wife, 19 August, 9 August 1917.

133 J. Cornes, 'The Village and Other Recollections', p. 11, private collection. I am grateful to David Brown for access to these memoirs.

134 Gwinnell memoir, p. 130.

135 G. Chapman, *A Passionate Prodigality. Fragments of Autobiography* (New York: Holt, Rinehart & Winston, 1966), p. 276.

136 Storm Jameson quoted in Tylee, *The Great War and Women's Consciousness*, p. 185.

137 Major Russell sent his ex-batman Leeks a Christmas gift in 1921, and a decade later Leeks wrote a long letter to Russell describing his family and their new life in Canada. Leeks to Russell, 16 January 1921; Leeks to Russell, 9 October 1931, in papers of R. D. Russell, IWM 88/18/1.

138 J. James to Stanley Wootton, 11 May 1920, in papers of S. Wootton, IWM Misc. 207/3002.

139 H. E. Miles, *Untold Tales of War-Time London* (London: Cecil Palmer, 1930), p. 111.

140 E. Leed, *No Man's Land. Combat and Identity in World War I* (Cambridge: Cambridge University Press, 1979), p. 185.

141 Templer memoir, p. 57.

142 Templer memoir, pp. 55–7.

143 Templer memoir, p. 27.

# Epilogue[1]

I am sitting on the garden bench by the kitchen lean-to on a clear spring Melbourne morning, looking out over my grand-parents' back yard towards the carefully tended vegetable patch with its sapling fence, and the lemon tree to the right, relieved on by three generations of Roper boys. My grandfather sits beside me, one arm across my back, the other across my little sister's, and he sings in a soft falsetto, 'Singing Tooral liooral liaddity/Singing Tooral liooral liay/Singing Tooral liooral liaddity/And we're bound for Botany Bay'. My sister and I are taking in the gentle warmth of the sun, nestled close to granddad's chest. Bion's idea of 'reverie' does not quite capture the mood, for this is a memory, not so much of my granddad's receptiveness to our feelings, as of the way his peace of mind, in his serene moments, spread over us too.

It was not always like this. We knew about granddad's war at Gallipoli and the Middle East from an early age. There was the unusual roan horse who hit a broomstick bomb and whose belly fell to the ground whilst he and his rider galloped on for a further 100 yards; the man who collapsed into the arms of a doctor with a bullet through his throat and a beautiful smile on his face; the man taking a break on a tunnelling party, chatting about winners of the Melbourne cup when the broken casing of a French 75 shell came right down the tunnel shaft and hit him. Once he got going my grand-father's stories would spill out one after another. When I was seven or eight I listened from the bedroom as granny ticked him off for telling me his war stories; they would give the boy nightmares. Playing hide-and-seek in the bush with my sister one holiday, granddad offered some advice: I must not peep out to see where my sister was, because if I did she would spot me. For Granddad this was no game, but a lesson in survival.

His life as a veteran had been comfortable after a pretty unpromising start. His father was farm bailiff for the lunatic asylum in Beechworth, a once prosperous gold mining town in rural North-Eastern Victoria, by then in decline. Money did not go far among the family of thirteen, although they never went hungry as there was usually fresh produce about. Granddad had very little of the maternal support that the men in this study counted on. His mother gave birth each year between 1893 and 1896 when granddad was born; the older siblings were not old enough to help with childcare and domestic tasks, and his mother was preoccupied by the seven younger children born between 1897 and 1907. According to him and his sisters, their mother had it in for granddad. She made him walk to school barefoot in the snow when the others were allowed to stay at home.

In 1908, at the age of twelve-and-a-half, granddad left home. He was given lodgings by a storekeeper's wife in Beechworth who got him work on local farms, shooting crows and rabbits. He began to travel further afield, working as a deck boy on coal ships plying the Eastern coast of Australia between Melbourne and Sydney; as a farm boy in the New South Wales outback; as a rouseabout during the shearing season in rural Victoria; and cutting prickly-pear in Queensland. Meanwhile his mother, probably depressed by her debts to local storekeepers, the recent death of her mother and the cumulative exhaustion of childbirth and childrearing, went to live in Melbourne around 1910. The care of the remaining children, the youngest of whom was three, fell to her husband and the elder daughters. Granddad returned to Beechworth for a while, perhaps to help his father out. Whilst back home he studied for a clerical qualification and got an office job in the mental asylum, then took a transfer to the Kew asylum in Melbourne but got fed up with white-collar work and returned to itinerant labouring in the outback. Granddad enlisted near Sydney on 24 April 1915. He was nineteen. The occupation listed on his attestation paper, 'clerk', though not his most recent, was the most respectable of the many he had pursued since leaving school. He was far from the stereotype of the urban British ranker, his pre-war life spent in the bosom of home and neighbourhood.

Granddad reached Gallipoli on 5 August 1915 and was plunged almost immediately into the bombardment that preceded the Battle of Lone Pine, one of the most bloody to be fought on the Peninsula. After going over the top he was directed to a sap and told to guard it and to use the three bodies lying nearby as a barricade. As his memoirs, written in the mid-1970s explain, he 'had a hell of a night. Rifle + machine gun fire, bursting of jam tin bombs + after a few hours trying to keep myself awake. Very lights (our own and enemy) were bursting in the air.' Nobody came to relieve him, and at daybreak when the battle started to get nasty again he was about to run back to their trenches when he was ordered in.[2] As he worked his way back through the trenches he heard his name called out, and he discovered 'Diggs' La Touche, a well-meaning ex-vicar who had signed on as a private and who had kept an eye on them all on the voyage from Australia, lying with blood all over the front of his tunic and in great pain. A machine gun had got him in the abdomen and groin.[3] Later that day granddad was ordered to the parados to throw jam tin bombs at the Turks and some of his mates were injured when the bombs blew up prematurely. After about three hours he was blown down by a small artillery shell and 'when I extricated myself from under three or four bodies my body was covered in blood + guts.'[4] The dead were sometimes scattered two and three deep in the crowded battlefield, wrote the official Australian war historian C. E. W. Bean, and the 'only respect which could be paid them was to avoid treading on their faces.'[5]

On re-grouping after battle, twenty-three of the 150 reinforcements for the 2nd Battalion who had landed 40 hours earlier with granddad answered the roll-call. The others were among the 2,000 Australian and 7,000 Turkish casualties in the five days of fighting.[6] Granddad was overjoyed to spot one of the men with whom he had shared a tent on his first night on the Peninsula, they 'kissed one another and we talked.'[7] He remembers feeling very tired. A Lance Corporal got him some soup and directed him to an open sap where he lay down among the dead. 'I just remember howling [long pause]. I don't know when I got over it; I went to sleep.'[8] Lone Pine was his baptism of fire, and its influence would show itself after the war in his politics, friendships and home life.

Like many in the hot climates of Turkey and the Middle-East, granddad suffered from repeated bouts of ill health including vomiting and diarrhoea, excruciatingly painful boils on his buttocks (granddad's mate Stan Mac could never understand how he managed to sit on his camel with them) and gingivitis; the latter two being associated with poor nutrition and stress. He was admitted to hospital on about a dozen occasions during his overseas service. A slim man on enlisting, five foot ten yet weighing only eight and three quarter stone, he would not have had much nourishment in reserve after three years of war.

Two days before the armistice he was admitted to hospital with malaria. He seems to have continued to suffer from poor health as on 23 March 1920 he was discharged from military service on the grounds of being 'medically unfit'.[9] It was in the twelve months between his disembarkation in Melbourne in early September 1919, and his discharge, that he met my grandmother. Both were working at the Victoria Barracks in Melbourne, my grandmother as a typist and my grandfather as a clerk, finalising the Australian Imperial Force records of the Egypt campaign that he had fought in. This marriage, like so many others, was conceived amid recuperation.

They were anxious to get their own home and start a family, but they waited until October 1923 to marry, when they had saved enough money to put a deposit on a house. Among my grand-father's records is a memorandum for the Inspector-General of the State Bank dated December 1923, setting out the war record which would entitle him to a mortgage at preferential rates. In 1924 their first son Lindsay was born, and my father Stanley in 1926. My grandmother had trouble breastfeeding Stan, and when they finally called the doctor out he found dad dangerously under-nourished. The similarity to granddad's own situation at the end of the war probably compounded the worry.

By then my grandfather was working for the Victorian Railways, beginning as a porter and being promoted to operating porter. He worked twelve-hour shifts but it was a steady job, and they kept a local grocer's chain in eggs and seasonal vegetables, which earned them an extra five bob a week. They didn't spend much money on themselves, mainly on furniture for the house and on going-out clothes for the boys. Granddad recalled proudly that 'they were better dressed than most of the kids in Frankston.' As a shift worker he saw more of his children than most fathers, and after school the boys used to like coming up to the signal box or station to keep him company. With help from granny's family they were able to pay off the house before the Great Depression, when granddads' wages were cut and he was demoted. Many of his veteran mates who became railway men lost their homes then and he could still list their names fifty years later.[10]

Having risen to become Assistant Station Master at Camberwell, a suburban station in Melbourne, granddad retired in 1961. He was a stout man in old age, the consequence of my grandmother's prodigious cooking and baking. The day began with porridge and toast, after morning tea there was a two-course meal at midday which he sometimes returned home from work to eat, and afternoon tea was followed by supper. Granny would cook for him no matter what time his shift, even if it was a 2 a.m. start. Until she had to go into a residential home in her mid-eighties, she would set the table complete with condiments last thing before going to bed. There was a strict division of labour between them. Granddad's job was to bring home the money and granny cooked and cleaned, though he did the washing up and he used to enjoy taking us out into the back garden to throw the scraps of porridge to the birds. The stability of his life with my grandmother – they lived in the same house for almost fifty years – presents a stark contrast to the disruption and dearth of his early years.

Nevertheless the war left its mark. You could see it in granddad's bearing. He wore a uniform for much of his life and his shoes were always mirror-shiny. His hand and arm were scarred from gunshot wounds which he got in Gaza. My father remembers his bouts of malaria, the high fevers that knocked him out for up to a week. He used to have nightmares, which granny found frightening; she would listen out when he talked in his sleep and thought some of it was war stuff. He was prone to angry outbursts and even we grandchildren sometimes trod on eggshells. One afternoon when my father was about five, Lindsay went missing, having told my father that he was going to run away from home. By late evening granny was very worried, and she called my grandfather back from work to look for Lindsay, a decision she would not have taken lightly in the Depression when an unreliable worker was easily replaced. When Lindsay was found curled up asleep in the privet hedge, granddad took a razor strop to him and granny had to get between the two of them. In granddad's experience, loved ones who went missing did not return: his mother had walked out of the family home never to be heard from again, and his best mate 'Spud' Tait never answered roll call after Lone Pine.[11] Unlike those veterans whose anger or madness made them impossible to live with, however, granddad's anger was never so much out of control as to risk the home life he worked so hard to secure.

Mostly his hatred was directed at enemies outside the home: right-wing politicians, class traitors like the Labour 'turncoat' Joe Lyons, and capitalist bosses like Keith Murdoch, whom he had overheard on Frankston station saying to his cronies "Well, gentlemen, we've got the bloody worker now where we want him. *See that we keep him there!*"[12] Granddad thought the war had changed him; he became 'a bit bitter'. He had resented the officers who bossed them around and after the war he transferred that resentment to the bosses. In the war 'we were mates, and we just got the wrong end of the stick. And we learned to hate'.[13] Beside his bed he kept a 'black book' of his officers' misdeeds during the war. Even in old age, on hearing of any injustice, he would fume away at the radio or TV.[14]

His closest mate Stan Mac (whose name my father bore), was less lucky in his home life than granddad. Unbeknown to each other at the time, they had been at opposite ends of the same sap that first night at the Battle of Lone Pine. Granddad thought that might explain 'why we became so pally.'[15] They might have been forgotten by their officers, but they would not let each other down and their hatred of the officer class was mutual. After the war Stan Mac had opted for a life in the bush on a soldier-settlement scheme, running a fruit farm, but they kept in touch and Stan would come and stay whenever he was in Melbourne. The bush life greatly appealed to my grandfather and he was sorely tempted, when Stan Mac's marriage broke up about 1940, to take over the fruit farm, but he was not sure how well granny, a city girl, would take to being away from her family. Yearn as he might for the outback and the freedom of his youth, forfeited so abruptly when he signed up, his wife and children came first. I don't have much memory of Stan Mac, but I do remember the occasions when his returned soldier friends would visit, and would sit in the front room swapping stories, filling up the mother-of-pearl ashtray.

Other traces of granddad's war were less obvious, but apparent to me now. Every winter from the mid-1960s to the early 1970s, he and granny would drive up the East coast of Australia to Queensland for their holidays. Granddad would write a regular supply of the most wonderful letters and postcards to each of his grandchildren, in a slightly arch but elegant style that was largely self-taught. We loved his letters. I suspect that the war showed him the value of letter-writing and honed his skills; he was very pleased after Lone Pine to receive letters from his father, brothers and sisters. Though most of his comrades had a mother and father who kept in touch, granddad's father and his 'Australian eleven' did not let him down.[16] He had kept a diary during the war and he used this as the basis for the war memoirs which he wrote in the early 1970s. I recall him incinerating these diaries after the memoirs were finished; there was some poisonous stuff in them, including descriptions of an attempted mutiny, which he felt were still too dangerous to pass on to posterity.

Shortly before my grandfather's death, when I was the age that he had been when he landed at Gallipoli, I interviewed him about the war for a university oral history project. Listening to that tape twenty-seven years on brings my grand-parents back to me with startling vividness. I can hear my grandmother in the background, whispering to my sister that they should go out and make tea for us. The recording is interspersed with rattles and clanks as the china is laid out. Granny's role is to support granddad's telling of his war story, as she had probably supported his recovery from the war.

Granny interrupts at one point, to explain how she knitted socks and helmets for the men, and stocked billies for their Christmas in 1915, upon which were stuck cardboard images of a kangaroo booting out the Turk from the Peninsula. Granddad remembers these billies too, and in a bitter laugh, remarks that it was the Turks who booted the ANZACs off the peninsula that Christmas ('ANZACs' was the name given during the war to the Australian and New Zealand Army Corps). The chasm between the fronts, in the form of well-intentioned but ignorant civilian support, still animates his memory of the war.

With tea out of the way Granddad suggests starting the story with Gallipoli, but I confound his attempt to organise his recollections in a historical sequence. I can see now what I was after, though I was not clear then: I want his anger about the war on tape, so I suggest that he starts with the Battle of Gaza, when the 'bastard' General Murray stayed behind in Cairo in his hotel 180 miles from the front. I lead him toward the ironic twist. As Murray headed by train for the front after the battle, the hospital train coming the other way was sent to a siding. The wounded lay in open trucks and the dead were being thrown over the side as Murray swept past.

My grand-father's voice is weak and he has trouble with his memory. He knows what he wants to say but often he just can't find the word. Granny, trying to be helpful, chips in with suggestions but these make him all the more frustrated. He will not have his war told by someone who was not there. I listen to his stories and exclaim at one point, all youthful naivety, 'I hope there is never another war.' My grandmother thinks war is not so bad, it gives young men a purpose and gets the unemployed off the streets. Granddad is deeply divided. He says nothing on the tape, but his words run through my mind. 'War is a terrible thing, man's inhumanity to man', he would say, and shake his head. But this did not stop him from trying to sign up for the Second World War. When I was about ten I went with him to a reunion on ANZAC day. Surrounded by his veteran mates near the Shrine of Remembrance in Melbourne, drinking tea, one of them asked me if I would become a soldier. 'Ruddy Salvation Army, more like', granddad quipped. I felt it as a sharp insult; I could never become the man he had been. But it was his views, and his stories, that turned me away from war.

My grandfather's family life and war were unlike the experiences of the men in this study in many respects. He never really forgave his mother and probably would not have cried out for her that night in the sap after Lone Pine. The physical and mental scars of Gallipoli were deep compared even with the Western Front, if those who saw service in both theatres, such as A. P. Herbert, are to be believed. Gratifying as it was to receive letters from his father, sisters and brothers, the news they contained was weeks old. Parcels of shop-bought goods were beyond his family's means, while any food with the taste of home about it would have been well and truly stale by the time it reached him. Men like my grandfather were left largely to their own resources. Not having had their letters home preserved by a mother or other loved one, the war experiences of these men are more likely to be lost to posterity.

If granddad's life up to the end of the war was unusually harsh, afterwards he probably enjoyed greater prosperity in the 'Lucky Country', and contentment in his family, than many British ex-rankers. But despite the differences there are striking similarities. War defined his generation in Australia in the same way it did the British men in this study. Most had felt anxiety which was beyond the capacity of another to calm. Fear, my grandfather wrote, is the 'most painful + horrible malady a human being can suffer from.'[17] Their distress made them angry towards those who should look after them, but it could also bring them close to each other. This book, in giving an account of the care that soldiers received and the care they tried to give each other, has sought to show how it was possible to survive a war unprecedented in the scale of its terror. It pays tribute to the ability of men like my grandfather and their families to love and look after others despite the injuries inflicted on them.

## Notes

1 Information on Robert Henry Roper's family background was compiled from his war memoirs, my father's recollections, and notes taken by me in 1980 while visiting his birthplace, Beechworth. I would particularly like to thank my father, William Stanley Roper, for his long-distance help in this research.

2 Robert Henry Roper, 'Gallipoli memoirs', p. 18.

3 Roper, 'Gallipoli memoirs', p. 19.

4 Roper, 'Gallipoli memoirs', p. 21.
5 Australian War Memorial, 'Lone Pine. Its Place in History, Casualties'; http://dev.links.com.au/diorama/subcat.asp?cat=3&subcat=25. Accessed 31 July 2007.
6 L. Carlyon, *Gallipoli* (Sydney: Macmillan, 2001), p. 357.
7 Robert Henry Roper interview, 'First World War', 1980.
8 Roper interview, 'First World War'.
9 14th Light Horse Regiment Casualty Form – Active Service; 'Memorandum for the Inspector-General, State Savings Bank, Melbourne', both from National Archives of Australia, Defence Records B2455, Roper R. 2198.
10 Robert Henry Roper interview, 'The Depression', 1980.
11 My grandfather did not re-establish contact with his mother until the 1950s.
12 Roper interview, 'The Depression'. Joe Lyons resigned from the Australian Labour Party in January 1931 to set up a rival party, the Australian United Party, of which he became leader.
13 Quoted in M. Roper, 'Memories of a Depression', *Melbourne Historical Journal*, Vol. 9 (1982), p. 25.
14 My grandfather's story fits with the analysis of Alistair Thomson, who notes how some Australian veterans developed a radical critique of the war as an imperialist project, substituting the militant worker for the rebellious digger, *Anzac Memories. Living With the Legend* (Melbourne: Oxford University Press, 1994, p. 171.
15 Roper interview, 'First World War'.
16 Roper 'Gallipoli memoirs', p. 32.
17 Roper 'Gallipoli memoirs', p. 15.

# Bibliography

## Primary sources

### *Letters and diaries*

*Imperial War Museum*

*Note*: Rank is given where known, and relates to dates of letters used rather than to final rank.

Anderton, E. H., letters to mother, 88/20/1

Arnold, A. J., letters to and from mother and sister, Con Shelf

Baker, A. G., letters to parents; to and from sister; condolence, 01/6/1

Best, Lieut. O. H., letters to family; mother's notes, 87/56/1

Bowser, Lieut. H. F., letters to mother and father, 88/56/1

Brown, S. E., letters to mother, 89/7/1

Burke, A., letters to family, Con Shelf

Buxton, B. G., letters to parents; aunt, 78/60/3

Carter, H., letters to and from parents; from sisters, 86/8/1

Chapman, B. F. J., letters to mother, brothers and sisters, 98/17/1

Chapman, 2nd Lieut. E. F. letters to mother and sisters, Con Shelf; 92/3/1

Christopher, W. C. and R., letters from brothers to mother and sisters, 88/11/1

Clarke, J. A. C., letters to family; from mother; photos; condolence 96/57/1

Connor, Rev. J. M., diary, 87/10/1

Corless, T., letters to grandmother and aunt, 81/13/1

Fenton, D. H., letters to father and brother; condolence, 87/13/1

Foulkes, Capt. R., letters to mother, 82/4/1

Gibbs, Capt. A., letters to mother and father, P317

Goodwin, W. A., letters to and from mother and father, Con Shelf

Hague, 2nd Lieut H. W., letters to mother and father, 98/33/1

Hall, 2nd Lieut. L., letters to mother and father, 96/57/1
Hannam, Capt. C. D., letters from batman, Misc. 8/165
Hate, W. T., letters to mother; diary, 86/51/1
Higginson, A., condolence letters, 95/1/1
Holroyd, Lieut. M., letters to parents, 97/37/1
Hoyle, W., letters from mother, 85/22/1
Hubbard, A. H., letters to mother and father, brothers, sisters, Con Shelf
Hutt, 2nd Lieut. E. R., letters to mother and father; condolence, 90/7/1; 90/7/1A
Knight, A., letters to and from mother; from sister, Con Shelf
Leland, Captain H. J. C., letters to wife, 96/51/1
'Ma' to 'My dear Sid', letters to son, Misc. 216
Marchant, E., letters to mother, father and sisters, DS/MISC/26
Mercer, 2nd Lieut. E. C., letters to and from mother; condolence. 92/52/1
Merivale, J. H., diary of Miss B. Merivale (aunt); letters of Jack, Vernon and Frank Merivale to family, P471
Middlebrook, J. B., letters to mother, father and sister, Con Shelf
Mountfort, R. D., letters to mother, father, sister, Con Shelf
Munro, Lieut. H. A., diary, P374
Nightingale, Capt. G. W., letters to mother and sister. P216
Nugee, G. T., diary of Edith Nugee, mother, 77/102/1
Parry-Okeden, Rev. C. E., letters; diary, 90/7/1
Payne, 2nd Lieut. H. S., letters to mother and sister; condolence, 90/1/1
Poole, E. J., letters to father and sister, 82/11/1
Ramsdale, C. W., letters to mother and sister, Con Shelf
Robinson, M., diary, 96/7/1
Russell, N. R., letters to mother and family, 01/21/1
Russell, Major R. D., letters from batman, 88/18/1
Savours, Lieut. H. J., letters to mother and father; from mother, PP/MCR/327
Smith, P., letter to parents, 01/21/1
Spencer, Lieut. W. B. P., letters to mother, father and sister, 87/56/1
Standrick, Capt. J. H., letters from mother; condolence, 96/23/1
Steavenson, Lieut. A. G., letters from mother, 86/77/1
Swettenham, A. H., letters to mother and brother, 83/31/1
Synge, Capt. R. M., letters to Lieut. R. Leverson-Gower from batman, 99/15/1
Taylor, Capt. N. A., letters to sisters, step-mother and father, 90/28/1
Thompson, Lieut. A., letters to mother from friends, 79/55/1
Timpson, L., diary, 92/3/1
Thorpe, T., letters to mother, father and sister, Con Shelf
Tomlinson, J. D., letters to mother and brother; condolence, 87/51/1
Unidentified London lady, diary, Misc. 29/522

Webb, M., letters to mother and father, 90/28/1

Wollocombe, 2nd Lieut. F., letters to mother and father; diaries, 95/33/1

Woodroffe, 2nd Lieut. N., letters to and from mother; condolence, 95/31/1

Wooton, S., letter from batman, Misc. 207/3002

*Liddle collection (1914–18) (Leeds University Library)*

Hooper, A., 2nd Lieut. (son), letters to brother; mother and father, GS0793

Hooper, K., Lieut. (son), letters to mother and father; diary, POW 036

Hooper, L. (mother), letters to K. Hooper (POW), DF066

McLeod, I., letters to Capt. N. M. McLeod from mother and wife, DF088

*Other collections*

The Bickersteth War Diaries and the Papers of John Burgon Bickersteth; diary and letters from sons. Churchill Archives Centre, GBR/0014/BICK

Dawson, Mrs S. J., letters to son, private collection

Stephens, Mrs E. D., correspondence of the Rifle Brigade Comfort Fund, condolence. National Army Museum, 8902–201–1043 to 1396

Trench, Capt. R. C., letters to mother, private collection

Tynan, K., correspondence and notes of, Tynan/Hinkson collection, John Rylands University Library of Manchester

Urwick, 2nd Lieut. L. F., letters to and from mother and father; 1914 diary of Henry Urwick, private collection

William, P. E., letters to mother, private collection

Wills, W. M., diary 1914–19, John Rylands University Library of Manchester

### *Unpublished memoirs and other retrospective sources*

*Imperial War Museum*

Bowser, Lieut. H. F., memoir, 88/56/1

Brady, J., memoir, 01/36/1

Brierley, R. W., memoir, P191

Brown, 2nd Lieut J. W., letter to Brown's son from his aunt, 01/52/1

Carpenter, Capt. A. G., photograph, 76/184/1

Clegg, H., memoir, 88/18/1

Cornes, F. J., memoir, 99/22/1

Fortune, G., memoir, 04/5/1

Gwinnell, R., memoir, 01/38/1

Harrison, E. J., memoir, 78/11/1

Hennesey, C. R., memoir, 03/31/1

Luther, R. M., memoir, 87/8/1

Middlebrook, J. B., memoir, Con Shelf

Miller, Capt. C. C., letter to daughters, 83/3/1

Starrett, D., memoir, 79/35/1

Taylor, C. W., memoir, 01/8/1
Templer, C. G., memoir, 86/30/1

*Other collections*

Cornes, J., 'The Village and Other Recollections', private collection
Roper, R. H., Memoir of Gallipoli, early 1970s, in author's possession
Roper R. H., Memoir of Egypt and Palestine, early 1970s, in author's possession
Roper R. H. interview, 'First World War', interviewed by M. Roper, 1980, in author's possession
Roper R. H. interview, 'The Depression', interviewed by M. Roper, 1980, in author's possession
Thompson, P. and T. Lummis, 'Family Life and Work Experience Before 1918, 1870-1973' [computer file], 5th edition (Colchester: UK Data Archive [distributor], April 2005. SN: 2000)
Urwick, L., 'Apprenticeship to Management. An Autobiography of Lt. Col. L. F. Urwick', 1970, private collection

*Military records*

*National Archives*

Brown, 2nd Lieut. J. W., Military Service Records, WO 339/13699
Leland, Capt. H. J. C., Military Service Records, WO 374/41657
Smith, 2nd Lieut. E. K., Military Service Records, WO 339/35618
War Diary of the 10th Battalion Royal Fusiliers, WO 95/2532
War Diary of 1st Battalion, The Buffs, WO 95/1608

*Imperial War Museum*

Company Roll Book, Capt. J. A. Bell, 1 Platoon, 'A' Coy, 7th Durham Light Infantry Reg't, April 1915, IWM 83/50/1
Section or Platoon Roll Book, 'D' Coy 8th Northamptonshire Reg't, 1916, IWM Misc. 60/911

**Published primary sources**

*Letters, diaries and other contemporary sources*

Asquith, C., *Diaries 1915–18* (London: Hutchinson, 1968)
Barbusse, H., *Under Fire* (London: Penguin, 2003)
Bell, J. (ed.), *Wilfred Owen. Selected Letters* (Oxford: Oxford University Press, 1985)
Bickersteth, J. (ed.), *The Bickersteth Diaries 1914–1918* (London: Leo Cooper, 1995)
Bishop, A. and M. Bostridge (eds.), *Letters From a Lost Generation. First World War Letters of Vera Brittain and Four Friends* (London: Abacus, 1999)

Bishop, A. with T. Smart (eds.), *Vera Brittain. War Diary 1913–1917, Chronicle of Youth* (London: Victor Gollancz, 1981)
Brophy, J. and E. Partridge (eds.), *The Long Trail. Soldiers' Songs & Slang 1914–18* (London: Sphere Books, 1969)
Carthew, N., *Voices from Trenches. Letters to Home* (Sydney: New Holland, 2002)
Churchill, Lady R. (ed.), *Women's War Work* (London: Arthur Pearson, 1916)
Clark, A., *Echoes of the Great War* (Oxford: Oxford University Press, 1985)
Drumont, Mme E., *A French Mother in War Time. Being the Journal of Madame Edouard Drumont* (London: Edward Arnold, 1916)
Greenwell, G., *An Infant in Arms. War Letters of a Company Commander 1914–1918* (London: Allen Lane, The Penguin Press, 1972)
Hankey, D., *A Student in Arms* (London: Andrew Melrose, 1917)
Hart-Davis, R. (ed.), *Siegfried Sassoon Diaries 1915–1918* (London: Faber & Faber, 1983)
Loane, M., *The Queen's Poor. Life as They Find it in Town and Country* (London: Middlesex University Press, 1998)
McDougall, W., 'Four Cases of "Regression" in Soldiers', *Journal of Abnormal Psychology*, Vol. 15 (1920–21), pp. 136–56
Nesham, F. (ed.), *Socks, Cigarettes and Shipwrecks. A Family's War Letters 1914–1918* (Gloucester: Alan Sutton, 1987)
Raemaekers, L., *The Great War. A Neutral's Indictment: One Hundred Cartoons* (London: Fine Art Society, 1916)
Reilly, C. (ed.), *Scars Upon My Heart. Women's Poetry & Verse of the First World War* (London: Virago, 1981)
Rivers, W. H. R., *Instinct and the Unconscious. A Contribution to a Biological Theory of the Psycho-Neuroses* (Cambridge: Cambridge University Press, 1920)
Rivers, W. H. R., *Conflict and Dream* (New York: Harcourt, Brace & Co., 1923)
Sassoon, S., *Siegfried Sassoon. The War Poems* (London: Faber & Faber, 1983)
Smith, E. K., *Letters Sent From France. Service with the Artists' Rifles and the Buffs, December 1914–December 1915* (London: J. Cobb, 1994)
Smith, G.E. and T. H. Pear, *Shell Shock and its Lessons* (Manchester: Manchester University Press, 1917)
Stallworthy, J. (ed.), *The Poems of Wilfred Owen* (London: Chatto & Windus, 1990)

*Memoirs, fiction and other retrospective sources*

Aldington, R., *Death of a Hero* (London: Consul, 1965)
Bion, W. R., *The Long Weekend 1897–1919. Part of a Life* (London: Free Association Books, 1986)
Bion, W. R., *War Memoirs 1917–19* (London: H. Karnac, 1997)
Bion, W. R., *All My Sins Remembered. Another Part of a Life and the Other Side of Genius. Family Letters* (London: H. Karnac, 1991)

Blunden, E., *Undertones of War* (London: Penguin, 2000)
Brittain, V., *Testament of Youth. An Autobiographical Study of the Years 1900–1925* (London: Virago, 1978)
Carrington, C., *Soldier From the Wars Returning* (London: Arrow Books, 1965)
Chapman, G., *A Passionate Prodigality. Fragments of Autobiography* (New York: Holt, Rinehart & Winston, 1966)
Church, R., *Over the Bridge. An Essay in Autobiography* (London: William Heinemann, 1955)
Cloete, S., *A Victorian Son. An Autobiography* (London: Collins, 1972)
Coppard, G., *With A Machine Gun to Cambrai. A Story of the First World War* (London: Cassell, 1980)
Crozier, F. P., Brig.-Gen., *A Brass Hat in No Man's Land* (London: Jonathan Cape, 1930)
Deeping, W., *No Hero – This* (London: Cassell, 1936)
Deeping, W., *Sorrell and Son* (London: Cassell, 1926)
Dunn, J. C. (ed.), *The War the Infantry Knew. A Chronicle of Service in France and Belgium* (London: Abacus, 1994)
Eden, A., *Another World 1897–1917* (London: Allen Lane, 1976)
Edmonds, C. (C. E. Carrington), *A Subaltern's War* (London: Anthony Mott, 1984)
Frankau, G., *Peter Jackson. Cigar Merchant* (London: Hutchinson & Co., 1922)
Fraser, R., *In Search of a Past. The Manor House, Amnersfield, 1933–1945* (London: Verso, 1984)
Fussell, P. (ed.), *The Ordeal of Alfred M. Hale. The Memoirs of a Soldier Servant* (London: Leo Cooper, 1975)
Gladden, N., *Ypres 1917* (London: William Kimber, 1967)
Graves, R., *Goodbye to All That* (Harmondsworth: Penguin, 1960)
Graves, R. and A. Hodge, *The Long Weekend. A Social History of Great Britain 1918–1939* (London: Faber & Faber, 1940)
Herbert, A. P., *A. P. H. His Life and Times* (London: Heinemann, 1970)
Herbert, A. P., *The Secret Battle* (Thirsk: House of Stratus, 2001)
Hewins, A. (ed.), *The Dillen. Memories of a Man of Stratford upon Avon* (Oxford: Oxford University Press, 1983)
Higgonet, M. (ed.), *Nurses at the Front. Writing the Wounds of the Great War* (Boston: Northeastern University Press, 2001)
Manning, F., *Her Privates We* (London: Serpent's Tail, 1999)
Miles, H. E., *Untold Tales of War-Time London* (London: Cecil Palmer, 1930)
Montague, C. E., *Disenchantment* (London: MacGibbon & Kee, 1968)
Moran, C., *The Anatomy of Courage* (London: Constable, 1945)
Mottram, R. H., *The Spanish Farm Trilogy 1914–1918* (Harmondsworth: Penguin, 1979)
Myers, C. S., *Shell Shock in France 1914–18* (Cambridge: Cambridge University Press, 1940)

Noakes, F. E., *The Distant Drum. The Personal History of a Guardsman in the Great War* (Tunbridge Wells: npub, 1952)

Owen, H. *Journey From Obscurity. Wilfred Owen 1893–1918. Vols I–III* (Oxford: Oxford University Press, 1965)

Peel, C. S., *How We Lived Then. 1914–1918. A Sketch of Social and Domestic Life in England During the War* (London: Bodley Head, 1929)

Reeves, M. P., *Round About a Pound a Week* (London: Virago, 1979)

Remarque, E. M., *All Quiet on the Western Front* (London: Vintage, 1996)

Richards, F., *Old Soldiers Never Die* (Uckfield: Naval and Military Press, 1994)

Roberts, R., *The Classic Slum. Salford Life in the First Quarter of the Century* (Harmondsworth: Penguin, 1971)

Sassoon, S., *The Complete Memoirs of George Sherston* (London: Faber & Faber, 1972)

Sassoon, S., *To My Mother . . . Drawings by Stephen Tennant* (London: Faber and Gwyer, 1928)

Sassoon, S., *The Old Century and Seven More Years* (London: Faber and Faber, 1937)

Sherriff, R. C., *Journey's End* (London: Heinemann, 1981)

Smith, H. Z., *Not So Quiet . . . Stepdaughters of War* (New York: Feminist Press, 1989)

Vaughan, E. C., *Some Desperate Glory. The Diary of a Young Officer 1917* (London: Leo Cooper, 1987)

West, R., *The Return of the Soldier* (London: Virago, 1980)

## *Memorial books*

Anon., *Boy of My Heart* (London: Hodder & Stoughton, 1916)

Charteris, M. C. W., *A Family Record* (London: Curwen Press, 1932)

Lubbock, A. A., *Eric Fox Pitt Lubbock, born 16th May 1893. Killed in Aerial Fight Near Ypres, 11th March 1917. A Memoir by his Mother* (London: A. L. Humphries, 1918)

Makeham, E. N., *These to his Memory. A Selection in Prose and Verse from the Writings of Eric Noel Makeham* (London: Finden Brown, 1917)

Mayo, W. C., *In Memoriam. William Charles Mayo* (Sherborne: Sawtell, 1916)

Murray, A. R., *In Memoriam. Alexander Roxburgh Murray* (npub, nd)

Parry, H., *In Memoriam: Harold Parry, Second Lieutenant, K.R.R.C.: Born at Bloxwich – December 13th, 1896. Fell in Flanders – May 6th, 1917* (London: W.H. Smith, n.d.)

Sanders, L., *A Soldier of England. Memorials of Leslie Yorath Sanders* (Dumfries: J. Maxwell, 1917)

Scott, J. M., *In Memoriam. Poems and Letters, With Two Sermons by the Late John Millar Scott* (Alloa: Buchan Bros, 1917)

Smith, E. and A., *Two Brothers. Eric and Arnold Miall Smith* (Edinburgh: Constable, 1918)
Talbot, G., *Gilbert Walter Lyttleton Talbot. Born September 1 1891. Killed in Action at Hooge, July 30 1915* (London: Chiswick Press, 1916)

### *Military sources*

'Basilisk', *Talks on Leadership Addressed to Young Artillery Officers* (London: Hugh Rees, 1921)
Hood, Capt. B., *Duties For All Ranks. Specially Compiled For the New Armies and Volunteer Training Corps from the C O. to the Private* (London: Harrison & Sons, 1915)
'Regular', *Customs of the Army. A Guide for Cadets and Young Offficers* (London: Harrison & Sons, 1917)
*Statistics of the Military Effort of the British Empire during the Great War, 1914–1920* (London: War Office, HMSO, 1922)
Trapmann, Capt. A. H., *Straight Tips for "Subs"* (London: Forester Groom, 1916)
War Office, Directorate of Graves Registration and Enquiries, *The Care of the Dead. An Account of the Work of the Directorate of Graves Enquiries* (London: Eyre & Spottiswoode, 1916)
War Office, General Staff, *British Trench Warfare 1917–1918. A Reference Manual* (London: Imperial War Museum Department of Printed Books in association with the Battery Press, 1997)
War Office, General Staff Censorship and Publicity Section, 'Censorship Orders For Troops in the Field' (London: Censorship and Publicity Section, General Staff, 1918)
War Office, General Staff Censorship and Publicity Section, 'Lecture on the Postal Censorship Orders' (London: Censorship and Publicity Section, General Staff, 1918)

## Secondary sources

Acton, C., 'Writing and Waiting: The First World War Correspondence between Vera Brittain and Roland Leighton', *Gender and History,* Vol. 11, No. 1 (April 1999), pp. 54–83
Acton, C., 'Bodies Do Count: American Nurses Mourn the Catastrophe of Vietnam', in P. Gray and K. Oliver, *The Memory of Catastrophe* (Manchester: Manchester University Press, 2004), pp. 158–71
Acton, C., *Grief in Wartime. Private Pain, Public Discourse* (Basingstoke: Palgrave, 2007)
Ashworth, T., *Trench Warfare 1914-1918. The Live and Let Live System* (London: Macmillan, 1980)

Audoin-Rouzeau, S., *Men at War 1914–1918. National Sentiment and Trench Journalism in France during the First World War* (Oxford: Berg, 1995)

Audoin-Rouzeau, S. and A. Becker, *1914–1918. Understanding the Great War* (London: Profile Books, 2002)

Barham, P., *Forgotten Lunatics of the Great War* (New Haven: Yale University Press, 2004)

Barker, P., *Regeneration* (Harmondsworth: Penguin, 1992)

Beckett, I., 'The British Army 1914–18: The Illusion of Change', in J. Turner, *Britain and the First World War* (London: Unwin Hyman, 1988)

Beckett, I., *Home Front, 1914–1918. How Britain Survived the Great War* (Kew: The National Archives, 2006)

Berkeley, R. S., W. W. Seymour, T. R. Eastwood and H. G. Parkyn, *The History of the Rifle Brigade in the War of 1914–1918* , 3 vols. (London: The Rifle Brigade Club, 1927–36)

Bet-El, I., *Conscripts. Forgotten Men of the Great War* (Stroud: Sutton Publishing, 2003)

Bick, E., 'The Experience of the Skin in Early Object Relations', in A. Briggs (ed), *Surviving Space. Papers on Infant Observation* (London: H. Karnac, 2002), pp. 55–9

Bick, E., 'Further Considerations on the Function of the Skin in Early Object Relations', in A. Briggs, (ed.), *Surviving Space. Papers on Infant Observation* (London: H. Karnac, 2002), pp. 60–71

Bion, W. R., 'Attacks on Linking', in W. R. Bion, *Second Thoughts. Selected Papers on Psychoanalysis* (London: H. Karnac, 1987), pp. 93–110

Bion, W. R., 'Development of Schizophrenic Thought', in W. R. Bion, *Second Thoughts. Selected Papers on Psychoanalysis* (London: H. Karnac, 1987), pp. 36–43

Bion, W. R., *Learning From Experience* (London: H. Karnac, 1991)

Bion, W. R., 'Notes on the Theory of Schizophrenia', in W. R. Bion, *Second Thoughts. Selected Papers on Psychoanalysis* (London: H. Karnac, 1987), pp. 23–36

Bion, W. R., 'A Theory of Thinking', in W. R. Bion, *Second Thoughts. Selected Papers on Psychoanalysis* (London: H. Karnac, 1987), pp. 110–20

Bion, W. R., "The War of Nerves": Civilian Reaction, Morale and Prophylaxis', in E. Miller (ed.), *The Neuroses in War* (London: Macmillan, 1940), pp. 180–200

Bond, B., *The Unquiet Western Front. Britain's Role in Literature and History* (Cambridge: Cambridge University Press, 2002)

Booth, A., *Postcards From the Trenches. Negotiating the Space between Modernism and the First World War* (Oxford: Oxford University Press, 1995)

Bourke, J., *Dismembering the Male. Men's Bodies and the Great War* (London: Reaktion Books, 1996)

Bourke, J., *An Intimate History of Killing. Face-To-Face Killing in Twentieth-Century Warfare* (London: Granta Books, 1999)

Bourke, J., 'In the Presence of Mine Enemies: Face-to-Face Killing in Twentieth Century Warfare', www.history.ac.uk/eseminars/sem21.html. Accessed 2 October 2006, pp. 1–17

Bourke, J., *Fear. A Cultural History* (London: Virago, 2005)

Bourne, J., *Britain and the Great War* (London: Edward Arnold, 1989)

Bourne, J., 'The British Working Man in Arms', in H. Cecil and P. Liddle, *Facing Armageddon. The First World War Experienced* (London: Pen & Sword, 1996), pp. 336–52

Boyden, P. B., *Tommy Atkins' Letters. The History of the British Army Postal Service From 1795* (London: National Army Museum, 1990)

Bracco, R. M., *Merchants of Hope. British Middlebrow Writers and the First World War* (Oxford: Berg, 1993)

Briggs, A., 'The Life and Work of Esther Bick', in A. Briggs (ed.), *Surviving Space. Papers on Infant Observation* (London: H. Karnac, 2002), pp. 1–23

Britton, R., *Belief and Imagination. Explorations in Psychoanalysis* (London: Routledge, 1998)

Brown, M., *The Imperial War Museum Book of the Western Front* (London: Pan, 2001)

Brown, M., *Tommy Goes to War* (Stroud: Tempus, 2005)

Buettner, E., *Empire Families. Britons and Late Imperial India* (Oxford: Oxford University Press, 2004)

Burnett, J., *Plenty and Want: A Social History of Diet in England from 1815 to the Present Day* (London: Scolar Press, 1979)

Burnett, J. (ed.), *Destiny Obscure. Autobiographies of Childhood, Education and Family from the l820s to the l920s* (London: Allen Lane, 1982)

Burnett, J., *A Social History of Housing, 1815–1985* (London: Methuen, 1986)

Caesar, A., *Taking It Like a Man. Suffering, Sexuality and the War Poets* (Manchester: Manchester University Press, 1994)

Caine, B., *Destined to be Wives. The Sisters of Beatrice Webb* (Oxford: Oxford University Press, 1988)

Campbell, P. *Siegfried Sassoon. A Study of the War Poetry* (Jefferson, NC: McFarland & Co., 1999)

Cannadine, D., 'War and Death, Grief and Mourning in Modern Britain', in J. Whaley (ed.), *Mirrors of Mortality. Studies in the Social History of Death* (London: Europa Publications, 1981), pp. 187–242

Carlyon, L., *Gallipoli* (Sydney: Macmillan, 2001)

Chamberlain, M. and R. Richardson, 'Life and Death', *Oral History*, Vol. 11, No. 1 (1983), pp. 31–43

Cohen, D., *The War Come Home: Disabled Veterans in Britain and Germany, 1914–1939* (Berkeley: University of California Press, 2001)

Cole, S., *Modernism, Male Friendship and the First World War* (Cambridge: Cambridge University Press, 2003)

Collini, S., *Public Moralists. Political Thought and Intellectual Life in Modern Britain* (Oxford: Clarendon, 1993)

Copelman, D. M., '"A New Comradeship Between Men and Women": Family, Marriage and London's Women Teachers 1870–1914', in J. Lewis (ed.), *Labour and Love. Women's Experience of Home and Family 1850–1940* (Oxford: Blackwell, 1986), pp. 175–95

Crossick, G., 'The Emergence of the Lower Middle Class in Britain': A Discussion', in G. Crossick (ed.), *The Lower Middle Class in Britain, 1870–1914* (London: Croom Helm, 1977), pp. 11–60

Damousi, J., *The Labour of Loss. Mourning, Memory and Wartime Bereavement in Australia* (Cambridge: Cambridge University Press, 1999)

Damousi, J., *Living With the Aftermath. Trauma, Nostalgia and Grief in Post-War Australia* (Cambridge: Cambridge University Press, 2001)

Das, S., *Touch and Intimacy in First World War Literature* (Cambridge: Cambridge University Press, 2005)

Davidoff, L., *Worlds Between. Historical Perspectives on Gender and Class* (Cambridge: Polity Press, 1995)

Davin, A., *Growing Up Poor. Home, School and Street in London, 1870–1914* (London: Rivers Oram Press)

Di Ceglie, G., 'Symbol Formation and the Construction of the Inner World', in S. Budd and R. Rushbridger (eds.), *Introducing Psychoanalysis. Essential Themes and Topics* (London: Routledge, 2005), pp. 95–105

De Groot, G. J., *The First World War* (Basingstoke: Palgrave, 2001)

Duffett, R., 'A War Unimagined: Food and the Rank and File Soldier of the First World War', in J. Meyer (ed.), *Popular Culture and the First World War* (Leiden: Brill, 2007)

Dyehouse, C., 'Mothers and Daughters in the Middle-Class Home c. 1870–1914', in J. Lewis (ed.), *Labour and Love. Women's Experience of Home and Family 1850–1940* (Oxford: Blackwell, 1986), pp. 27–49

Earle, R., 'Introduction: Letters, Writers and the Historian', in R. Earle (ed.), *Epistolary Selves. Letters and Letter-Writers, 1600–1945* (Aldershot: Ashgate, 1999), pp. 1–15

Egremont, M., *Siegfried Sassoon. A Biography* (London: Picador, 2005)

Ellis, J., *Eye Deep in Hell. Trench Warfare in World War I* (Baltimore: Johns Hopkins University Press, 1976)

Englander, D., 'Soldiering and Identity: Reflections on the Great War', *War in History*, Vol. 1, No. 3, pp. 300–18

Ferguson, N., *The Pity of War* (London: Penguin, 1998)

Fitzpatrick, D., *Oceans of Consolation. Personal Accounts of Irish Migration to Australia* (Cork: Cork University Press, 1994)

Fletcher, A., 'An Officer on the Western Front', *History Today*, Vol. 54, No. 8 (August 2004), pp. 31–7

Fletcher, A., 'Patriotism, Identity and Commemoration: New Light on the Great War from the Papers of Major Reggie Chenevix Trench', *History*, Vol. 90, No. 300 (October 2005), pp. 532–49

Frances, M., 'The Domestication of the Male? Recent Research on Nineteenth and Twentieth-Century British Masculinity', *The Historical Journal*, Vol. 45, No. 3 (2002), pp. 637–52

Freud, S., 'Beyond the Pleasure Principle', *The Standard Edition of the Complete Psychological Works of Sigmund Freud* tr. J. Strachey, Vol. 18 (London: Vintage, 2001), pp. 7–64

Freud, S., 'Family Romances', *The Standard Edition of the Complete Psychological Works of Sigmund Freud*, tr. J. Strachey, Vol. 9 (London: Vintage, 2001), pp. 235–41

Freud, S., 'Mourning and Melancholia', *The Standard Edition of the Complete Psychological Works of Sigmund Freud*, tr. J. Strachey, Vol. 14 (London: Vintage, 2001) pp. 243–59

Freud, S., 'Thoughts for the Times on War and Death', *The Standard Edition of the Complete Psychological Works of Sigmund Freud*, tr. J. Strachey, Vol. 14 (London: Vintage, 2001), pp. 273–302

Fuller, J. G., *Troop Morale and Popular Culture in the British and Dominion Armies* (Oxford: Clarendon Press, 1991)

Fussell, P., *The Great War and Modern Memory* (Oxford: Oxford University Press, 1975)

Garland, C. (ed.), *Understanding Trauma. A Psychoanalytical Approach* (London: H. Karnac, 2002)

Garton, S., 'Longing For War: Nostalgia and Australian Returned Soldiers after the First World War', in T. G. Ashplant, G. Dawson and M. Roper (eds.), *The Politics of War Memory and Commemoration* (London: Routledge, 2000), pp. 222–40

Gathorne-Hardy, J., *The Rise and Fall of the British Nanny* (London: Arrow, 1972)

Gillis, J. R., *A World of Their Own Making. Myth, Ritual and the Quest for Family Values* (New York: Basic Books, 1996)

Grayzel, S., *Women's Identities at War. Gender, Motherhood and Politics in Britain and France during the First World War* (Chapel Hill, NC: University of North Carolina Press, 1999)

Gregory, A., *The Silence of Memory. Armistice Day 1919–1946* (Oxford: Berg, 1994)

Grieves, K. (ed.), *Sussex in the First World War* (Lewes: Sussex Record Society, 2004)

Grotstein, J., 'Towards the Concept of the Transcendent Position: Reflections on some of "The Unborns" in Bion's "Cogitations"', *The Journal of Melanie Klein and Object Relations*, Vol. 11, No. 2 (1993), pp. 55–73

Gullace, N., *The Blood of Our Sons. Men, Women and the Renegotiation of British Citizenship in the Great War* (Basingstoke, Hamps.: Palgrave, 2002)

Hagermann, K., 'Home/Front: The Military, Violence and Gender Relations in the Age of the World Wars', in K. Hagermann and S. Schüler-Springorum (eds.), *The Home Front. The Military, War and Gender in Twentieth-Century Germany* (Oxford: Berg, 2002)

Hämmerle, C., '"You Let a Weeping Woman Call you Home?": Private Correspondences During the First World War in Austria and Germany', in R. Earle (ed.), *Epistolary Selves. Letters and Letter-Writers, 1600–1945* (Aldershot: Ashgate, 1999), pp. 152–82

Hammerton, J., 'Pooterism or Partnership? Marriage and Masculine Identity in the Lower Middle Class, 1870–1920', *The Journal of British Studies*, Vol. 38, No. 3 (July 1999), pp. 291–321

Hanna, M., 'A Republic of Letters: The Epistolary Tradition in France during World War I', *The American Historical Review* Vol. 108, No. 5 (2003), www.historycooperative.org/journals/ahr/108.5/hanna.html. Accessed 25 May 2007

Harrison, T., *Bion, Rickman, Foulkes and the Northfield Experiments* (London: Jessica Kingsley, 2000)

Hartley, J., '"Letters are Everything These Days": Mothers and Letters in the Second World War', in Earle, R. (ed.), *Epistolary Selves. Letters and Letter-Writers, 1600–1945* (Aldershot: Ashgate, 1999), pp. 183–224

Hendrick, H., *Children, Childhood and English society 1880–1990* (Cambridge: Cambridge University Press, 1997)

Hibberd, D., *Wilfred Owen. A New Biography* (London: Weidenfeld & Nicolson, 2002)

Hibberd, D. *Wilfred Owen. The Last Year* (London: Constable, 1992)

Hibberd, D. (ed.), *Poetry of the First World War. A Casebook* (London: Macmillan, 1981)

Hinshelwood, R. D., *A Dictionary of Kleinian Thought* (London: Free Association, 1991)

Hinshelwood, R. D., 'The Elusive Concept of "Internal Objects" (1934–1943). Its Role in the Formation of the Klein Group', *International Journal of* Psychoanalysis, Vol. 78 (1997), pp. 877–97

Holmes, R., *Tommy. The British Soldier on the Western Front 1914–1918* (London: Harper Perennial, 2005)

Holt, T., *Major and Mrs Holt's Battlefield Guide to the Somme* (London: Leo Cooper, 1996)

Holt, T. and V., *'My Boy Jack'. The Search for Kipling's Only Son* (London: Pen & Sword, 1998)

Horne, J., 'Soldiers, Civilians and the Warfare of Attrition: Representations of Combat in France, 1914–1918', in F. Coetzee and M. Shevin-Coetzee (eds.), *Authority, Identity and the Social History of the Great War* (Oxford: Berghahn Books, 1995), pp. 223–50

Hughes, C., 'The New Armies', in F. W. Beckett and K. Simpson, *A Nation in Arms* (Manchester: Manchester University Press, 1985), pp. 100–25

Hynes, S., *A War Imagined. The First World War and English Culture* (London: Pimlico, 1992)

Hynes, S., *The Soldier's Tale. Bearing Witness to Modern War* (London: Pimlico, 1998)

Jalland, P., *Death in the Victorian Family* (Oxford: Oxford University Press, 1996)

Jamieson, L., 'Limited Resources and Limiting Conventions: Working-Class Mothers and Daughters in Urban Scotland c. 1890–1918', in J. Lewis (ed.), *Labour and Love. Women's Experience of Home and Family 1850–1940* (Oxford: Blackwell, 1986), pp. 73–99

Joseph, B., 'Transference: The Total Situation', *International Journal of Psycho-Analysis*, Vol. 66 (1985), pp. 447–54

Keegan, J., *The Face of Battle* (London: Jonathan Cape, 1976)

Kent, S., *Making Peace. The Reconstruction of Gender in Interwar Britain* (Princeton, NJ: Princeton University Press, 1993)

Khan, N., *Women's Poetry of the First World War* (Hemel Hempstead: Harvester–Wheatsheaf, 1988)

Klein, M., *Love, Guilt and Reparation and Other Works 1921–1945* (London: Virago, 1994)

Klein, M., *Envy and Gratitude and Other Works 1946–1963* (London: Vintage 1997)

Koven, S., 'Remembering and Dismemberment: Crippled Children, Wounded Soldiers and the Great War in Great Britain', *The American Historical Review*, Vol. 99, No. 4 (October 1994), pp. 1167–1202

Kudrus, B., 'Gender Wars: The First World War and the Construction of Gender Relations in the Weimar Republic', in K. Hagermann and S. Schüler-Springorum (eds.), *The Home Front. The Military, War and Gender in Twentieth-Century Germany* (Oxford: Berg, 2002)

LaCapra, D., *Writing History, Writing Trauma* (Baltimore: Johns Hopkins University Press, 2001)

Leed, E., *No Man's Land. Combat and Identity in World War I* (Cambridge: Cambridge University Press, 1979)

Leese, P., 'Problems Returning Home: The British Psychological Casualties of the Great War', *The Historical Journal*, Vol. 40, No. 4 (December 1997), pp. 1055–67

Liddle, P., *The Soldier's War 1914–1918* (London: Blandford Press, 1988)

Lifton, R. J., *The Broken Connection. On Death and the Continuity of Life* (New York: Simon & Schuster, 1979)

Light, A., *Forever England. Femininity, Literature and Conservatism Between the Wars* (London: Routledge, 1991)

Lloyd, D., *Battlefield Tourism. Pilgrimage and the Commemoration of the Great War in Britain, Australia and Canada* (Oxford: Berg, 1998)

López-Corvo, R. E., *The Dictionary of the Work of W. R. Bion* (London, H. Karnac, 2003)

Luckins, T., *The Gates of Memory. Australian People's Experiences and Memories of Loss and the Great War* (Freemantle, WA: Curtin University Books, 2004)

McCartney, H., *Citizen Soldiers. The Liverpool Territorials in the First World War* (Cambridge: Cambridge University Press, 2005)

Michel, S., 'Danger on the Home Front: Motherhood, Sexuality and Disabled Veterans in American Postwar Films', in M. Cooke and A. Woollacott (eds.), *Gendering War Talk* (Princeton, NJ: Princeton University Press, 1993), pp. 260–82

Moody, R. S. H., *Historical Records of the Buffs East Kent Regiment 1914–1919* (London: The Medici Society, 1922)

Moriaty, C., '"Though in a Picture Only". Portrait Photography and the Commemoration of the First World War', in G. Braybon (ed.), *Evidence, History and the Great War* (Oxford: Berghahn Books, 2003), pp. 30–47

Mosse, G., *Fallen Soldiers. Reshaping the Memory of the World Wars* (Oxford: Oxford University Press, 1990)

Mosse, G., *The Image of Man. The Creation of Modern Masculinity* (Oxford: Oxford University Press, 1996)

Nelson, C., *Boys Will Be Girls. The Feminine Ethic and British Children's Fiction 1857–1917* (New Brunswick: Rutgers University Press, 1991)

Ouditt, S., *Fighting Forces, Writing Women. Identity and Ideology in the First World War* (London: Routledge, 1994)

Pederson, S., 'Gender, Welfare, and Citizenship in Britain during the Great War', *American Historical Review*, Vol. 95, No. 4 (1990), pp. 983–1006

Petter, M., '"Temporary Gentlemen" in the Aftermath of the Great War: Rank, Status and the Ex-Officer Problem', *The Historical Journal*, Vol. 37, No. 1 (March, 1994), pp. 127–52

Pick, D., *War Machine. The Rationalisation of Slaughter in the Modern Age* (New Haven: Yale University Press, 1993)

Pound, R., *A. P. Herbert. A Biography* (London: Michael Joseph, 1976)

Prior, R. and T. Wilson, *The Somme* (New Haven: Yale University Press, 2005)

Proud, E. B., *History of the British Army Postal Service. Volume II, 1903–1927* (Dereham: Proud–Bailey, 1982)

Puttowski, J. and J. Sykes, *Shot at Dawn. Executions in World War One by Authority of the British Army Act* (London: Leo Cooper, 1999)

Reznick, J., S., *Healing the Nation. Soldiers and the Culture of Caregiving in Britain during the Great War* (Manchester: Manchester University Press, 2004)

Robb, G., *British Culture and the First World War* (Basingstoke: Palgrave, 2002)

Roberts, J. S., *Siegfried Sassoon 1886–1967* (London: Richard Cohen Books, 1999)

Roper, M., 'Between Manliness and Masculinity: The "War Generation" and the Psychology of Fear in Britain, 1914–1970', *Journal of British Studies*, Vol. 44, No. 2 (2005), pp. 343–63

Roper, M., 'Maternal relations: moral manliness and emotional survival in letters home during the First World War', in S. Dudink, K. Hagermann and J. Tosh (eds.), *Masculinity in Politics and War: Re-writings of Modern History* (Manchester: Manchester University Press, 2004), pp. 295–315

Roper, M. 'Memories of a Depression', *Melbourne Historical Journal*, Vol. 9 (1982), pp. 22–8

Roper, M., 'Re-Remembering the Soldier Hero: The Composure and Re-Composure of Masculinity in Memories of the Great War', *History Workshop Journal*, Vol. 50 (Spring 2000), pp. 181–205

Roper, M., 'Slipping Out of View: Subjectivity and Emotion in Gender History', *History Workshop Journal*, Vol. 59 (Spring 2005), pp. 57–73

Ross, E., *Love and Toil. Motherhood in Outcast London 1870–1918* (Oxford: Oxford University Press, 1993)

Ross, E., 'Labour and Love: Re-Discovering London's Working-Class Mothers, 1870–1918', in J. Lewis (ed.), *Labour and Love. Women's Experience of Home and Family 1850–1940* (Oxford: Blackwell, 1986), pp. 73–99

Roth, S., 'Projective Identification', in S. Budd and R. Rushbridger (eds.), *Introducing Psychoanalysis. Essential Themes and Topics* (London: Routledge, 2005), pp. 200–11

Ruderman, J., *D. H. Lawrence and the Devouring Mother* (Durham, NC: Duke University Press, 1984)

Sandler, P., 'Bion's War Memoirs: A Psychoanalytical Commentary', http://psychematters.com/papers/psandler2.htm. Accessed 21 January 2005

Scates, B., *Return to Gallipoli. Walking the Battlefields of the Great War* (Cambridge: Cambridge University Press, 2006)

Scates, B., 'The Unknown Sock Knitter: Voluntary Work, Emotional Labour, Bereavement and the Great War', *Labour History*, Vol. 81 (2001), pp. 29–49

Schulte, R., 'Käthe Kollwitz's Sacrifice', *History Workshop Journal* Vol. 41 (Spring 1996), pp. 193–221

Segal, H. 'Notes on Symbol Formation', in Bott-Spilius, E., *Melanie Klein Today Vol 1: Mainly Theory* (London: Routledge, 1996), pp. 160–78

Sheffield, G., *Forgotten Victory. The First World War: Myths and Realities* (London: Headline Book Publishing, 2001)

Sheffield, G., *Leadership in the Trenches. Officer–Man Relations, Morale and Discipline in the British Army in the Era of the First World War* (Basingstoke: Palgrave, 2000)

Shephard, B., *A War of Nerves. Soldiers and Psychiatrists 1914–1994* (London: Jonathan Cape, 2000)

Simkins, P., *Kitchener's Army. The Raising of the New Armies, 1914–16* (Manchester: Manchester University Press, 1988)

Simpson, A., *Hot Blood and Cold Steel. Life and Death in the Trenches of the First World War* (London: Tom Donovan, 1993)

Simpson, K., 'Dr James Dunn and Shell-Shock', in H. Cecil and P. Liddle, *Facing Armageddon. The First World War Experienced* (London: Pen & Sword, 1996), pp. 502–20

Simpson, K., 'The Officers' in I. Beckett and K. Simpson, *A Nation in Arms. A Social Study of the British Army in the First World War* (Manchester: Manchester University Press, 1985), pp. 64–97

Smith, L., 'Paul Fussell's *The Great War and Modern Memory*: Twenty-Five Years Later', *History and Theory*, Vol. 40, No. 2 (May 2001), pp. 241–60

Smith, M., 'The War and British Culture', in S. Constantine, M. W. Kirby and M. B. Rose (eds.), *The First World War in British History* (London: Edward Arnold, 1995), pp. 168–84

Stacke, H., *The Worcestershire Regiment in the Great War* (Kidderminster: G. T. Cheshire & Sons Ltd, 1928)

Strange, J.-M., *Death, Grief and Poverty in Britain 1870–1914* (Cambridge: Cambridge University Press, 2005)

Strange, J.-M., '"She Cried a Very Little": Death, Grief and Mourning in Working-Class Culture c. 1880–1914', *Social History* Vol. 27, No. 2 (May 2002), pp. 143–61

Stryker, L., 'Mental Cases. British Shellshock and the Politics of Interpretation', in G. Braybon (ed.), *Evidence, History and the Great War* (Oxford: Berghahn Books, 2003), pp. 154–71

Symington, J. and N., *The Clinical Thinking of Wilfred Bion* (London: Routledge, 1996)

Tate, T., *Modernism, History and the First World War* (Manchester: Manchester University Press, 1998)

Tebbutt, M., *Women's Talk? A Social History of 'Gossip' in Working Class Neighborhoods 1880–1960* (Aldershot: Scolar Press, 1995)

Thompson, P., *The Edwardians. The Remaking of British Society* (London: Routledge, 1992)

Thorpe, M., *Siegfried Sassoon. A Critical Study* (London: Oxford University Press, 1966)

Todman, D., *The Great War. Myth and Memory* (London: Hambledon, 2005)

Tonnessman, M., 'Transference and Countertransference: An Historical Approach', in S. Budd and R. Rushbridger (eds.), *Introducing Psychoanalysis. Essential Themes and Topics* (London: Routledge, 2005), pp. 185–200

Tooley, H., *The Western Front. Battle Ground and Home Front in the First World War* (Basingstoke: Palgrave, 2003)

Tosh, J., *A Man's Place. Masculinity and the Middle-Class Home in Victorian England* (New Haven: Yale University Press, 1999)

Travers, T., *The Killing Ground. The British Army, the Western Front and the Emergence of Modern Warfare 1900–1918* (Barnsley: Pen & Sword, 2003)

Tylee, C., *The Great War and Women's Consciousness. Images of Militarism and Womanhood in Women's Writings 1914–1964* (Iowa City: University of Iowa Press, 1990)

Van Emden, R. and S. Humphries, *All Quiet on the Home Front* (London: Headline Publishing, 2003)

Vincent, D., *Bread, Knowledge and Freedom: A Study of Nineteenth-Century Working Class Autobiography* (London: Europa, 1981)

Vincent, D., *Literacy and Popular Culture. England 1750–1914* (Cambridge: Cambridge University Press, 1989)

Vincent, D., *The Rise of Mass Literacy. Reading and Writing in Modern Europe* (Cambridge: Polity, 2000)

Ward, P., 'Empire and the Everyday: Britishness and Imperialism in Women's Lives in the Great War', in P. Buckner and R. Douglas Francis, *Re-Discovering the British World* (Calgary: Calgary Press, 2005), pp. 267–83

Ward, P., 'Women of Britain Say Go: Women's Patriotism in the First World War', *Twentieth Century British History*, Vol. 12, No. 1 (2001), pp. 23–46

Watson, J., *Fighting Different Wars. Experience, Memory and the First World War in Britain* (Cambridge: Cambridge University Press, 2004)

Weisbrod, D., 'Military Violence and Male Fundamentalism: Ernst Jünger's Contribution to the Conservative Revolution', *History Workshop Journal*, Vol. 49, (Spring 2000), pp. 68–94

Wells, E., *Mailshot. A History of the Forces Postal Service* (London: Defences Postal and Courier Service, Royal Engineers, 1987)

Wild, J., 'A Merciful, Heaven-Sent Release?: The Clerk and the First World War in British Literary Culture', *Cultural and Social History* Vol. 4, No. 1 (March 2007), pp. 73–95

Wilson, J. M., *Siegfried Sassoon. The Making of a War Poet. A Biography 1886–1918* (London: Duckbacks, 1998)

Wilson, T., *The Myriad Faces of War. Britain and the Great War, 1914–1918* (Cambridge: Polity, 1986)

Winter, D., *Death's Men. Soldiers of the Great War* (London: Penguin, 1979)

Winter, J. M., 'Britain's "Lost Generation" of the First World War', *Population Studies*, Vol. 31, No. 3 (November 1977), pp. 449–66

Winter, J. M., 'Forms of Kinship and Remembrance in the Aftermath of the Great War', in J. M. Winter and E. Sivan, *War and Remembrance in the Twentieth Century* (Cambridge: Cambridge University Press, 1999), pp. 40–60

Winter, J. M., *The Great War and the British People* (Basingstoke: Macmillan, 1985)

Winter, J. M., *Sites of Memory, Sites of Mourning. The Great War in European Cultural History* (Cambridge: Cambridge University Press, 1995)

Wohl, A., *The Generation of 1914* (Cambridge, MA: Harvard University Press, 1979)

Woollacott, A., 'Sisters and Brothers in Arms: Family, Class and Gendering in World War I Britain', in M. Cooke and A. Woollacott (eds.), *Gendering War Talk* (Princeton, NJ: Princeton University Press, 1993), pp. 128–47

Wright, P., *Tank. The Progress of a Monstrous War Machine* (London: Faber & Faber, 2000)

Young, A., 'W. H. R. Rivers and the War Neuroses', *Journal of the History of the Behavioural Sciences*, Vol. 35, No. 4 (Fall 1999), pp. 359–78

Young, R. M., 'Bion and Experiences in Groups', http://human-nature.com/rmyoung/papers/pap148h.html. Accessed 7 May 2007, pp. 1–17

### *Internet sources*

Australian War Memorial – Lone Pine. Its Place in History, Casualties', http://dev.links.com.au/diorama/subcat.asp?cat=3&subcat=25. Accessed 31 July 2007

bbc.co.uk, 'World War One, The Last Tommy Gallery', www.bbc.co.uk/history/worldwars/wwone/last_tommy_gallery-03.shtml. Accessed 13 June 2007

Commonwealth War Graves Commission, www.cwgc.org/search/casualty_details.aspx?casualty=291770. Accessed 19 July 2007

Oxford Dictionary of National Biography, www.oxforddnb.com/view/printable/3166. Accessed 20 September 2005

Pro Patria Mori: Gommecourt – The Battle, www.gommecourt.co.uk/battle.htm. Accessed 26 March 2007

Shot at Dawn Website, 'Shot Unjustly, Unlawfully', www.shotatdawn.org.uk/page15.html. Accessed 5 May 2007

The Long, Long Trail. The British Army in the Great War, www.1914-1918.net/dukes.htm. Accessed 16 April, 3 July 2007

### *Unpublished work*

Corr, C., 'Killing and Dying: The Experience of Shell and Sniper-Fire in the First World War', unpublished MA dissertation, Department of Sociology, University of Essex, 2004

Duffett, R., '"I believe 'e'd sell 'imself for a tin o' toffee": The Significance of Food in the Memoirs of the Rank and File Soldiers of the First World War', MA dissertation, Department of History, University of Essex, 2005

Fletcher, A., 'Richard Chenevix Trench and his Legacy: An Appreciation by Anthony Fletcher'

Fletcher, A., 'The Western Front 1918: March 21st'

Fletcher, A., 'Writing Home in the First World War: What and How Much to Tell'

Fletcher, D., 'Isabel Chenevix Trench: A Fond Memory from her Grand-Daughter'

Peters, H., '"Unmanned Men": In What Ways Did the Experience of Shell Shock Challenge Early Twentieth Century Notions of Masculinity?', MA Dissertation, Department of History, University of Essex, 2004

# Index

Lightning Source UK Ltd.
Milton Keynes UK
UKOW03f1003211113

221530UK00003B/142/P